ATLAS OF TUMOR PATHOLOGY

Second Series
Fascicle 28

TUMORS OF THE HEMATOPOIETIC SYSTEM

by

ROBERT J. LUKES, M.D.

Professor of Pathology, Emeritus
University of Southern California School of Medicine
Los Angeles, California 90033

Head, Division of Hematopathology
Scripps Clinic and Research Foundation
La Jolla, California 92037

and

ROBERT D. COLLINS, M.D.

Professor of Pathology and
Director of Hematopathology
Vanderbilt University School of Medicine
Nashville, Tennessee 37232

Published by the
ARMED FORCES INSTITUTE OF PATHOLOGY
Washington, D.C.

Under the Auspices of
UNIVERSITIES ASSOCIATED FOR RESEARCH AND EDUCATION IN PATHOLOGY, INC.
Bethesda, Maryland
1992

Submitted for Publication
1988

For sale by the Armed Forces Institute of Pathology
Washington, D.C. 20306-6000
ISBN 1-881041-04-2

ATLAS OF TUMOR PATHOLOGY

Sponsored by

AMERICAN CANCER SOCIETY
ARMED FORCES INSTITUTE OF PATHOLOGY
NATIONAL CANCER INSTITUTE, NATIONAL INSTITUTES OF HEALTH
UNIVERSITIES ASSOCIATED FOR RESEARCH AND EDUCATION IN PATHOLOGY, INC.

EDITOR
WILLIAM H. HARTMANN, M.D.
Department of Pathology
Memorial Medical Center
Long Beach, California 90801

COEDITOR
LESLIE H. SOBIN, M.D.
Armed Forces Institute of Pathology
Washington, D.C. 20306-6000

EDITORS' NOTE

The Atlas of Tumor Pathology was originated by the Committee on Pathology of the National Academy of Sciences – National Research Council in 1947. The form of the Atlas became the brainchild of the Subcommittee on Oncology and was shepherded by a succession of editors. It was supported by a long list of agencies; many of the illustrations were made by the Medical Illustration Service of the Armed Forces Institute of Pathology; the type was set by the Government Printing Office; and the final printing was done by the Armed Forces Institute of Pathology. The American Registry of Pathology purchased the Fascicles from the Government Printing Office and sold them at cost, plus a small handling and shipping charge. Over a period of 20 years, 15,000 copies each of 40 Fascicles were produced. They provided a system of nomenclature and set standards for histologic diagnosis that received worldwide acclaim. Private contributions by almost 600 pathologists helped to finance the compilation of an index by The Williams & Wilkins Company to complete the original Atlas.

After the preparation of the final Fascicle of the first Atlas, the National Academy of Sciences – National Research Council handed over the task of further pursuit of the project to Universities Associated for Research and Education in Pathology, Inc. Grant support for a second series was generously made available by both the National Cancer Institute and the American Cancer Society. The Armed Forces Institute of Pathology has expanded and improved its press facilities to provide for a more rapid and efficient production of the new series. A new Editor and Editorial Advisory Committee were appointed, and the solicitation and preparation of manuscripts continued.

This second series of the Atlas of Tumor Pathology is not intended as a second edition of the first Atlas, and, in general, there is variation in authorship. The basic purpose remains unchanged in providing an Atlas setting standards of diagnosis and terminology. Throughout this series, the terminology chosen for the World Health Organization's series "International Histological Classification of Tumours" has been used when available. Hematoxylin and eosin stained sections still represent the keystone of histologic diagnosis; therefore, most of the photomicrographs are of sections stained by this technique, and sections prepared by other techniques are specifically designated in the legends. It is hoped that in many of the new series a broader perspective of tumors may be offered by the inclusion of special stains, histochemical illustrations, electron micrographs, data on biologic behavior, and other pertinent information when indicated for a better understanding of the disease.

The format of the new series is changed to allow better correlation of the illustrations with the text, and a more substantial cover is provided. An index is included in each Fascicle.

It is the hope of the Editors, past and present, the Editorial Advisory Committees, past and present, and the Sponsors that these changes will be welcomed by the readers. Constructive criticisms and suggestions will always be appreciated.

William H. Hartmann, M.D.
Leslie H. Sobin, M.D.

Permission to use copyrighted illustrations has been granted by:

American Association of Pathologists, Inc.:
Am. J. Pathol. 122:562-572, 1986. For figures 97-102.

Grune & Stratton Inc.:
Blood 52:311-322, 1978. For figures 3 and 11.
Progress in Clinical Pathology, Vol. IX, 1983. For figures 19 and 20.

J.B. Lippincott Company:
Am. J. Clin. Pathol. 58:607-617, 1972. For plate LVII-E and F.
Am. J. Clin. Pathol. 61:382-392, 1974. For figures 21-23.
Am. J. Clin. Pathol. 73:459-470, 1980. For plate XLIX-D.
Am. J. Clin. Pathol. 85:739-744, 1986. For figures 103-106.
Am. J. Clin. Pathol. 87:121-128, 1987. For figures 33-38.

John Wiley & Sons Ltd.:
Hematol. Oncol. 2:319-347, 1984. For plate LIII-A and figures 126-130.

Macmillan Press Ltd.:
Br. J. Cancer 31(Suppl. 2):1-28, 1975. For figures 39, 40, and 42.

Plenum Publishing Corporation:
The Reticuloendothelial System, 1983. For figures 90-92 and 95.

Raven Press Ltd.:
Am. J. Surg. Pathol. 14:1047-1060, 1990. For figures 51 and 52.

Dr. Bertram Schnitzer, University of Michigan:
Letter to the Editor. Lancet 2:649, 1974. For figure 26.

Waverly Press Inc.:
Cancer Res. 26:1063-1083, 1966. For plate XXXIX-B and C and figures 57, 67, 70, 72, 73, 75, and 77.
Cancer Res. 31:1755-1767, 1971. For figures 54-56, 74, 79, 81, and 83.

ACKNOWLEDGMENTS

We are particularly indebted to the many physicians in the United States and abroad who have contributed cases for study. Specific credits are given for those cases that are prototypic examples of certain entities described by the contributor.

Work by the members of the University of Southern California and Vanderbilt hemato-pathology groups has been used as the scientific base for this Fascicle. Individual publications by these collaborators are referenced throughout the text. In particular, we are indebted to Dr. John Parker for his contributions to the biology of the immune system and the markers of normal and neoplastic cells; Dr. Clive Taylor for his work on the relationship of lymphoma pathology to lymphocyte distribution patterns and the application of immunoperoxidase methods to lymphoid neoplasms; Dr. Alexandra Levine for contributing the clinical section of each cell type; Dr. Alan Glick for providing illustrations and most of the electron micrographs; Dr. John Cousar for contributions in the B cell areas; and Dr. Steve Bennett for literature analysis of the lymphoproliferative disorders. We are also indebted to Drs. Richard Brunning and Robert McKenna for providing textual material and key illustrations in the leukemia section.

We are most appreciative for the assistance, support, and guidance provided by Dr. William H. Hartmann, Chief of Pathology at Memorial Medical Center, Long Beach, California.

We are indebted for photomicrography to Mr. Andy Gero, R.B.P., Director of Medical Photography at Los Angeles County/USC Medical Center, and to the staff of Medical Illustrations of the Armed Forces Institute of Pathology.

We thank Ms. Donna Posey, Bronna Scoggins, Gloria Jenkins, Connie Singleton, Ruth Ann House, and Jean Kolodziej for typing the manuscript and Ms. Elizabeth Collins for proofreading and copyediting.

Robert J. Lukes, M.D.
Robert D. Collins, M.D.

TUMORS OF THE HEMATOPOIETIC SYSTEM

Contents

TUMORS OF THE HEMATOPOIETIC SYSTEM

GENERAL COMMENTS

The hematopoietic system comprises several tissues in which erythrocytes, granulocytes, platelets, lymphocytes, and monocytes are produced and function. In this Fascicle, hematopoietic tumors are considered according to these three inter-related functioning systems: (1) lymphoid; (2) mononuclear phagocyte; and (3) myeloid (production of erythroid, granulocytic, and megakaryocytic components).

Many functions and sites of action are shared by these systems. In adults, the bone marrow produces the basic elements of all three systems. Since the origin, sites of action, and functions of the systems are shared, and since their neoplasms may be similar both clinically and pathologically, there is a considerable practical and conceptual advantage in initially discussing these systems and their diseases in a unified fashion before examining their neoplasms individually.

The hematopoietic system is understood in a general way, but many details about the cellular interactions and functions, as well as mechanisms of disease production, are yet to be learned. Some lymphoid and mononuclear phagocyte subpopulations are imprecisely defined in terms of function and criteria for recognition. There are also conspicuous gaps in our knowledge of hematopoietic neoplasms, despite intensive investigation over the last 15 years. Not all of the tumors have been completely defined in terms of diagnostic criteria, clinical manifestations,

and natural history, and additional hematopoietic neoplasms will be recognized in the near future. For example, neoplasms of natural killer cells have been described only in the recent past. The level of our understanding about these neoplasms may be summarized briefly as follows: (1) Neoplasms have been demonstrated in all of the anatomic compartments of the hematopoietic system. In many neoplasms the neoplastic cells closely resemble a normal subpopulation. (2) Most lymphoid neoplasms have B features. T neoplasms in the United States and Europe are infrequent but may be more diverse than B neoplasms. (3) Mononuclear phagocyte system malignant neoplasms are predominantly of marrow origin in adults, and extramarrow mononuclear phagocyte system neoplasms are very rare. (4) Relatively specific structural and functional criteria for diagnosing many lymphomas have been established. Analyses based on these combined criteria have allowed the recognition or confirmation of various morphologic features diagnostic of certain neoplasms and therefore predictive of immunologic type (Lukes et al.). (5) Due to the enhanced precision of analyses of lymphoid neoplasms, it has become feasible to use the relatively homogeneous populations of neoplastic cells to study the functions of the normal immune system.

This Fascicle deals mainly with neoplasms of the hematopoietic system, as well as reactive processes resembling or progressing to neoplasms. The criteria for diagnosis are given for each neoplasm. This section describes the general features of hematopoietic neoplasms and our approach to their diagnosis and classification.

GENERAL CHARACTERISTICS

Hematopoietic neoplasms resemble neoplasms of other tissues in several important ways. Most neoplasms are clonal. For lymphomas and leukemias, there is abundant immunologic, karyotypic, or enzymatic evidence indicating they contain clonal expansions of a single functional subpopulation. Some lymphomas and leukemias are readily recognizable on histologic sections or smears. Others show only subtle variations from one another in growth pattern or cytologic features. Carcinomas also exhibit enormous variation in their ease of recognition. The etiology and pathogenesis of most neoplasms (including leukemias and lymphomas) are generally unknown.

Neoplasms of the hematopoietic system differ from neoplasms of other tissues in the following ways. First, hematopoietic neoplasms are often widespread at presentation, presumably due to the innate capacity of these cell types to circulate. Another difference is that they often change in appearance and clinical behavior during the course of illness due to an alteration in cell cycle or differentiation dynamics. Hematopoietic neoplasms are broadly categorized by light microscopic examination, as are other neoplasms. Precise categorization of lymphomas and leukemias, however, often requires an evaluation of cytochemical, ultrastructural, karyotypic, or immunologic results since

currently recognized light microscopic features of some neoplasms are not diagnostic. Several lymphoid neoplasms differing in appearance and behavior may arise from individual functional subpopulations. For example, follicular center cells may produce neoplasms of indolent behavior (cleaved follicular center cell lymphomas) or aggressive behavior (small noncleaved follicular center cell/Burkitt's lymphoma). The potential for such diverse neoplasms to arise from single subpopulations greatly amplifies the number of neoplastic clinico-pathologic entities developing from the hematopoietic system. The actual number of different lymphoid neoplasms is unknown, but 40 to 50 is a reasonable estimate of the important entities. The diversity of neoplasms arising from non-hematopoietic cell lines is not as apparent. Most cells in some hematopoietic neoplasms (i.e., Hodgkin's disease) appear to be reactive, in contrast to the small number of reactive cells in epithelial neoplasms. Another unusual feature is that most neoplastic cells in some hematopoietic neoplasms (i.e., chronic lymphocytic leukemia) may be in a Go or dormant phase of the cell cycle. Benign proliferations of hematopoietic cells are common, but benign hematopoietic neoplasms are rare and even debated, in contrast to the frequency of benign neoplasms of other tissues.

FACTORS AFFECTING APPEARANCE AND BEHAVIOR OF HEMATOPOIETIC NEOPLASMS

Most neoplasms are classified on the basis of an evaluation of their histopathologic appearance. Several factors affecting the appearance of lymphomas and leukemias are also predictive of their behavior. These factors are crucial in classification and are becoming increasingly subject to analysis.

The mixture of neoplastic and reacting cells is one factor that determines appearance. In some cases (e.g., Hodgkin's disease), neoplastic cells may be in the minority. In most cases, clonal expansion of a population results in aggregates of similar cells resembling one another in appearance and functional characteristics. Reacting cells usually include fibrovascular elements and various components of the hematopoietic system.

The appearance of hematopoietic neoplasms is also affected by the mix of dividing, dormant, or differentiating neoplastic cells. Neoplasms in all cases have a component of dividing cells, but the percentage of cells in division varies widely from disease to disease and may vary in individual patients at different times. In some cases, most of the neoplastic cells will be in a dividing pool, whereas in others, only a minority will be dividing. Partial or complete differentiation to effector cells is seen in some neoplasms. Others may show incomplete or no differentiation and may contain a large population of dormant cells in addition to a small dividing component. For example, Burkitt's lymphoma is composed predominantly of dividing cells, chronic lymphocytic leukemia of dormant cells, and multiple myeloma of differentiated cells.

The inherent cytologic characteristics of the neoplastic clone are also important. Lymphocytes in some lymphoid neoplasms are characteristic in their light microscopic appearance. Small lymphocytes differ in appearance from transformed lymphocytes or immunoblasts (plate I-A,B). The immunologic subtype of some lymphocytes may be reliably predicted on light microscopy. Plasma cells, some follicular center cells, and cerebriform T cells may be recognized using this method. However, light microscopy may be most reliably used to predict the immunologic type in neoplasms by less subtle features such as growth pattern or pattern of nodal involvement.

The distinctive distribution of neoplastic and reacting cells in affected tissues may be the major factor affecting the histologic appearance of hematopoietic neoplasms. The production of neoplastic follicular nodules by follicular center cell lymphomas is a specific marker of this type of lymphoma. The growth pattern of neoplasms as detected by low magnification examination is often characteristic and in some cases is actually diagnostic.

The behavior of neoplasms is determined in part by the proportion of dividing and dormant cells. Neoplasms with a large dividing pool (e.g., Burkitt's lymphoma) are likely to be aggressive and rapidly growing. Neoplasms with a large dormant pool (e.g., chronic lymphocytic leukemia) are indolent processes, although they may be widespread at presentation. Tumor products in some neoplasms with prominent differentiation cause important clinical and pathologic effects (i.e., those of immunoglobulin production in myeloma).

Since differentiation and growth in the hematopoietic system are normally controlled in part by complex interactions between the various members of these systems, it is likely that their neoplasms are similarly regulated. Reacting components might therefore have important regulatory capacities for growth and differentiation in lymphomas and leukemias. Certain presently undefined features of reactive elements may be as predictive of clinical behavior as inherent characteristics of the neoplastic component.

CHANGES IN APPEARANCE AND BEHAVIOR OF HEMATOPOIETIC NEOPLASMS

In contrast to epithelial neoplasms in which histopathologic features appear to persist in a relatively stable form throughout the illness, some leukemias and lymphomas show striking changes in their morphologic appearance (York et al.). Such changes are often associated with a deteriorating clinical status and are typically unresponsive to therapy. Multiparameter analyses have shown that these changes in appearance are due, in approximately equal frequency, to either the development of a second hematopoietic neoplasm or to changes in the morphology of the original neoplasm. In either instance, the mechanisms of the transformative process are unknown. These phenomena are clearly of great importance in terms of patient welfare, often provoke considerable confusion in diagnostic histopathology, and are of fundamental biologic significance.

Transformation with evidence of persistence of the original clone usually involves neoplasms in which there is well-developed differentiation (plasmacytoid lymphocytic neoplasms, multiple myeloma, chronic myelogenous leukemia) or in which the predominant cell is a dormant lymphocyte (small cell lymphoid neoplasms, cleaved follicular center cell lymphomas). In the former group, transformation apparently involves the loss of capacity to differentiate since karyotypic and immunologic evidence indicates the original clone is still involved in the neoplastic process. In blast transformation of chronic myelogenous leukemia, the neoplastic blasts or stem cells have either shown slight differentiation along granulocytic or monocytic lines or, rarely, have features indicating a B or T lymphocytic phenotype. In both circumstances, a pluripotential stem cell was probably involved. In contrast to these situations involving a loss of capacity to differentiate, transformation of cleaved follicular center cell lymphomas is probably due to clonal evolution. High growth fractions develop in which there is apparently limited capacity to feed into the dormant pool of tumor cells.

Transformation also occurs in a variety of hematopoietic neoplasms in which multiparameter studies indicate that a second neoplasm has developed. Examples of such a circumstance include myelomonocytic leukemia arising in patients with Hodgkin's disease or non-Hodgkin's lymphoma developing in patients with Hodgkin's disease. Evaluation of this phenomenon is hampered by the absence of specific markers of Reed-Sternberg cells, and some transformations of this type might simply represent development of a high growth fraction in the initial Hodgkin's disease component. Therapy is generally implicated as the cause for most of the transitions in this group since transformative changes usually occur in patients receiving chemotherapy and radiotherapy.

Finally, it should be noted that second neoplastic clones arising in some patients may be particularly difficult to recognize when the second neoplasm closely resembles the first morphologically. Patients with leukemia and Burkitt's lymphoma at relapse have rarely been shown to have tumors differing in karyotype or G6PD type from the original process. This phenomenon is certainly more common than appreciated since it has only been detected by sophisticated analyses of the initial material and all "relapses."

SPECIAL INFORMATION REQUIRED TO PRACTICE HEMATOPATHOLOGY

Hematopathology has traditionally been considered a difficult area of study for the following reasons. (1) The biology of the hematopoietic system is inherently complex, with many interacting components. Techniques for the recognition of structural or functional features of its components are imperfect. (2) Hematopoietic neoplasms are likewise complex, with the full extent of their diversity yet to be defined. Reliable diagnostic criteria are not available for every neoplasm. Relatively subtle morphologic differences must be evaluated to distinguish clinical and pathologic entities with quite different prognoses or treatments. (3) Some hematopoietic neoplasms may be mimicked closely by reactive states. Some of these reactive states may develop into neoplasms, and some reactive conditions are inherently life threatening. (4) Technical problems in the fixation, sectioning, and staining of hematopoietic tissues may significantly and adversely affect interpretation of histopathologic material (plate I-C,D). (5) Most pathologists have limited experience with the less common hematopoietic neoplasms or reactions. Thus, it is understandable why this area of pathology has proved to be so difficult, particularly in light of differences in conceptual approach and classification systems.

In contrast to general impressions and with full recognition of all of the problems above, there is an order and predictability to hematopoietic neoplasms and reactions. Certain neoplasms are usually responsible for specific clinical presentations. Once certain distinctive features are recognized, the pattern of anatomic involvement of hematopoietic tissue is very specific. Thus, hematopathology is comparable to other branches of pathology, and the general approach used in other areas is fully applicable to hematopathology.

The purpose of this Fascicle is to describe the histopathologic and immunologic features of hematopoietic neoplasms, as well as reactive states closely resembling neoplasms or those likely to develop into neoplasms. Furthermore, we intend to describe an approach to the pathologic analysis of hematopoietic processes that illustrates the order and predictability of hematopoietic diseases and improves diagnostic capability.

Pathologists need to be aware of the following basic information to successfully practice hematopathology: (1) the key clinical features of the most common hematopoietic neoplasms (Table 1); (2) the most common neoplasms in frequently affected sites (Table 2); (3) the distribution of neoplasms in relation to key anatomic features (as detected by low magnification examination) particularly helpful in differential diagnosis (Tables 3-6); (4) the histopathologic, cytologic, karyotypic, and immunologic diagnostic criteria for the most common neoplasms (given for each cell type); (5) the valuable antibodies and their expected patterns of reactivity, because certain immunoperoxidase and other methods for marking cells have become indispensable in the practice of hematopathology (plate II; Tables 7, 8); and (6) a conceptual basis for classifying hematopoietic neoplasms.

5

APPROACH TO DIAGNOSIS
AND CLASSIFICATION

Hematopoietic neoplasms should be classified in a manner comparable to the neoplasms of other tissues, specifically by presumed site of origin, phenotype of neoplastic cell, and cell cycle or differentiation stage of the predominant neoplastic cell. For the purposes of classification, histopathologic features are the cornerstone of diagnostic hematopathology. Immunologic, cytochemical, and other functional studies must be integrated with histopathologic analyses to produce a single final diagnosis. "Diagnoses" made prematurely on the basis of partial analyses of the available studies are often re-evaluated subsequently. There seems to be increasing pressure for a quick diagnosis so that treatment may begin, although all parties but the patient are aware that such diagnoses are more likely to be erroneous.

Uncommon or complicated cases should be sent to a consultant for diagnosis or confirmation. Consultants should be prepared to perform appropriate immunologic or other sophisticated studies and should have the opportunity to interpret immunologic results in light of histopathologic changes.

The diagnostic criteria for many leukemias, lymphomas, and histiocytoses vary in specificity and reproducibility. This condition is due in part to the fact that the techniques for diagnosis and classification of hematopoietic neoplasms have changed dramatically in the last few years as their complexities have become more apparent. It is now clear that precise categorization of these neoplasms requires an integrated approach using histopathologic, cytologic, immunologic, and histochemical techniques. The following findings have had

the greatest influence in changing the diagnostic approach in hematopathology. (1) Distinct subpopulations of lymphocytes and monocytes have been demonstrated and have been shown to interact in many immune functions and diseases. (2) Techniques for recognition of normal hematopoietic subpopulations may be used to identify neoplastic derivatives of these populations. For lymphocytes, studies of membrane characteristics of living cells are often necessary for subpopulation identification. For derivatives of the myeloid and mononuclear phagocyte system, histochemical or ultrastructural techniques are essential at this time, but surface antigenic features will become important in the future. (3) Lymphocytes may undergo striking morphologic changes in vitro after mitogenic stimulation and in vivo during immune responses, changing from small "mature" or "well-differentiated" lymphocytes to large blasts (plate I-A,B). Lymphocyte transformation has become so completely ingrained in our perceptions of lymphocyte biology that its significance is almost obscured. The morphologic changes documented in these figures facilitated the recognition of similar transformation in vivo and precipitated major terminology changes in the classification of lymphoid neoplasms.

Our approach is to establish the diagnosis of neoplasia using histopathologic and cytologic criteria and then to determine the cell line involved by correlating functional and morphologic studies (plate II-C–F). The integration of histopathologic and multiparameter analyses seems essential, as isolated interpretations of various components of the examination may lead to misinterpretation of the case as a whole. The diagnosis of neoplasia is based primarily on traditional morphologic evaluation. In the future, it will be tempting to turn to more quantitative analyses when the data generated might be less subject to interpretive error, the criteria for diagnosis more rigidly controlled, and sequential analyses more helpful in evaluating response to therapy. However, the traditional histopathologic approach not only provides essential diagnostic information but is also available in all community hospitals.

Microscopy may be utilized at its full potential in hematopathology only if tissues have been well fixed, the sections are one cell thick, and a battery of properly stained sections are available for study. Improper fixation causes major variations in cytologic detail (plate I-C,D). In thick sections, these details are obscured, and large cells may be "hidden" by overlying smaller cells. The routine use of periodic acid Schiff-hematoxylin, methyl-green pyronine (MGP), and Giemsa stains greatly enhances the diagnostic potential of light microscopy in hematopathology. The microscopic analysis of tissue sections begins with a detailed low magnification examination to detect the distribution of lesions. The low magnification features that are particularly useful and may be reliably recognized are summarized in Table 6. This information is often predictive of the ultimate diagnosis (Tables 3-5). Examination by intermediate and high magnifications is directed toward evaluation of cytologic features that are described and illustrated for each neoplasm. Judgments about the information gained from these evaluations determine most diagnoses. Relative size, nuclear configuration, and the amount of cytoplasm are compared for the common T and B cell neoplasms in the schematics shown in figures 1 and 2.

The histopathologic features that establish the malignancy of a lymphoid, myeloid, or histiocytic process vary from neoplasm to neoplasm in their ease of recognition. Many of these features are similar to those seen in other cancers—mass lesions, destruction of architecture, invasive tendencies, and cytologic atypia. Generally, the most reliable criterion for establishing that a lymphoproliferative or myeloproliferative process is a malignant neoplasm is the presence of a mass lesion containing a relatively homogeneous population of cells. Normally, hematopoietic cells are intermingled and homogeneous populations tend to be neoplastic. The establishment of homogeneity of a cell product (e.g., immunoglobulin) or the demonstration of a clonal population of lymphocytes by immunologic studies supports the possibility of a neoplastic disorder.

Invasion is more difficult to evaluate in leukemias and lymphomas because of the wide distribution of myeloid and lymphoid elements. There are, however, relatively specific distribution patterns of these cells, and the recognition of abnormal distributions may serve as an adjunct to the other more reliable diagnostic criteria. Familiarity with the extremes of reactive patterns in optimally prepared material is necessary to minimize false diagnoses of neoplasia.

A low magnification evaluation of tissue sections is a critical part of microscopic examination. It is particularly useful in establishing the general nature of neoplastic processes by detecting the growth patterns of neoplasms and in defining the relationship of mass lesions to residual architectural features. The diagnosis of many types of lymphoma and leukemia may be accurately predicted after low magnification examination (Table 6).

7

PLATE I

A. NORMAL IN VITRO LYMPHOCYTE TRANSFORMATION
Normal lymphocytes separated by gradient density centrifugation from the peripheral blood (top) are shown for comparison with the phytohemagglutinin transformed lymphocytes (bottom) 72 hours postexposure to phytohemagglutinin. The nuclei of the transformed lymphocytes are large and primitive in appearance, with finely dispersed acidophilic chromatin. Nucleoli are prominent, and the cytoplasm is abundant and azurophilic. Wright's stain. X600.

B. IN VITRO TRANSFORMED LYMPHOCYTES
This is a histologic section of in vitro transformed lymphocytes 72 hours postexposure to phytohemagglutinin. Normal transformed lymphocytes in sections have large nuclei, one or more nucleoli, and a moderate amount of dense cytoplasm. H&E. X625.

C. EFFECT OF FIXATION ON APPEARANCE OF SECTIONS
(Plate I-C and D are from the same patient)
This tissue was allowed to stand in tissue culture media (RPMI) for several hours before fixation. It shows the dramatic changes that may be produced in tissue by improper handling. This small noncleaved follicular center cell lymphoma is almost unrecognizable. H&E. X600.

D. EFFECT OF FIXATION ON APPEARANCE OF SECTIONS
A section from the same lymphoma specimen in Plate I-C fixed promptly in B-5 shows the typical morphology. H&E. X600.

PLATE I

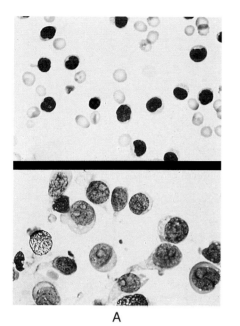

A

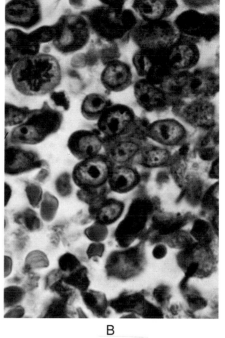

B

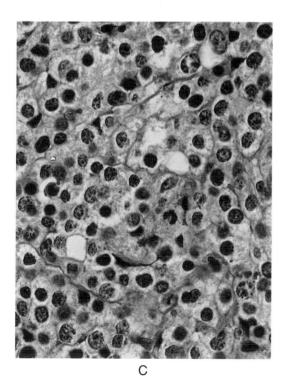

C

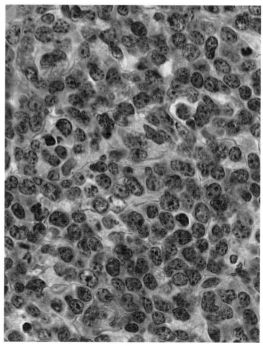

D

PLATE II

A. TONSIL, PIP, WITH CDw75 (LN-1)
Paraffin immunoperoxidase techniques with labeled antibodies are extremely helpful in studying hematopoietic tissues. This section shows the dramatic marking of follicular centers with LN-1, a follicular center cell marking antibody. X130.

B. TONSIL, PIP, WITH CD45RO (UCHL-1)
Staining with pan-T antibody UCHL-1 shows that the follicular centers are negative, while most T cells are found in the mantle zone and in the interfollicular area. X80.

C. LYMPH NODE, NODULAR SCLEROSING HODGKIN'S DISEASE,
PLASTIC IMMUNOPEROXIDASE, WITH CD15
(Plate II-C and D are from the same patient)
Characteristic membranous and Golgi-associated positivity is shown. This pattern of positivity is frequently seen in Hodgkin's disease but is not diagnostic per se. X40.

D. LYMPH NODE, NODULAR SCLEROSING HODGKIN'S DISEASE,
PLASTIC IMMUNOPEROXIDASE, WITH CD3
In this illustration, Reed-Sternberg cells show definite positivity with antibodies against a T cell antigen. X40.

E. SKIN, CEREBRIFORM T CELL LYMPHOMA, PLASTIC IMMUNOPEROXIDASE, WITH CD5
(Plate II-E and F are from the same patient)
Both small and large cerebriform cells marked with this pan-T antibody. X40.

F. SKIN, CEREBRIFORM T CELL LYMPHOMA, PLASTIC IMMUNOPEROXIDASE, WITH CD4
The smaller tumor cells mark as T helper cells, but positivity is not detected as expected on the larger tumor cells. X40.

PLATE II

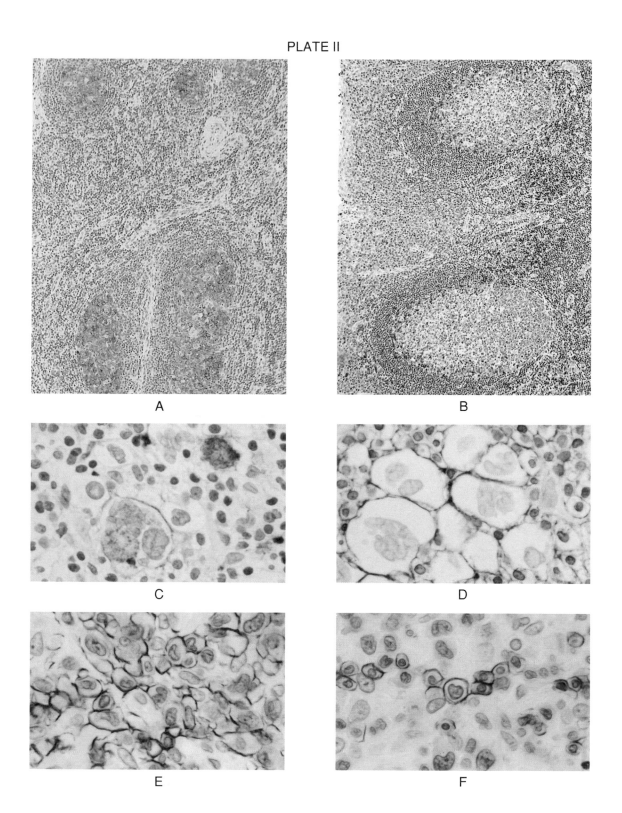

A

B

C

D

E

F

Table 1

RELATIONSHIP OF KEY CLINICAL FEATURES
(Age, Sex, Location of Hematopoietic System Tumor)
TO MOST LIKELY DIAGNOSIS

Key Clinical Features	Likely Diagnosis
Young (<30 years of age) male, mediastinal mass ± cervical adenopathy ± leukemic phase	Convoluted (lymphoblastic) T lymphoma
Young (5-15 years of age) male/female, abdominal mass	Follicular center cell, small noncleaved cell
Young (3-5 years of age) male/female, leukemia	Acute lymphocytic leukemia (often pre-B)
Teenage male, isolated cervical adenopathy	Hodgkin's disease, lymphocyte predominant
Teenage/young adult female, mediastinal mass	Hodgkin's disease, nodular sclerosing Malignant lymphoma, large B cell
Adult male >50 years of age, fever, pancytopenia, abnormal liver function tests; disease mostly below the diaphragm	Hodgkin's disease, lymphocyte depletion
Adult >55 years of age, with lymphocytic leukemia	Small B cell neoplasms (chronic lymphocytic leukemia)
Adult, generalized adenopathy ± splenomegaly ± leukemic phase	Follicular center cell, small cleaved cell
Adult, retroperitoneal adenopathy often with sclerosis ± inguinal adenopathy	Follicular center cell, large cleaved cell/ small cleaved cell
Adult, single or multiple masses in central nervous system	Follicular center cell, small noncleaved cell/ immunoblastic lymphoma B ? AIDS associated
Adult, isolated conjunctival mass	Plasmacytoid lymphocytic lymphoma; small B cell neoplasms
Adult, Hashimoto's disease and thyroid mass	Follicular center cell, large noncleaved cell; immunoblastic lymphoma B
Adult, salivary gland mass	Follicular center cell; plasmacytoid lymphocytic lymphoma
Adult, isolated lung mass	Plasmacytoid lymphocytic lymphoma; small B cell neoplasms; follicular center cell
Adult, multiple lung masses	Lymphomatoid granulomatosis
Adult, stomach mass	Follicular center cell, large noncleaved cell
Child/young adult, ilial mass	Follicular center cell, small noncleaved cell
Adult, small intestinal tumor	Follicular center cell, large noncleaved cell
Adult, skin lesions with epidermis involved	Cerebriform T cell lymphoma
Adult, skin lesions with dermis involved	Small B cell neoplasms; follicular center cell, cleaved cell

Table 2

MOST COMMON HEMATOPOIETIC SYSTEM NEOPLASMS IN VARIOUS TISSUES

Tissue	Most Common Neoplasms
Bone marrow	Acute lymphocytic leukemia*; acute myelomonocytic leukemia; small B cell neoplasms; multiple myeloma
Node	
High cervical	Hodgkin's disease, lymphocytic predominant*
Mid cervical	Follicular center cell, small cleaved cell; Hodgkin's disease, nodular sclerosing; Hodgkin's disease, mixed cellularity
Supraclavicular	Hodgkin's disease, nodular sclerosing
Axillary	Follicular center cell, small cleaved cell
Mediastinal	Hodgkin's disease, nodular sclerosing; convoluted (lymphoblastic) T lymphoma
Mesenteric	Follicular center cell, small cleaved cell/large cleaved cell with and without sclerosis
Retroperitoneal	Follicular center cell, small cleaved cell/large cleaved cell with sclerosis
Inguinal	Follicular center cell, small cleaved cell
Spleen	Hodgkin's disease, nodular sclerosing; follicular center cell, small cleaved cell; hairy cell leukemia; acute myelomonocytic leukemia; chronic myelogenous leukemia
Waldeyer's ring	Follicular center cell, small cleaved cell/large cleaved cell/large noncleaved cell
Thymus	Hodgkin's disease, nodular sclerosing; convoluted (lymphoblastic) T lymphoma*
Gonads	Follicular center cell, small noncleaved cell; immunoblastic lymphoma B
Lung	Follicular center cell, small cleaved cell; plasmacytoid lymphocytic lymphoma
Stomach	Follicular center cell, large noncleaved cell; immunoblastic lymphoma B; plasmacytoid lymphocytic lymphoma
Small intestine	Follicular center cell, small noncleaved cell*; immunoblastic lymphoma B
Large intestine	Follicular center cell, large noncleaved cell
Rectum, anus	Immunoblastic lymphoma B
Skin	Cerebriform T; immunoblastic lymphoma T; small B and T cell neoplasms
Conjunctiva	Follicular center cell, small cleaved cell; plasmacytoid lymphocytic lymphoma
Thyroid	Follicular center cell, large noncleaved cell; immunoblastic lymphoma B; plasmacytoid lymphocytic lymphoma
Salivary gland	Follicular center cell, small cleaved cell/large noncleaved cell
Lacrimal gland	Follicular center cell, small cleaved cell; plasmacytoid lymphocytic lymphoma
Bone	Follicular center cell, small noncleaved cell (Burkitt's)*; acute lymphocytic leukemia*
Central nervous system	
Intracerebral	Immunoblastic lymphoma B; follicular center cell, small noncleaved cell
Meningeal	Acute lymphocytic leukemia T; convoluted (lymphoblastic) T lymphoma

* Patients under 16 years of age

Table 3

LYMPH NODE: DIAGNOSTIC APPROACH USING LOW MAGNIFICATION

Nodulation*			Interfollicular*	Sinuses*	Effaced Architecture*	
Nonfollicular	Follicular	Pseudofollicular			Partial	Diffuse
BENIGN LYMPHOPROLIFERATIONS						
Dermatopathia	Hyperplasia		Reactive, non-specific		Dermatopathia	Reactive, non-specific
	Progressive follicular transformation		Immunoblastic reactions			Immunoblastic reactions
	Persistent generalized adenopathy					Immunoblastic lymphadenopathy
MALIGNANT LYMPHOPROLIFERATIONS						
Hodgkin's disease, nodular sclerosing	Hodgkin's disease, L&H nodular	Malignant lymphoma	Hodgkin's disease, all types	Malignant lymphoma, Ki-1 (+)	Malignant lymphoma, large cell	Hodgkin's disease, all types
	Malignant lymphoma, follicular center cell, all types	Small B/T cell neoplasms	Malignant lymphoma, convoluted (lymphoblastic) T	Microvillous lymphoma		Malignant lymphoma, follicular center cell, all types
	Mantle zone lymphoma	Plasmacytoid lymphocytic lymphoma	Small B/T cell neoplasms			Small B/T cell neoplasms
		Malignant lymphoma, parafollicular B	Hairy cell leukemia			Malignant lymphoma, immunoblastic lymphoma B/T
						Malignant lymphoma, lympho-epithelioid lymphoma T

MYELOPROLIFERATIONS

Extramedullary hematopoiesis

Leukemia, myeloid

Mastocytosis

Acute myeloid leukemia

MONONUCLEAR PHAGOCYTE SYSTEM PROLIFERATIONS

Reactive

Eosinophilic granuloma

Malignant histiocytosis

Histiocytosis X

Acute monocytic leukemia

Malignant histiocytosis

OTHER

Metastases

Metastases

Metastases

Metastases

* Abnormal area

15

Table 4

BONE MARROW: DIAGNOSTIC APPROACH USING LOW MAGNIFICATION

| Diffuse | Medullary* | | Peritrabecular | Trabecular* | |
	Focal	Patchy		*Sclerosis*	Bony *Erosion*
BENIGN LYMPHOPROLIFERATIONS					
	Lymphoid nodule				
	Immunoblastic lymphadenopathy				
MALIGNANT LYMPHOPROLIFERATIONS					
Acute lymphocytic leukemia, all types					
Small B/T cell neoplasms, including chronic lymphocytic leukemia	Small B/T cell neoplasms, including chronic lymphocytic leukemia			Small T cell neoplasms	
Plasmacytoid lymphocytic lymphoma	Plasmacytoid lymphocytic lymphoma				
Malignant lymphoma, follicular center cell, small noncleaved cell	Malignant lymphoma, immunoblastic lymphoma B/T		Malignant lymphoma, follicular center cell, small cleaved cell		
Hodgkin's disease, nodular sclerosing, mixed cellularity, lymphocyte depletion	Hodgkin's disease, nodular sclerosing, mixed cellularity, lymphocyte depletion				
Hairy cell leukemia	Hairy cell leukemia				
Multiple myeloma	Multiple myeloma				Multiple myeloma

MYELOPROLIFERATIONS

Myeloproliferative disorders, reactive	Mastocytosis	Mastocytosis
Myeloproliferative disorders, with/without fibrosis		Myeloproliferative disorders
Myeloid leukemias		Myeloid leukemias

MONONUCLEAR PHAGOCYTE SYSTEM PROLIFERATIONS

Acute monocytic leukemia	Malignant histiocytosis

OTHER

Metastatic carcinoma	Metastatic carcinoma	Metastatic carcinoma
Metastatic melanoma	Metastatic melanoma	

* Abnormal area

17

Table 5

SPLEEN: DIAGNOSTIC APPROACH USING LOW MAGNIFICATION

White Pulp*		Red and White Pulp*	Red Pulp*		
Uniform Involvement	Random Involvement		Billroth Cords	Sinuses	Both Cords and Sinuses
BENIGN LYMPHOPROLIFERATIONS					
Hyperplasia		Immunoblastic reactions			
MALIGNANT LYMPHOPROLIFERATIONS					
Small B/T cell neoplasms	Hodgkin's disease, all types	Small B/T cell neoplasms	Hairy cell leukemia		
Plasmacytoid lymphocytic lymphoma	Malignant lymphoma, large B/T cell	Plasmacytoid lymphocytic lymphoma			
Malignant lymphoma, follicular center cell, small cleaved cell	Malignant lymphoma, marginal zone lymphoma				
Malignant lymphoma, lympho-epithelioid lymphoma T	Malignant lymphoma, lympho-epithelioid lymphoma T				
Malignant lymphoma, immuno-blastic lymphoma T					
MYELOPROLIFERATIONS					
Mastocytosis	Myeloid leukemia		Myeloid leukemia		Extramedullary hematopoiesis
					Myeloproliferative disorders
MONONUCLEAR PHAGOCYTE SYSTEM PROLIFERATIONS					
	Granulomas		Malignant histiocytosis	Benign histiocytosis	Malignant histiocytosis
			Acute monocytic leukemia		
OTHER					
	Metastatic tumors				

* Abnormal area

Table 6

LOW MAGNIFICATION FEATURES HELPFUL IN THE RECOGNITION OF SPECIFIC HEMATOPOIETIC SYSTEM NEOPLASMS

Low Magnification Pattern	Likely Diagnosis
NODE	
Neoplastic follicular nodules, in part or entire node, ± intrafollicular or extrafollicular sclerosis	Follicular center cell lymphoma, usually cleaved cell type
Diffusely effaced architecture, homogeneous appearance ± proliferation centers (mounds)	Small B cell neoplasm
Infiltrative, marked architectural distortion; high mitotic rate and numerous macrophages	Convoluted (lymphoblastic) T lymphoma; small noncleaved cell (Burkitt's or non-Burkitt's)
Large irregular nodules ± compressed adjacent node	Hodgkin's disease, L&H nodular
Thick capsular ± intranodal polarizing bands outlining polymorphous nodules	Hodgkin's disease, nodular sclerosing
SPLEEN	
Scattered large nodules in white pulp	Hodgkin's disease, nodular sclerosing
Uniform increase in lymphoid tissue, diffuse or white pulp nodules	Follicular center cell, small cleaved cell; small B cell neoplasm; plasmacytoid lymphocytic lymphoma
Small follicles Interfollicular growth	Hairy cell leukemia; leukemic infiltrates
MARROW	
Nodules or sheets of cytoplasmic tumor cells	Multiple myeloma
Paratrabecular lymphocytic infiltrates	Follicular center cell, small cleaved cell
Large lymphocytic nodules, or diffuse effacement, small lymphocytes	Small B cell neoplasm; plasmacytoid lymphocytic lymphoma
Diffuse effacement, blasts	Acute lymphocytic leukemia; Acute myelomonocytic leukemia

19

Table 7

IMMUNOPHENOTYPING ANTIBODIES USEFUL IN
PARAFFIN-EMBEDDED HEMATOPOIETIC TISSUE

CD Designation	Reactivity	Frequently Used Reagents
LEUKOCYTES		
CD45[‡]	Pan-leukocyte	Leukocyte Common Antigen
CD45RB	Pan-leukocyte	PD7/26
*	Immature T and B cells, some myeloid leukemias	TdT
B LYMPHOCYTES		
CDw75[‡]	Follicular B cells, some T cells, erythrocytes, many epithelial cells	LN-1
CD74[‡]	Pan-B cells, histiocytes, some T cells, Reed-Sternberg cells, some epithelial cells	LN-2
Unclustered	Anti-HLA-DR B cells and activated T cells, histiocytes	LN-3
Unclustered	Mantle zone lymphocytes and histiocytes	LN-5
Unclustered but known to be CD20-associated[‡]	Pan-B cells, some Reed-Sternberg cells	L26
CD45R	Pan-B cells, some T cells, monocytes	MB-1, 4KB5, 4RB5
Unclustered	Pan-B cells, some T cells, many epithelial cells, endothelial cells	MB-2
CD45-like	Pan-B cells, some T cells, monocytes	KiB3
*	Cytoplasmic immunoglobulin	IgG, IgM, IgA, Kappa, Lambda
T LYMPHOCYTES		
CD3[‡]	Pan-T cells, some Reed-Sternberg cells	Anti-CD3
CD43[‡]	Pan-T cells, granulocytes, macrophages, some B cells	MT-1, Leu-22
CD45R[‡]	T cells, mantle zone and marginal zone B cells	MT-2
CD45RO[‡]	Subset of activated T cells, histiocytes, granulocytes	UCHL-1
CD57	Natural killer cells	Leu-7
MONONUCLEAR PHAGOCYTE SYSTEM CELLS		
*	Histiocytes	α_1-antitrypsin, -antichymotrypsin
*	Histiocytes/monocytes	Lysozyme
*	Langerhans histiocytes, melanoma, neural crest derivatives	S-100
CD68	Histiocytes/monocytes, mast cells	KP1
REED-STERNBERG CELLS		
CD15[‡]	Reed-Sternberg cells, granulocytes	Leu-M1
CD30[‡]	Reed-Sternberg cells and variants, some T and rare B cell neoplasms, embryonal carcinoma	Ber H2
*	Some lymphocytic and/or histiocytic variants of Reed-Sternberg cells, anaplastic large cell lymphomas	EMA

* Will not be assigned a CD number.
‡ May be used in frozen or plastic-embedded sections.

Table 8

IMMUNOPHENOTYPING ANTIBODIES FREQUENTLY USEFUL IN FROZEN OR PLASTIC-EMBEDDED HEMATOPOIETIC TISSUE

CD Designation	Reactivity	Frequently Used Reagents
B LYMPHOCYTES		
CD19	Pan-B cells	Leu-12, B4
CD20	B cells	B1
CD22	Pan-B cells	Leu-14
CD10	Common ALL antigen	CALLA, J5, BA-3
*	Demonstration of surface or cytoplasmic immuno-globulin	IgG, IgM, IgA, Kappa, Lambda
T LYMPHOCYTES		
CD1	Cortical thymocytes, Langerhans cells, interdigitating cells	Leu-6, T6, OKT6
CD2	Pan-T cells	Leu-5, T11, OKT11
CD3	Pan-T cells	Leu-4, T3, OKT3
CD5	Pan-T cells	Leu-1, T1, OKT1
CD7	Pan-T cells, NK cells, some myeloid leukemias	Leu-9
CD4	Helper/inducer subset	Leu-3, T4, OKT4
CD8	Suppressor/cytotoxic subset	Leu-2, T8, OKT8
*	Immature T cells	TdT
MONONUCLEAR PHAGOCYTE SYSTEM CELLS		
CDw14	Monocytes	Leu-M3, MY4
CD13	Myelomonocytes	MY7
CD15	Reed-Sternberg cells, granulocytes	Leu-M1
CD33	Myelomonocytes	MY9
*	Macrophages	Anti-macrophages
OTHER MARKERS OF INTEREST		
CD30	Reed-Sternberg cells, certain anaplastic lymphomas	RSC-II (Ki-1)
*	Immature T and B cells, some myeloid leukemias	TdT
*	Nuclear proliferation Ag	Proliferating cell (Ki-67)

* Will not be assigned a CD number.

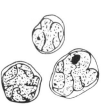
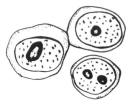

SMALL LYMPHOCYTIC
LYMPHOMA - T CELL

CONVOLUTED (LYMPHOBLASTIC)
LYMPHOMA

IMMUNOBLASTIC LYMPHOMA, T CELL

Figure 1
T CELL NEOPLASMS

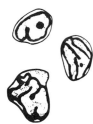
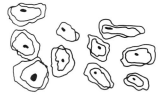

CEREBRIFORM (CUTANEOUS)
T CELL LYMPHOMA

LYMPHOEPITHELIOID LYMPHOMA

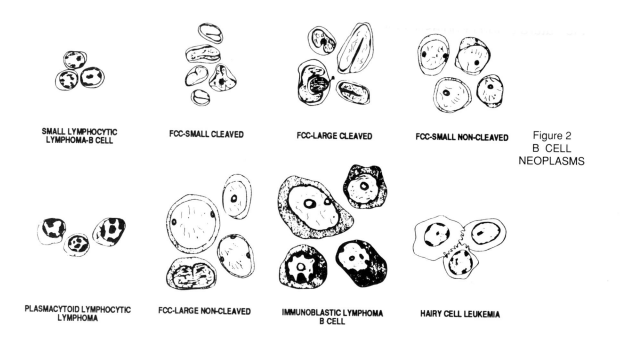

SMALL LYMPHOCYTIC
LYMPHOMA-B CELL

FCC-SMALL CLEAVED

FCC-LARGE CLEAVED

FCC-SMALL NON-CLEAVED

Figure 2
B CELL
NEOPLASMS

PLASMACYTOID LYMPHOCYTIC
LYMPHOMA

FCC-LARGE NON-CLEAVED

IMMUNOBLASTIC LYMPHOMA
B CELL

HAIRY CELL LEUKEMIA

The relative size and nuclear configuration of various T and B cell neoplasms are illustrated in these camera lucida drawings. This type of schematic is valuable in portraying cell size, nuclear size, and the configuration in the various lymphomas.

INFORMATION USED TO CLASSIFY HEMATOPOIETIC NEOPLASMS

Six pieces of information are generally useful in classifying hematopoietic neoplasms: (1) the presumed site of origin; (2) the phenotype of the neoplastic cell; (3) the stage of cell cycle of predominant cell or predominant differentiation phase; (4) the nature of the reacting component; (5) the preceding immunologic or dysmyelopoietic syndrome, if present; and (6) the DNA features or abnormality in karyotype.

The site of origin may be difficult to determine if the neoplasm is widespread at presentation. In other cases, the originating site of the neoplasm may usually be determined by evaluating the clinical history, the distribution of the tumor, the histologic appearance of affected tissues, and the nature of the neoplastic cell.

The phenotype of neoplastic cells is determined by varying combinations of histopathologic, cytologic, cytochemical, ultrastructural, and immunologic data (including evaluating the rearrangement of immunoglobulin or T-receptor genes). For some neoplasms, histopathologic and cytologic evaluations are sufficient to establish the phenotype. For other neoplasms, cytochemical, ultrastructural, or immunologic analyses are required. The stage of cell cycle or differentiation sequence is usually determined on cytologic evaluation by microscopically assaying the percentages of blasts, small cells, or differentiating cells. Flow cytometric and immunologic evaluation of differentiation antigens are useful techniques in quantitating the cell cycle phenomena.

Reacting components are most apparent in Hodgkin's disease but are also seen in many non-Hodgkin's lymphomas. Reacting macrophages are readily appreciated in some of the T lymphomas, but our most detailed information on reacting cells concerns the T lymphocytes in certain B lymphomas. As many as 40 percent of the cells in follicular center cell lymphomas have T cell features. By frozen section immunoperoxidase techniques, these T cells are distributed in both neoplastic follicles and interfollicular areas. Helper T lymphocytes generally predominate in both locations, but the T helper/suppressor ratio may be lower in these lymphomas than in reactive nodes. The functional capacities of T cells that react either with the neoplastic B component or normal B cells are being evaluated.

Lymphomas/leukemias evolving from previous immunologic abnormalities or dysmyelopoietic syndromes may have a different pathogenesis and natural history from similar-appearing neoplasms arising de novo. Documentation of the nature of disorders preceding neoplasms may have an important predictive value, as well as an intrinsic significance in developing strategies to prevent neoplasia.

Some karyotypic abnormalities have specific associations with individual lymphomas or leukemias (Yunis). Such specific relationships are likely to be recognized with increasing frequency. Small cleaved cell lymphomas of the Burkitt's type are universally associated with abnormalities in chromosome 8, usually t(8;14) and less frequently t(2;8) or t(8;22). Follicular center cell lymphomas, usually small cleaved cell type, often have a t(14;18) abnormality. A diagnostic criterion for chronic myelogenous leukemias is the t(9;22) abnormality. Virtually all acute leukemias have demonstrable karyotypic abnormalities (Yunis et al.) that in some cases are highly predictable. For example, acute promyelocytic leukemia usually shows a t(15;17). DNA analysis may well become the most specific indicator of tumor cell differentiation.

This background information indicates why our classification terminology specifies the following items: (1) the tissue sampled; (2) the type of neoplasm, such as leukemia, lymphoma, or malignant histiocytosis (if type is uncertain, more general terms such as lymphoid neoplasm or hematopoietic neoplasm are used); (3) the subpopulation of origin (e.g., follicular center cell, T cell, myelomonocytic); (4) the cell cycle or differentiation state of the predominant cell (qualifying terms of varying logic and descriptiveness, such as acute, chronic, cleaved, small, or noncleaved, are often applied to indicate the cell cycle or differentiation stage); and (5) the reacting component, preceding abnormality, or karyotypic abnormalities are given if known.

LEUKEMIAS

Leukemias are seen infrequently in community hospitals. Nevertheless, it is important for pathologists to be familiar with the principles of both marrow examination and classification of leukemias in order to correctly process marrow and blood from these patients. Due to the availability of overnight transportation, leukemic cases can be worked up thoroughly with samples obtained in community hospitals. Because leukemias are classified in part on the differentiation of tumor cells, the different types are discussed under the T cell, B cell, mononuclear phagocyte system, and myeloid cell areas. This discussion is focused on the nature of leukemia and how tissue should be processed.

Leukemias are hematopoietic neoplasms that arise in the marrow and often show prominent involvement of the peripheral blood. Marrow origins have not been proven for hairy cell leukemia and chronic lymphocytic leukemia, which in some or all cases may arise outside the marrow but spread quickly to it. Leukemias are clonal processes that can develop de novo, after marrow injury (chemotherapy, radiation), or in myelodysplastic states. Most patients with leukemia present with extensive marrow involvement and by diagnosis have begun passing through a phase of marrow insufficiency to overt marrow failure. Therefore, random marrow biopsies are rarely negative in symptomatic leukemic patients. Very rarely, leukemic patients present with extramarrow tumorous lesions (chloromas), and marrow lesions may not be apparent for several years.

Marrow examinations are crucial in diagnosing leukemia. In most patients, material obtained from the marrow is abundant and provides all the cells necessary for routine and specialized studies. In some cases, however, marrows may be packed and difficult to aspirate, or samples may be marginal due to the paucity of leukemic cells, artifactual damage from crushing, or poor viability.

In all types of leukemia, marrow particles or biopsies usually show effaced architecture and are hypercellular. Although histologic examination of the marrow particles or biopsy provides guidance in terms of the classification of leukemia, diagnosis is usually dependent on a multiparameter examination of tumor cells obtained from either the marrow and/or the peripheral blood. Marrow particle smears, touch preparations of marrow biopsies, cells blown from the aspirating needle in dry taps, or peripheral blood films are all processed in a similar fashion: Wright's-stained peripheral blood and marrow films remain essential components of the diagnostic procedure. However, numerous slides should be preserved unstained for cytochemistry and immunocytochemistry. Cytochemistry should be performed in all cases, and many myelocytic, monocytic, and promyelocytic leukemias may be diagnosed with assurance after examining cytochemical preparations. All Sudan black/peroxidase negative, esterase negative cases should be phenotyped. Flow cytometry is essential for precise categorization of acute lymphoid leukemias and for recognition of hybrid processes. For flow examination, peripheral blood or aspirated marrow particles anticoagulated with acid citrate dextrose can be sent by overnight carrier in containers protected from temperature extremes. These samples should not be frozen. Comparable phenotypic analyses can be performed on cytocentrifuge preparations of blood and marrow smears with alkaline phosphatase immunoperoxidase preparations. Electron microscopy remains an essential component of the diagnostic armamentarium of many laboratories and can be performed on glutaraldehyde-fixed buffy coats, aspirated marrow particles, or the 1 mm distal tip of marrow biopsies. Karyotypic analysis is performed routinely in many centers and in some cases is essential for the diagnosis. Molecular biologic techniques can be particularly valuable in recognizing cases of chronic myeloid leukemia without a detectable Philadelphia chromosome and some cases of T and B cell leukemia.

EXTRANODAL LYMPHOMAS

Most lymphomas begin in nodal tissue, but they may arise in many extranodal sites as well. Lymphomas originating in the gastrointestinal tract (particularly the stomach), thyroid, skin, and lung are sufficiently common to be important. Such processes are often confused with benign proliferations and generally have been thought to have a more indolent course than their histologic counterpart arising in nodal tissue.

Some extranodal lymphomas probably arise after a preceding prolonged immunologic reaction resulting in the accumulation of reacting lymphoid tissue. For example, lymphomas of the thyroid develop in patients with Hashimoto's disease, lymphomas of the bowel occur in some patients with a sprue-like illness, and some lymphomas of the skin (cerebriform T cell lymphoma) possibly develop following long-standing immunologic reactions in the skin. Thus, many extranodal lymphomas develop as complications of prolonged immunologic reactions. Paradoxically, some extranodal lymphomas (e.g., central nervous system) are more frequent in patients on immunosuppressive therapy or in immune-deficient states (e.g., AIDS).

Lymphomas may also begin in lymphoid tissue that is normally present in organs such as the spleen, tonsil, small intestine, and bone. The pathogenesis of these "extranodal" processes is probably similar to that of processes arising in nodes and does not necessarily involve previous immunologic reactions.

COMPOSITE LEUKEMIAS, LYMPHOMAS, AND HISTIOCYTOSES

A few patients with neoplasms of the hematopoietic, lymphoid, and mononuclear phagocyte systems may also have carcinomas detected at presentation or during their illness. Others exhibit transformation in the morphology and clinical character of their leukemia or lymphoma, usually due to a change in the growth fraction of the original neoplasm (van den Tweel et al.; York et al., 1984). A composite neoplasm has been detected in a very small group of patients. In these cases, evidence has been developed suggesting that the two neoplasms arose from different cell lines in the hematopoietic system.

Most of these cases have had acute leukemia, presumably developing as a complication of treatment of myeloma or Hodgkin's disease. In our experience, composite lymphomas have consisted of peripheral T cell lymphomas that developed in patients under treatment for follicular center cell lymphomas (York et al., 1985), and malignant histiocytoses in patients with a follicular center cell lymphoma or malignant lymphoma, small B cell type. Rare cases of Hodgkin's disease and non-Hodgkin's lymphoma have been reported to coexist.

MELANOMAS, CARCINOMAS, OR SARCOMAS CONFUSED WITH LYMPHOMAS

Metastatic melanomas, carcinomas, and sarcomas are usually easily recognized by their histopathologic features or are strongly suspected on clinical grounds. However, lymphomas in unusual clinical pathologic settings (involving the breast, thyroid, and central nervous system) are often misdiagnosed as small cell carcinomas.

Cohesion of tumor cells and sinusal involvement are reliable indicators of metastatic tumors, but poorly differentiated carcinomas, sarcomas, and melanomas are easily mistaken for malignant lymphoma or malignant histiocytosis and vice versa. Electron microscopy often provides specific information about the phenotype of the neoplastic cells, although most laboratories now rely on PIP procedures.

Immunoperoxidase techniques are appealing because of their availability to community hospitals and their claimed specificity, but their reliability must be established by the usual quality controls and the experience of studying known neoplasms. Very few antibodies are as specific as claimed, although an exception seems to be the leukocyte common antigen. There are few false negatives with this antibody, and false positives are rare. A battery of antibodies should be used for the characterization of neoplasms because the use of a single antibody is hazardous. Table 9 shows antibodies that are particularly useful in differentiating lymphomas from other neoplasms.

There are several specific neoplasms in which node metastases may closely mimic malignant lymphoma. Nasopharyngeal carcinoma may occur in children and young adults. Patients often present with cervical adenopathy without a readily apparent mass in the nasopharynx. Nodal involvement by nasopharyngeal carcinoma may be misinterpreted as nodular sclerosing Hodgkin's disease due to its fibrotic tissue reaction, eosinophilia, and small clusters of tumor cells. Metastatic melanoma may be mistaken for immunoblastic lymphoma B

Table 9

IMMUNOPEROXIDASE PROCEDURES USEFUL IN SEPARATING LYMPHOMAS FROM MALIGNANT HISTIOCYTOSES, CARCINOMAS, SARCOMAS, AND MELANOMAS

	CD45	CD68 (KP-1)	Keratin	Epithelial Membrane Antigen	S-100	HMB45
Malignant Lymphoma	+	$-^1$	−	±	−	−
Malignant Histiocytosis	±	+	−	±	±	−
Carcinoma	−	−	+	+	−	−
Sarcoma	−	$-^2$	$-^3$	$-^3$	$±^4$	−
Melanoma	−	−	−	−	+	+

1   CD68 may be reactive in lymphomas but positivity is focal in comparison to strong extensive positivity in histiocytes.

2   Some malignant fibrous histiocytoses may be positive.

3   Epithelioid sarcoma and synovial sarcoma may be keratin (+) or EMA (+).

4   Malignant schwannoma may be S-100 (+).

cells or lymphocyte-depleted Hodgkin's disease.

Breast carcinoma, particularly lobular carcinoma, often infiltrates the nodes without evidence of gland formation and can be confused with malignant lymphoma or malignant histiocytosis. Inguinal and abdominal nodes are frequent sites for metastasis by seminoma. Seminoma cells resemble transformed lymphocytes; however, the cytoplasm of seminoma cells, unlike most lymphomas, is rich in PAS positive glycogen, and nodal stroma may show a characteristic granulomatous response to metastatic seminoma.

CLASSIFICATION OF HEMATOPOIETIC NEOPLASMS

Hematopoietic neoplasms are listed according to lymphoid, mononuclear phagocyte, and myeloid systems, even though these systems are closely interrelated anatomically and functionally (Table 10). It is generally thought that there are no benign neoplasms in these systems, although it is acknowledged that clonal proliferations of limited clinical aggressiveness do exist. Finally, only those conditions accepted as malignant neoplasms are included, and all processes considered to be dysplastic or preneoplastic are excluded.

These neoplasms are arranged in Table 11 in relation to their probable site of origin. This table is intended to provide a conceptual framework for relating hematopoietic neoplasms to the normal cellular elements from which they arise. In practice, there are difficulties in establishing the tissue of origin for specific hematopoietic neoplasms, although diagnostic and therapeutic approaches to hematopoietic neo-

plasms are often based on assumptions as to point of origin. Assumptions about cell of origin are even more tenuous since specific cells have never been identified as the source of an individual patient's neoplasm. Nevertheless, we know most lymphomas and leukemias are clonal and therefore did develop from a single deranged cell.

Basically, hematopoietic neoplasms are classified by the phenotype of the predominant cell; however, the presumed cell of origin may differ from the predominant cell. The prime example of this discrepancy is chronic myelogenous leukemia, a neoplasm of pluripotential stem cells. The capacity for differentiation is retained in chronic myelogenous leukemia, and the predominant cell is a mature granulocyte. It is remarkable that this neoplasm arising from stem cells has the appearance of a differentiating process. In blast transformation, the capacity to differentiate is lost, and the neoplasm changes dramatically in appearance and clinical behavior. The natural history of chronic myelogenous leukemia, with its tendencies toward blast transformation, is understandable only by an appreciation of its presumed origin from a pluripotential stem cell.

Multiple myeloma is an example of a similar phenomenon involving the B cell system. Although most tumor cells are differentiated plasmacytic cells, multiple myeloma actually arises from a stem cell at the pre-B level. The capacity to differentiate is retained by this tumor as well, and the phenotype of the predominant cell is quite different from that of the presumed cell of origin. There is evidence that multiple myeloma spreads from its point of origin by the homing of small circulating tumor cells to foci throughout the marrow. Although the mechanism of production of

Table 10

CLASSIFICATION OF HEMATOPOIETIC SYSTEM NEOPLASMS

UNDEFINED CELL NEOPLASMS

Acute undefined leukemia

LYMPHOID NEOPLASMS

T Cell Neoplasms
   T cell acute lymphocytic leukemia
   Adult T cell leukemia
   Small T cell neoplasms, including chronic lymphocytic leukemia T
   Convoluted T lymphoma/lymphoblastic (thymic lymphoma)
   Immunoblastic T cell lymphoma, including peripheral T cell lymphomas
   Other T cell neoplasms, including lymphoepithelioid T lymphocytic lymphoma (Lennert's lymphoma), T-zone lymphoma
   Cerebriform T cell lymphoma (mycosis fungoides and Sézary syndrome)
   Extranodal T lymphomas

B Cell Neoplasms
   B cell acute lymphocytic leukemias, including B cell precursor acute leukemia
   Prolymphocytic leukemia
   Small B cell lymphoid neoplasms, including chronic lymphocytic leukemia
   B cell neoplasms with plasmacytic differentiation, including plasmacytoid lymphocytic lymphoma and multiple myeloma
   Hairy cell leukemia (leukemic reticuloendotheliosis)
   Mantle zone lymphomas
   Marginal zone lymphomas
   Parafollicular (monocytoid) B cell lymphomas
   Follicular center cell lymphomas, including Burkitt's lymphoma and non-Burkitt's types
   Immunoblastic lymphoma of B cells
   Large B cell lymphomas

HODGKIN'S DISEASE(S)*

Lymphocytic and histiocytic, nodular
Lymphocytic and histiocytic, diffuse
Nodular sclerosis
Mixed
Diffuse fibrosis
Reticular

MONONUCLEAR PHAGOCYTE SYSTEM NEOPLASMS

Marrow based
   Acute myelomonocytic leukemia
   Acute monocytic leukemia
   Chronic myelomonocytic leukemia

Tissue based
   Macrophage/histiocytic type neoplasms
      Histiocytic medullary reticulosis
      Splenic histiocytic type
   Follicular dendritic cell type
   Interdigitating cell type
   Langerhans cell type

MYELOID NEOPLASMS

Acute granulocytic leukemia
Promyelocytic leukemia
Erythroleukemia
Acute megakaryocytic leukemia
Chronic myelogenous leukemia
Granulocytic sarcoma
Mast cell disease

COMPOSITE HEMATOPOIETIC SYSTEM NEOPLASMS

* Reed-Sternberg cells in some types of Hodgkin's disease have B or T features.

Table 11

HEMATOPOIETIC NEOPLASMS IN RELATION TO
PROBABLE SITE AND PROBABLE CELL OF ORIGIN

T CELL		B CELL		MYELOID/MONONUCLEAR PHAGOCYTE SYSTEM		UNKNOWN CELL OF ORIGIN
Type	Cell of Origin	Type	Cell of Origin	Type	Cell of Origin	
MARROW						
Acute lymphocytic leukemia T*	Prothymocytes	Acute lympho-cytic leukemia, B cell precursor	Pluripotential stem cell	Acute myelo-monocytic leukemia	Pluripotential stem cell	Acute undefined leukemia
				Acute granulo-cytic, promyelo-cytic leukemia	Multipotential stem cell	
				Chronic myeloge-nous leukemia	Pluripotential stem cell	
		Lymphoplasma-cytic neoplasms Multiple myeloma	Multipotential stem cell	Chronic myelo-monocytic leukemia	Multipotential stem cell	
		Plasmacytoid lymphocytic lymphoma	Unknown B cell			
THYMUS						
Acute lymphocytic leukemia, T*	Cortical thymo-cytes	Large B cell neoplasms	Immunocompe-tent B cells (?)			Hodgkin's dis-ease, nodular sclerosing (some cases)
Convoluted (lymphoblastic) T lymphoma	Cortical thymo-cytes, medullary thymocytes					
Hodgkin's dis-ease, nodular sclerosing (some cases)	Thymocyte					

* Uncertainty as to site of origin

Table 11 (cont.)

T CELL		B CELL		MYELOID/MONONUCLEAR PHAGOCYTE SYSTEM		UNKNOWN CELL OF ORIGIN
Type	Cell of Origin	Type	Cell of Origin	Type	Cell of Origin	
NODE, SPLEEN, TONSIL, GUT						
Immunoblastic lymphoma T cell and other peripheral T cell lymphomas	Immunocompetent T cell	Follicular center cell, all types	Immunocompetent B cell	Granulocytic sarcoma	Undefined precursor	Hodgkin's disease, nodular sclerosing (some cases) Hodgkin's disease, mixed cellularity, lymphocyte depletion
		Immunoblastic lymphoma B	Immunocompetent B cell	Malignant histiocytosis	Macrophage or various dendritic cell types	
Hodgkin's disease, nodular sclerosing (some cases)	Immunocompetent T cell	Plasmacytoid lymphocytic lymphoma	Immunocompetent B cell			
		Mantle zone lymphoma	Immunocompetent B cell			
		Parafollicular B cell lymphoma	Immunocompetent B cell			
		Marginal zone lymphoma	Immunocompetent B cell			
		Hodgkin's disease, lymphocyte predominant	Immunocompetent B cell			
SKIN						
Cerebriform T	Immunocompetent T cell, organ specific (?)	Follicular center cell, various types	Immunocompetent B cell	Granulocytic sarcoma	Undefined precursor	
				Malignant histiocytosis	Macrophage or various dendritic cell types	
Peripheral T cell lymphoma	Immunocompetent T cell	Plasmacytoid lymphocytic lymphoma	Immunocompetent B cell			
		Immunoblastic lymphoma B	Immunocompetent B cell			
UNKNOWN SITE OF ORIGIN						
Small T cell lymphoma, including chronic lymphocytic leukemia T	Immunocompetent T cell	Small B cell lymphoma, including chronic lymphocytic leukemia	Immunocompetent B cell			
Adult T cell leukemia/lymphoma	Immunocompetent T cell	Prolymphocytic leukemia	Immunocompetent B cell			
		Angiotropic lymphoma	Immunocompetent B cell			
		Hairy cell leukemia	Immunocompetent B cell			

these circulating elements is unclear, an appreciation of the relationships between the presumed cell of origin (pre-B cell), the circulating tumor cells, and the phenotype of the predominant cell allows an understanding of the growth of myeloma in the marrow and of its pathogenesis.

THE WORKING FORMULATION FOR CLINICAL USAGE IN RELATION TO THE LUKES-COLLINS CLASSIFICATION

The Working Formulation evolved from a National Cancer Institute study (The Non-Hodgkin's Lymphoma Pathologic Classification Project) that attempted to resolve the controversy arising from differences in the numerous classifications of malignant lymphomas. The Working Formulation was proposed as a basis for translating between classifications to facilitate the comparison of data generated by the usage of any of the classifications.

In comparing the Working Formulation and the Lukes-Collins classification, a major difference becomes apparent. As illustrated in Table 12, the Working Formulation is subdivided according to clinical aggressiveness, whereas tumor grade is inherent in the definition of each cytologic type in the Lukes-Collins classification. Although many of the cytologic terms are derived from the Lukes-Collins classification, there are no immunologic terms or connotations in the Working Formulation. As a result, there are fundamental differences in the usage of terms in the Lukes-Collins classification and the Working Formulation. For example, small lymphocyte is considered separately under both B cell and T cell types, each with subtypes, in the Lukes-Collins classification but is a single type in

the Working Formulation. Furthermore, the plasmacytoid lymphocytic type is split off from the small B lymphocyte type in the Lukes-Collins approach, whereas plasmacytoid is listed as a modifier of small lymphocyte in the Working Formulation. This de-emphasis in the Working Formulation obscures the significance of this lymphoma. Plasmacytoid lymphocytic lymphomas are already underdiagnosed, particularly if MGP and Giemsa stains are not consistently employed.

A number of seemingly minor differences between the Working Formulation and Lukes-Collins classification involve the terms cleaved and noncleaved in which the designation follicular center cell is omitted. This difference in terms eliminates the important designation of the cell of origin and the implication of its B cell nature. For the term convoluted T cell under the Lukes-Collins classification, the Working Formulation uses lymphoblastic, convoluted, or nonconvoluted. More than 90 percent of these cases actually exhibit convolutions when reviewed. Thus, the term nonconvoluted is inappropriate, and lymphoblastic is not descriptive of the cytologic features. The cerebriform T cell of Lukes-Collins is an immunologic and cytologic type associated with two clinical syndromes: mycosis fungoides and Sézary syndrome. The Working Formulation does not use a cytologic term for this neoplasm; instead it uses the name of a clinical syndrome (mycosis fungoides) and omits Sézary syndrome.

Major problems are created in placing lymphoepithelioid, T lymphocytic, and immunoblastic lymphoma of T cell types in the Working Formulation. Both processes have a range of expressions and require a number of categories in the Working

Table 12

THE LUKES-COLLINS CLASSIFICATION OF NON-HODGKIN'S LYMPHOMAS IN RELATION TO THE WORKING FORMULATION

Working Formulation	Lukes-Collins Equivalents
LOW GRADE	
Malignant lymphoma, small lymphocytic	
consistent with chronic lymphocytic leukemia	Malignant lymphoma, small lymphocyte B or T
plasmacytoid	Malignant lymphoma, plasmacytoid lymphocytic
Malignant lymphoma, follicular	
Predominantly small cleaved cell	Malignant lymphoma, small cleaved follicular center cell, follicular
diffuse areas	Follicular and diffuse
sclerosis	Sclerosis
Malignant lymphoma, follicular	
Mixed, small cleaved and large cell	Malignant lymphoma, small cleaved follicular center cell, follicular
diffuse areas	Follicular and diffuse
sclerosis	Sclerosis
INTERMEDIATE GRADE	
Malignant lymphoma, follicular	
Predominantly large cell	Malignant lymphoma, large cleaved and large noncleaved
diffuse areas	follicular center cell, follicular or follicular and diffuse
sclerosis	Sclerosis
Malignant lymphoma, diffuse	
Small cleaved cell	Malignant lymphoma, small cleaved follicular center cell, diffuse
sclerosis	Sclerosis
Malignant lymphoma, diffuse	
Mixed small and large cell	Malignant lymphoma, large cleaved follicular center cell, diffuse
sclerosis	Sclerosis
epithelioid cell component	Malignant lymphoma, lymphoepithelioid T cell
Malignant lymphoma, diffuse	
Large cell	
cleaved cell	Malignant lymphoma, large cleaved follicular center cell, diffuse
noncleaved cell	Large noncleaved follicular center cell, diffuse
sclerosis	Sclerosis
HIGH GRADE	
Malignant lymphoma, large cell, immunoblastic	Malignant lymphoma, immunoblastic lymphoma
Plasmacytoid	Immunoblastic lymphoma B
Clear cell	Immunoblastic lymphoma T
Polymorphous	
Epithelioid cell component	Malignant lymphoma, lymphoepithelioid with immunoblastic lymphoma T
Malignant lymphoma, lymphoblastic	Malignant lymphoma, convoluted (lymphoblastic) T cell
Convoluted cell	
Nonconvoluted cell	
Malignant lymphoma, small noncleaved cell	Malignant lymphoma, small noncleaved follicular center cell
Burkitt's	Burkitt's or non-Burkitt's
Follicular areas	Follicular or diffuse
MISCELLANEOUS	
Composite	
Mycosis fungoides	Cerebriform T cell of mycosis fungoides and Sézary syndrome
Histiocytic	Histiocytic (genuine)
Extramedullary plasmacytoma	Plasmacytoma
Unclassifiable	Unclassifiable
Other	

Formulation since no single category exists for direct translation. Depending on the number of large cells, the lymphoepithelioid type may be categorized as diffuse mixed, diffuse large cell, or large cell immunoblastic. Immunoblastic lymphoma of T cells may also fall into the same categories as the lymphoepithelioid T lymphocytic type, depending on the number of large cells. Obviously, neither of these terms, lymphoepithelioid or immunoblastic lymphoma T, are directly translatable into the Working Formulation.

It is readily apparent that the goal of the Working Formulation to provide a useful basis for translation between classifications has not succeeded. The categories are essentially not equivalent between the Lukes-Collins classification and the Working Formulation. In addition, because it lacks a biologic conceptual basis, the Working Formulation is neither adaptable nor readily expanded in a logical fashion.

COMPARISON OF THE LUKES-COLLINS AND KIEL CLASSIFICATIONS

The Kiel classification, based on the approach of Lennert and associates, is immunologic in nature and in close concordance with the Lukes-Collins classification, even though many of the terms are not identical. A comparison of the Kiel and Lukes-Collins classifications is outlined in Table 13, as modified from a comparative analysis of the two classifications (Lennert et al.).

In this comparison, only one term, lymphoepithelioid, is common to both. Many terms are almost identical, and several are completely different, even though most of the cytologic categories are accurately trans-latable. Small lymphocytic B or T cell, plasmacytoid lymphocytic, and immunoblastic lymphoma B or T cells have almost identical counterpart terms in both classifications. The small cleaved follicular center cell (diffuse) of the Lukes-Collins classification is closely related to the small centrocytic type, and the diffuse large cleaved follicular center cell fits well with the large centrocytic type. The centrocytic-centroblastic category of Kiel includes both small cleaved follicular center cell and large cleaved follicular center cell. Two other follicular center cell terms of the Lukes-Collins classification, small non-cleaved follicular center cell and large non-cleaved follicular center cell, are quite dissimilar to B lymphoblastic and centroblastic, but these are corresponding cytologic categories. Similarly, in the T cell group, the convoluted lymphocytic and cerebriform lymphocytic of the Lukes-Collins classification correspond closely to the T lymphoblastic and lymphocytic type of the mycosis fungoides/Sézary syndrome of the Kiel classification. The Kiel term T-zone lymphoma is not apparent in the Lukes-Collins classification but is included in T immunoblastic lymphoma.

COMPARISON OF THE LUKES-COLLINS AND THE MODIFIED RAPPAPORT CLASSIFICATIONS

In Table 14, the Lukes-Collins classification is shown in relation to the modified Rappaport classification. The Lukes-Collins classification, which uses morphologic descriptive terms primarily, is based on an immunologic approach and composed of T and B cell types. A U cell type is included to describe primitive

Table 13

THE LUKES-COLLINS CLASSIFICATION OF NON-HODGKIN'S LYMPHOMAS AND EQUIVALENT ENTITIES IN THE KIEL CLASSIFICATION, WITH DESIGNATIONS BY WORKING FORMULATION

Lukes-Collins Classification	Kiel Equivalent	Working Formulation
Undefined	*U Cell*	
Undefined	Lymphoblastic, unclassified*	
B Cell	*B Cell*	
Small lymphocyte B chronic lymphocytic leukemia	Lymphocytic, B chronic lymphocytic leukemia	Malignant lymphoma, small lymphocytic (chronic lymphocytic leukemia)
Plasmacytoid lymphocyte	Lymphoplasmacytic/lymphoplasmacytoid (lymphoplasmacytic immunocytoma)	Malignant lymphoma, small lymphocytic plasmacytoid
Follicular center cell types ‡		
Small cleaved	Centrocytic; centroblastic-centrocytic ‡	Malignant lymphoma, follicular/diffuse, small cleaved
Large cleaved	Centrocytic; centroblastic-centrocytic ‡	Malignant lymphoma, follicular/diffuse, large cell, or mixed small cleaved and large cell
Small noncleaved	B lymphoblastic	Malignant lymphoma, small noncleaved cell
Burkitt's	Burkitt type	Burkitt's
Non-Burkitt's	Others	
Large noncleaved	Centroblastic	Malignant lymphoma, large noncleaved cell
Immunoblastic lymphoma B	B immunoblastic	Malignant lymphoma, large cell immunoblastic, plasmacytoid
T Cell	*T Cell*	
Small lymphocyte T chronic lymphocytic leukemia	Lymphocytic, T chronic lymphocytic leukemia	Malignant lymphoma, small lymphocyte
Convoluted lymphocyte	T lymphoblastic (convoluted cell type and others)	Malignant lymphoma, lymphoblastic (convoluted or nonconvoluted)
Cerebriform lymphocyte (mycosis fungoides and Sézary syndrome)	Lymphocytic, mycosis fungoides, and Sézary syndrome	Mycosis fungoides
Lymphoepithelioid lymphocyte	[Lymphoepithelioid] §	
		Malignant lymphoma, diffuse mixed small and large cell with epithelioid cells
Immunoblastic lymphoma (T cell) including peripheral T cell lymphoma	T immunoblastic	Malignant lymphoma, large cell, immunoblastic, clear cell, polymorphous
	T-zone lymphoma	

* This category contains all lymphoblastic lymphomas that are immunologically undefined or cannot be typed for any of several reasons.

‡ Follicular, follicular and diffuse, or diffuse; with or without sclerosis.

§ This category was not included in the Kiel classification because at present, many cases cannot be distinguished from Hodgkin's disease with a large number of T lymphocytes and very few Reed-Sternberg cells.

35

Table 14

COMPARISON OF THE LUKES-COLLINS
AND THE MODIFIED RAPPAPORT CLASSIFICATIONS

LUKES-COLLINS	MODIFIED RAPPAPORT*
U CELL	
B CELL TYPES	
Small B lymphocytic	Lymphocytic, well differentiated
Plasmacytoid lymphocytic	Lymphocytic, well differentiated with plasmacytoid features
Follicular center cell Follicular or diffuse With or without sclerosis	
Small cleaved follicular center cell	Nodular, poorly differentiated lymphocytic Nodular, mixed lymphocytic-histiocytic Diffuse lymphocytic, poorly differentiated
Large cleaved follicular center cell	Nodular, histiocytic Diffuse mixed lymphocytic-histiocytic
Small noncleaved follicular center cell Burkitt's variant Non-Burkitt's variant	Undifferentiated, Burkitt's and non-Burkitt's
Large noncleaved follicular center cell	Nodular, histiocytic Diffuse, histiocytic with/without sclerosis
B immunoblastic	Diffuse histiocytic
T CELL TYPES	
Small lymphocytic	Lymphocytic well differentiated
Cerebriform lymphocytic	Mycosis fungoides
Convoluted lymphocytic	Lymphoblastic; convoluted/nonconvoluted
Lymphoepithelioid lymphocytic	‡
Immunoblastic	Diffuse histiocytic
GENUINE HISTIOCYTIC (see malignant histiocytosis)	

* In the modified Rappaport classification, four types had nodular growth pattern: lymphocytic, well and poorly differentiated; mixed lymphocytic and histiocytic; and histiocytic.

‡ No definite counterpart in the modified Rappaport classification.

lymphocytes that lack detectable morphologic or immunologic evidence of differentiation. According to the Lukes-Collins approach, because lymphomas are considered to be neoplasms of lymphocytes, the tumors of genuine histiocytes are included with the tumors of the monocyte/macrophage system under the malignant histiocytoses. In the B and T cell types, there are small lymphocytic types and immunoblastic types. Each of the four follicular center cell lymphomas may have follicular and/or diffuse expressions, and each also may be associated with sclerosis. The T cell types exhibit an unusual array of configurations, and the terms for four of the five cytologic types are descriptive of their appearance, whereas the fifth term, T immunoblastic, indicates the high proliferative state of a transformed T lymphocyte.

The modified Rappaport classification is based entirely on morphology and lacks any immunologic designations. The five cytologic types of the original classification were considered to have both nodular or diffuse expressions, whereas in the modified classification, four types (lymphocytic, well and poorly differentiated; mixed lymphocytic and histiocytic; and histiocytic) have nodular expressions, and 9 have diffuse expressions. Both well differentiated and poorly differentiated lymphocytic types in the modified classification can be associated with plasmacytoid features. The lymphoblastic type may be convoluted or nonconvoluted. The histiocytic type is found in both the original and modified classifications in nodular and diffuse forms. However, it is currently agreed that cases of verified histiocytic neoplasms are extremely uncommon.

The modified Rappaport classification was reported as a part of the International Formulation Study published in 1982. The comparisons shown in Table 14 are based on that study.

OTHER CLASSIFICATIONS

During the 1970s, the classification of Rappaport was updated and several others were proposed, namely those by the British National Lymphoma Investigative Group and Dorfman. These classifications are acknowledged by the authors to be morphologic classifications and lack any immunologic framework. Each classification added several terms for use in the National Cancer Institute study.

References

Dorfman, R.F. Classification of non-Hodgkin's lymphoma. Lancet 1:1295, 1974.

Lennert, K., Collins, R.D., and Lukes, R.J. Concordance of the Kiel and Lukes-Collins classifications of non-Hodgkin's lymphomas. Histopathology 7:549-559, 1983.

Lukes, R.J. and Collins, R.D. New approaches to the classification of the lymphomata. Br. J. Cancer 31(Suppl.2):1-28, 1975.

_____ , Taylor, C.R., and Parker, J.W. Multiparameter Studies in Malignant Lymphoma Based on Studies in 1186 Cases, pp. 203-213. In: 13th International Cancer Congress, Part E. Cancer Management. Mirand, E.A., Hutchinson, W.B., and Mihich, E. (Eds.). New York: Alan R. Liss, Inc., 1983.

The Non-Hodgkin's Lymphoma Pathologic Classification Project. National Cancer Institute sponsored study of classification of non-Hodgkin's lymphomas: summary and description of a working formulation for clinical usage. Cancer 49:2112-2135, 1982.

Rappaport, H. Tumors of the Hematopoietic System. Fascicle 8, First Series. Atlas of Tumor Pathology. Washington: Armed Forces Institute of Pathology, 1966.

van den Tweel, J.G., Lukes, R.J., and Taylor, C.R. Pathophysiology of lymphocyte transformation. A study of so-called composite lymphomas. Am. J. Clin. Pathol. 71:509-520, 1979.

York, J.C., Glick, A.D., Cousar, J.B., and Collins, R.D. Changes in the appearance of hematopoietic and lymphoid neoplasms: clinical, pathologic and biologic implications. Hum. Pathol. 15:11-38, 1984.

_____ , Cousar, J.B., Glick, A.D., et al. Morphologic and immunologic evidence of composite B- and T-cell lymphomas. A report of three cases developing in follicular center cell lymphomas. Am. J. Clin. Pathol. 84:35-43, 1985.

Yunis, J.J. The chromosomal basis of human neoplasia. Science 221:227-236, 1983.

_____ , Brunning, R.D., Howe, R.B., and Lobell, M. High-resolution chromosomes as an independent prognostic indicator in adult acute nonlymphocytic leukemia. N. Engl. J. Med. 311:812-818, 1984.

Additional References

Baer, M.R., Krantz, S.B., Cousar, J.B., Glick, A.D., and Collins, R.D. Malignant histiocytoses developing in patients with B-cell lymphomas. Cancer 57:2175-2184, 1986.

Bennett, M.H., Farrer-Brown, G., Henry, K., et al. Classification of non-Hodgkin's lymphomas. Lancet 2:405-406, 1974.

Collins, R.D., Bennett, B., and Glick, A.D. Neoplasms of the Mononuclear Phagocyte System, pp. 1-33. In: The Reticuloendothelial System, Vol. 5. Herberman, R.B. and Friedman, H. (Eds.). New York: Plenum Press, 1983.

Kim, H., Hendrickson, R., and Dorfman, R.F. Composite lymphoma. Cancer 41:959-976, 1977.

Lennert, K. Malignant Lymphomas Other Than Hodgkin's Disease: Histology, Cytology, Ultrastructure, Immunology. New York: Springer-Verlag, 1978.

_____ , Mohri, N., Stein, H., and Kaiserling, E. The histopathology of malignant lymphoma. Br. J. Cancer 31(Suppl.):193-203, 1975.

_____ , Kaiserling, E., and Muller-Hermelink, H.K. Malignant Lymphomas: Models of Differentiation and Cooperation of Lymphoreticular Cells, pp. 897-913. In: Differentiation of Normal and Neoplastic Hematopoietic Cells. Clarkson, B., Marks, P.A., and Till, J.E. (Eds.). Cold Spring Harbor, New York: Cold Spring Harbor Laboratory, 1978.

Lukes, R.J. and Collins, R.D. Immunologic characterization of human malignant lymphomas. Cancer 34(Suppl. 4):1488-1503, 1974.

Mann, R.B., Jaffe, E.S., and Berard, C.W. Malignant lymphoma — a conceptual understanding of morphologic diversity. Am. J. Pathol. 94:105-191, 1979.

Shackney, S.E., Levine, A.M., Fisher, R.I., et al. The biology of tumor growth in the non-Hodgkin's lymphomas. J. Clin. Invest. 73:1201-1214, 1984.

Vogler, L.B., Glick, A.D., and Collins, R.D. B cell neoplasms: correlation of recent developments with the biology of normal B lymphocytes. Prog. Clin. Pathol. 9:197-223, 1983.

T CELL NEOPLASMS

Immunologic studies of leukemias and lymphomas have shown that some of these neoplasms originate from the T arm of the immune system. Fifteen to 25 percent of acute lymphocytic leukemias and 10 to 20 percent of non-Hodgkin's lymphomas have T features (Foon and Todd; Lennert; Lukes et al.). T cell neoplasms seem to be far more complex than indicated by any of the classifications now used. It should be recognized that their heterogeneity may have a more biologic than clinical significance. These facts have significant implications for the classification of T cell neoplasms.

Although individual T cells circulate widely and probably constantly, T cells as a group are operationally distributed among certain anatomic sites, particularly the marrow, thymus, lymph nodes, spleen, gastrointestinal tract, and skin. T-precursor stem cells are incompletely defined in terms of markers but are apparently undeveloped immunologically. These cells migrate to the thymus, where functionally competent T cells evolve. The most immature thymocytes are found in the thymic cortex and constitute approximately 10 percent of the total lymphoid population. Common thymocytes, comprising approximately 50 percent of the lymphoid cells, are also principally located in the cortex. Late thymocytes are found in the medulla, where they segregate into helper/inducer and suppressor/cytotoxic subsets; these thymocytes migrate to peripheral compartments as immunologically competent effector T cells.

Peripheral T cells are found in the paracortex of nodes and the periarterial lymphoid sheaths of the spleen; minor populations also exist in the skin and the gastrointestinal and respiratory tracts.

Some T cell lymphomas, such as cerebriform and convoluted (lymphoblastic) T lymphomas, are distinct clinicopathologic entities with well-defined diagnostic criteria and clinical expressions. Other T cell lymphomas are very heterogeneous in their clinical, morphologic, and immunologic features. Nevertheless, most T cell neoplasms may be grouped in relation to the anatomic compartments described above (see Table 11). It is of interest that some T cell neoplasms in at least one compartment (thymus) may have a fetal phenotype (Stein et al.). Clear-cut immunologic differences have been described for T cell neoplasms within each anatomic compartment, as anticipated from the functional differences in normal T populations. However, many T cell neoplasms have phenotypes that differ from those of recognized T cell populations, and these discrepancies have even been cited as evidence of malignancy.

In contrast to B cell neoplasms, in which histopathologic findings alone are often diagnostic, immunophenotypic analyses provide important adjunctive or diagnostic information in T cell proliferations. Immunophenotypic criteria for the diagnosis of T cell neoplasms have been reviewed by Knowles and Picker and colleagues. Phenotypes associated with T cell malignancy include loss of pan-T antigens and anomalous T cell subset antigen expression. Analysis of T cell receptor β-chain gene rearrangement is an apparently accurate and sensitive indicator of T lineage and clonality (Knowles). While admitting the importance of immunophenotypic data in diagnosing T cell neoplasms, it is also our experience that Hodgkin's disease and certain B cell lymphomas are misdiagnosed as T cell lymphomas as a result of imprecise interpretation of flow data or frozen section immunoperoxidase. Reactive T lymphocytes may obscure the underlying process unless paraffin immunoperoxidase is also available to evaluate large cells for Reed-Sternberg or B cell features.

Initial Sites of Presentation. The marrow, thymus, nodes, or skin are the usual sites of involvement by T cell neoplasms at the time of presentation. In the marrow, 15 to 25 percent of acute lymphocytic leukemias demonstrate T-immunologic features. Separation of these neoplasms from convoluted (lymphoblastic) T lymphomas is often difficult clinically and pathologically. In both groups of neoplasms, there is a considerable overlap in the clinical features (predilection for young males, high incidence of mediastinal masses, frequent involvement of marrow and peripheral blood), as well as pathologic and immunologic characteristics. These similarities are reflected in a common clinical approach to the management of these patients.

Approximately 10 percent of the non-Hodgkin's lymphomas are T cell neoplasms. Peripheral T cell lymphomas arising in the nodes generally show a diffuse process that varies considerably in its histology, indicating the presence of several clinicopathologic entities. If a parallel may be drawn between peripheral T cell lymphomas and follicular center cell lymphomas in which the histopathology has been reasonably well established, then each nodal T population may yield neoplasms in

which the predominant cell is in various stages of the cell cycle or shows varying capacities for differentiation to effector cells. The term immunoblastic lymphoma of T cells has been used for those T neoplasms in which there is a prominent component of large or transformed T cells, but small lymphocytes may predominate in other peripheral T lymphomas. Currently, there are no effective techniques for distinguishing effector from dormant T cells, in contrast to the easy recognition of effector B cells (plasma cells).

T cell neoplasms may be presumed to be of cutaneous origin if the skin is the major site of involvement at presentation, the histopathologic changes are typical of cerebriform T cell lymphomas, and the neoplastic cells have the characteristic cerebriform convolutions. Recognition of the early stages of cutaneous T lymphomas has been difficult in part due to the presence of similar-appearing infiltrates in various reactive states. Cerebriform T cell lymphomas certainly appear to involve the skin primarily, although they ultimately develop a disseminated phase in which neoplastic cells may be demonstrated in the blood, nodes, marrow, and viscera. Despite the clinical and pathologic evidence indicating a cutaneous origin for these neoplasms, proliferation kinetics suggest that the neoplastic cells migrate from the blood to the skin (Miller et al.), with a production site in lymphatic tissue (Schwarzmeier et al.). There is karyotypic evidence in cerebriform T cell lymphomas suggesting an origin from a single clone rather than a multifocal process (Edelson et al.). Studies of most cutaneous T lymphomas have shown that the neoplastic cells express helper functions, although morphologically similar neoplasms have had suppressor activity (Hopper and Haren). A case of cerebriform T cell lymphoma exhibiting blastic transformation was shown to have helper activity immunologically, indicating a change in the dividing fraction of the original tumor (Lawrence et al.).

Lymphomas that are otherwise similar in histopathologic and immunologic features to the peripheral T cell lymphomas described above have occasionally been detected in sites other than the skin and nodes. In particular, peripheral T cell lymphomas have been described in the nasopharynx and rarely in liver and spleen.

Microscopic Features. Acute lymphocytic leukemia T and convoluted (lymphoblastic) T lymphomas are relatively uniform, densely cellular, and contain few reacting elements. The mitotic rate in both neoplasms may be very high, although cells with distinct nucleoli are generally not apparent. Peripheral T cell lymphomas arising in nodes are more heterogeneous with mixtures of neoplastic cells in varying stages of the cell cycle and intermixed reacting histiocytes and small lymphocytes. Some of these processes are associated with hypervascularity. Peripheral T cell lymphomas arising in the skin contain relatively monomorphic populations of cerebriform T cells intermixed with Langerhans cells. Transformed T lymphocytes may be found in these neoplasms even at the time of presentation. A significant percentage of cerebriform T cell processes undergo cytologic transformation during their course.

Plasma cells and eosinophils are infrequent in T cell lymphomas, although there are exceptions to this rule. Admixed reactive small B lymphocytes are present in very few numbers in peripheral T cell lymphomas, in contrast to the high frequency of reactive T cells in most B cell lymphomas.

Clinical Features. Differentiation to effector T cells must occur in some T cell neoplasms, but clinical effects from lymphokines or altered T cell functions have not been recognized. This situation contrasts sharply with the significant effects of immunoglobulin production in certain B cell neoplasms.

Some T cell neoplasms [acute lymphocytic leukemia T and convoluted (lymphoblastic) T lymphomas] are rapidly growing, extremely infiltrative processes that disseminate early and widely. Most of the clinical effects are probably due directly to tumorous growth. Cerebriform T cell lymphomas often have an indolent phase, but other small cell processes (chronic lymphocytic leukemia T) seem more aggressive than their B counterparts. Convoluted (lymphoblastic) T lymphomas and certain peripheral T cell lymphomas are distinguished by their extraordinary sensitivity to chemotherapeutic agents. Although rapid tumor lysis occurs shortly after induction, dissemination and resistant relapses remain the rule.

References

Edelson, R.L., Berger, C.L., Raafat, J., and Warburton, D. Karyotype studies of cutaneous T cell lymphoma: evidence for clonal origin. J. Invest. Dermatol. 73:548-550, 1979.

Foon, K.A. and Todd, R.F., III. Immunologic classification of leukemia and lymphoma. Blood 68:1-31, 1986.

Hopper, J.E. and Haren, J.M. Studies on a Sézary lymphocyte population with T-suppressor activity. Suppression of Ig synthesis of normal peripheral blood lymphocytes. Clin. Immunol. Immunopathol. 17:43-54, 1980.

Knowles, D.M. Immunophenotypic and antigen receptor gene rearrangement analysis in T cell neoplasia. Am. J. Pathol. 134:761-785, 1989.

Lawrence, E.C., Broder, S., Jaffe, E.S., et al. Evolution of a lymphoma with helper T cell characteristics in Sézary syndrome. Blood 52:481-492, 1978.

Lennert, K. Malignant Lymphomas Other Than Hodgkin's Disease: Histology, Cytology, Ultrastructure, Immunology. New York: Springer-Verlag, 1978.

Lukes, R.J., Parker, J.W., Taylor, C.R., et al. Immunologic approach to non-Hodgkin's lymphoma and related leukemias. Semin. Hematol. 15:322-351, 1978.

Miller, R.A., Coleman, C.N., Fawcett, H.D., Hoppe, R.T., and McDougall, I.R. Sézary syndrome: a model for migration of T lymphocytes to skin. N. Engl. J. Med. 303:89-92, 1980.

Picker, L.J., Weiss, L.M., Medeiros, L.J., Wood, G.S., and Warnke, R.A. Immunophenotypic criteria for the diagnosis of non-Hodgkin's lymphoma. Am. J. Pathol. 128:181-201, 1987.

Schwarzmeier, J.D., Paietta, E., Radaszkiewicz, T., Konrad, K., and Marosi, L. Proliferation kinetics of Sézary cells. Blood 57:1049-1054, 1981.

Stein, H., Petersen, N., Gaedicke, G., Lennert, K., and Landbeck, G. Lymphoblastic lymphoma of convoluted or acid phosphatase type—a tumor of T precursor cells. Int. J. Cancer 17:292-295, 1976.

Additional References

Barcos, M.P. and Lukes, R.J. Malignant lymphoma of convoluted lymphocytes: a new entity of possible T-cell type, pp.147-178. In: Conflicts in Childhood Cancer: An Evaluation of Current Management, Vol. 4. Sinks, L.F. and Godden, J.O. (Eds.). New York: Alan R. Liss, Inc., 1975.

Bernard, A., Boumsell, L., Reinherz, E.L., et al. Cell surface characterization of malignant T cells from lymphoblastic lymphoma using monoclonal antibodies: evidence for phenotypic differences between malignant T cells from patients with acute lymphoblastic leukemia and lymphoblastic lymphoma. Blood 57:1105-1110, 1981.

Broder, S., Uchiyama, T., and Waldmann, T.A. Current concepts in immunoregulatory T-cell neoplasms. Cancer Treat. Rep. 63:607-612, 1979.

Brouet, J.C., Valensi, F., Daniel, M.T., et al. Immunological classification of acute lymphoblastic leukaemias. Br. J. Haematol. 33:319-328, 1976.

Collins, R.D., Waldron, J.A., and Glick, A.D. Results of multiparameter studies of T-cell lymphoid neoplasms. Am. J. Clin. Pathol. 72(Suppl. 4):699-707, 1979.

Gramatzki, M., Dolan, M.F., Fauci, A.S., et al. Immunologic characterization of a helper T-cell lymphoma. Blood 59:702-708, 1982.

Greer, J.P., York, J.C., Cousar, J.B., et al. Peripheral T-cell lymphoma. J. Clin. Oncol. 2:788-798, 1984.

Haynes, B.F., Metzgar, R.S., Minna, J.D., and Bunn, P.A. Phenotypic characterization of cutaneous T-cell lymphoma. N. Engl. J. Med. 304:1319-1323, 1981.

Nadler, L.M., Reinherz, E.L., Weinstein, H.J., D'Orsi, C.J., and Schlossman, S.F. Heterogeneity of T-cell lymphoblastic malignancies. Blood 55:806-810, 1980.

Nossal, G.J. Current concepts: immunology. The basic components of the immune system. N. Engl. J. Med. 316:1320-1325, 1987.

Reinherz, E.L., Kung, P.C., Goldstein, G., Levey, R.H., and Schlossman, S.F. Discrete stages of human intrathymic differentiation: analysis of normal thymocytes and leukemic lymphoblasts of T-cell lineage. Proc. Natl. Acad. Sci. USA 77:1588-1592, 1980.

Royer, H.D. and Reinherz, E.L. T lymphocytes: ontogeny, function, and relevance to clinical disorders. N. Engl. J. Med. 317:1136-1142, 1987.

Suchi, T., Lennert, K., Tu, L.Y., et al. Histopathology and immunohistochemistry of peripheral T cell lymphomas: a proposal for their classification. J. Clin. Pathol. 40:995-1015, 1987.

ACUTE LYMPHOCYTIC LEUKEMIA, T CELL TYPE

SYNONYMS AND RELATED TERMS: Acute lymphoblastic leukemia T.

Definition. Acute lymphocytic leukemia T is a marrow-based neoplasm that arises from cells with T features and differs from other types of acute lymphocytic leukemia in certain membrane characteristics and in clinical and therapeutic implications.

Clinical Features. Acute lymphocytic leukemia T comprises approximately 15 to 25 percent of childhood acute lymphocytic leukemia in the United States. Most of the patients are between 10 and 20 years of age at the time of diagnosis, with a median age of approximately 12 years. Most of these patients are somewhat older than those with common childhood acute lymphocytic leukemia. Males are affected 2 to 3 times more frequently than females. The clinical features overlap with convoluted (lymphoblastic) T lymphomas (Greaves et al.), and the pathologic and immunologic features of these neoplasms are also similar.

Patients first seek medical attention with symptoms or signs of bone marrow failure:

weakness secondary to anemia, bleeding or bruising due to thrombocytopenia, and infection due to granulocytopenia. Mediastinal masses are found in approximately 50 percent of the patients. Superior vena cava syndrome, pleural effusions, or cardiac decompensation due to pathologic involvement of myocardium or pericardium have been frequently noted.

Physical examination may reveal pallor, evidence of bruising, or infection. Bony tenderness is often elicited. Hepatosplenomegaly is found in 80 to 90 percent of the patients, whereas peripheral lymphadenopathy is reported in approximately 50 percent of the patients.

Extreme leukocytosis is expected in this disease, with over 50 percent of the patients presenting with white blood cell counts in excess of 100,000/μL, and median white blood cell counts reported at 141,000/μL. The hemoglobin is less than 9 g/μL in approximately 50 percent, and a platelet count below 90,000/μL is also expected in 50 percent of the patients at the time of diagnosis. Peripheral blood terminal deoxynucleotidyl transferase is elevated.

With combination chemotherapy directed against this specific subtype of acute lymphocytic leukemia, complete remission is expected in approximately 80 percent of the patients. A significant percentage of these patients may achieve long-term, disease-free survival.

Pathologic Features (Table 15). The marrow shows sheets of cells with a high nuclear/cytoplasmic ratio, scant cytoplasm, and primitive nuclear chromatin. Nuclear convolutions are often prominent. There is a wide range in nuclear and cell size. In cytochemical reactions, the leukemic cells are Sudan black negative, with insignificant esterase activity but often with focal acid phosphatase positivity. Periodic acid Schiff (PAS) stain shows coarse granular and/or block positivity against a negative background in approximately 30 percent of the cases; however, most cases are PAS negative. Electron microscopy shows primitive cells with nuclear folding, often larger than the predominant cell in common acute lymphocytic leukemia (fig. 3).

Immunologic Features. Although initially identified by reactivity of tumor cells with sheep erythrocytes, most cases of acute lymphocytic leukemia are now recognized by CD7 reactivity (Foon and Todd). Most cases show CD2 positivity as well. Some cases express differentiation antigens. Clinical correlations have not been established with any immunologic features. A rearrangement of the T β-receptor gene has been described in most cases.

References

Foon, K.A. and Todd, R.F., III. Immunologic classification of leukemia and lymphoma. Blood 68:1-31, 1986.
Greaves, M.F., Janossy, G., Peto, J., and Kay, H. Immunologically defined subclasses of acute lymphoblastic leukaemia in children: their relationship to presentation features and prognosis. Br. J. Haematol. 48:179-197, 1981.

Additional References

Bernard, A., Boumsell, L., Reinherz, E.L., et al. Cell surface characterization of malignant T cells from lymphoblastic lymphoma using monoclonal antibodies: evidence for phenotypic differences between malignant T cells from patients with acute lymphoblastic leukemia and lymphoblastic lymphoma. Blood 57:1105-1110, 1981.
Bradstock, K.F., Janossy, G., Pizzolo, G., et al. Subpopulations of normal and leukemic human thymocytes: an analysis with the use of monoclonal antibodies. J.N.C.I. 65:33-42, 1980.
Broder, S., Uchiyama, T., and Waldmann, T.A. Current concepts in immunoregulatory T-cell neoplasms. Cancer Treat. Rep. 63:607-612, 1979.

Table 15

ACUTE LYMPHOCYTIC LEUKEMIA, T CELL TYPE

PATTERN	
• Marrow — diffuse, homogeneous effacement • Other sites — infiltrative, noncohesive	
CYTOLOGY — NEOPLASTIC	**MARKERS — NEOPLASTIC**

• Wide range in nuclear and cell size; nuclear convolutions prominent
 	
• High nuclear/cytoplasmic ratio, scant cytoplasm, primitive nuclear chromatin
	• Flow:
	  CD7 positive, all cases
	  CD2 positive, most cases
	  Phenotypes of acute lymphocytic leukemia T usually resemble early or intermediate thymocytes
	
	• Cytochemistry:
	  Sudan Black B (-)
	  PAS (+), block (30%)
	  Acid phosphatase (+)

INVOLVED SITES	**CLINICAL FEATURES**
• Marrow • Central nervous system • Mediastinum • Testes	• Affects teenagers, young adults — often males • Often have widespread disease at presentation, with mediastinal masses, hepatosplenomegaly, lymphadenopathy • Leukocytosis common
REACTIVE COMPONENTS	**DIFFERENTIAL DIAGNOSIS**
• Not described	• Convoluted (lymphoblastic) T lymphoma • Acute lymphocytic leukemia, common • Acute undefined leukemia • Acute myeloid leukemia • Neuroblastoma

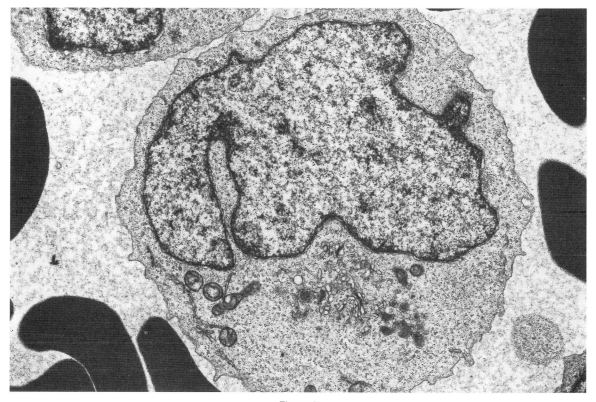

Figure 3
ACUTE LYMPHOCYTIC LEUKEMIA T, MARROW
In this electron microphotograph the nucleus is irregular, and cytoplasmic polysomes, sparse rough endoplasmic reticulum, and Golgi-associated dense granules are present. X13,800. (Fig. 6 from Glick, A.D., Vestal, B.K., Flexner, J.M., and Collins, R.D. Ultrastructural study of acute lymphocytic leukemia: comparison with immunologic studies. Blood 52:311-322, 1978.)

Janossy, G., Tidman, N., Papageorgiou, E.S., Kung, P.C., and Goldstein, G. Distribution of T lymphocyte subsets in the human bone marrow and thymus: an analysis with monoclonal antibodies. J. Immunol. 126:1608-1613, 1981.

Koziner, B., Gebhard, D., Denny, T., et al. Analysis of T-cell differentiation antigens in acute lymphatic leukemia using monoclonal antibodies. Blood 60:752-757, 1982.

Nadler, L.M., Reinherz, E.L., Weinstein, H.J., D'Orsi, C.J., and Schlossman, S.F. Heterogeneity of T-cell lymphoblastic malignancies. Blood 55:806-810, 1980.

Thiel, E., Rodt, H., Huhn, D., et al. Multimarker classification of acute lymphoblastic leukemia: evidence for further T subgroups and evaluation of their clinical significance. Blood 56:759-772, 1980.

ADULT T CELL LEUKEMIA

SYNONYMS AND RELATED TERMS: Adult T cell leukemia/lymphoma; HTLV-associated leukemia/lymphoma.

Clinical Features. Adult T cell leukemia or human T cell leukemia is very common in Japan, where it has been reported in endemic fashion in the southwestern portions of the country. Outbreaks of this disease have also occurred in the Caribbean.

In all geographic regions, adult T cell leukemia has been associated with a unique type C retrovirus. First isolated from an American patient with cerebriform T cell lymphoma, the virus, termed human T leukemia virus, has been found budding from leukemic T cells and is distinct from previously known animal retroviruses.

Specific antibodies to human T leukemia virus have been found in over 90 percent of all Japanese patients with adult T cell leukemia living in the endemic regions of Japan. Approximately 10 to 20 percent of the healthy individuals in this region have significant antibody titers to the retrovirus, although mean titers of antibody are higher in the patient group. Specific antibodies to human T leukemia virus have also been reported in adult T cell leukemia patients from the West Indies and, occasionally, from the United States.

Adult T cell leukemia in Japan occurs primarily in the fifth decade, with patients ranging in age from 28 to 71 years. Males and females are equally affected. Lymphadenopathy is seen in approximately 80 percent at the time of diagnosis, whereas 50 percent have hepatomegaly and/or splenomegaly. Skin lesions (erythroderma or nodules) are present in 60 percent of the patients. The peripheral white blood cell count is approximately 25,000/μL (with a range of 6000-480,000/μL), with a relative normality of hemoglobin and platelet counts and a minor degree of marrow involvement. Significant hypercalcemia is reported in 30 to 40 percent of the patients. Response to therapy is quite poor, and survival is less than 1 year.

Adult T cell leukemia in the United States shares many clinical characteristics with those cases reported in Japan (Yanagihara et al.). The age of onset is somewhat younger, with a mean of 33 years and a range of 24 to 62 years. Males

may be affected more commonly than females. Prominent involvement of peripheral and retroperitoneal nodes is expected, with sparing of the mediastinum. The skin, central nervous system, lungs, and gastrointestinal tract may also be involved. Hypercalcemia, increased bone turnover, x-ray evidence of osteoporosis/lytic bone lesions, and normal serum parathormone levels are observed in the majority of the patients. Despite multiagent chemotherapy, survival has been approximately 1 year.

Pathologic Features. (Table 16). Peripheral blood and marrow involvement are present in most cases at presentation and in all cases as the disease runs its course. Cells in the peripheral blood vary considerably in size but usually show marked variation in nuclear configuration, with cloverleaf forms (plate III). Lytic bone lesions may not contain recognizable tumor (Jaffe et al.).

Histopathologic changes in nodes are similar in HTLV-positive cases, regardless of the ethnic population affected. Growth patterns are diffuse, without follicular nodulation. Sinuses often contain numerous loosely scattered neoplastic cells (plate III; figs. 4, 5). Predominant cells range from a small cell type to a large pleomorphic variant, but most cases have medium (5-9 μm in nuclear diameter) or larger cells. Microscopically similar peripheral T cell lymphomas may be HTLV negative (Jaffe et al.), although Lennert and colleagues feel that HTLV-associated T cell lymphomas are invariably pleomorphic.

Immunologic Features. The tumor cells in most cases express pan-T antigens CD3, CD5, and CD2; lack CD7; and are CD4 positive, CD8 negative (Knowles). Most cases are CD25 (anti-TAC) positive,

Table 16

ADULT T CELL LEUKEMIA/LYMPHOMA

PATTERN
• Nodes — diffuse effacement of architecture; sinuses contain numerous loosely scattered neoplastic cells • Skin — may contain dermal infiltrate and Pautrier's abscesses

CYTOLOGY — NEOPLASTIC	MARKERS — NEOPLASTIC

• > small lymphocyte in size; nuclear configuration extremely irregular and lobated; may have cloverleaf configuration
 	
• Occasional blasts may be present
	• Flow:
	   T helper phenotype usual
	   CD7 negative, most cases
	   CD25 (anti-TAC) positive, most cases
	
	• Karyotype:
	   no characteristic abnormalities described

INVOLVED SITES	CLINICAL FEATURES
• Blood • Nodes • Liver, spleen • Skin	• Adults are affected in fourth-fifth decade of after • Patients often have skin lesions, lymphadenopathy, or hepatosplenomegaly • Hypercalcemia is common in patients seen in the United States

REACTIVE COMPONENTS	DIFFERENTIAL DIAGNOSIS
• Few reactive components	• Cerebriform (cutaneous) T cell lymphoma usually has chronic premycotic phase • Non-Hodgkin's lymphoma, intermediate to high grade

PLATE III
ADULT T CELL LEUKEMIA TYPE
(Plate III is from the same patient)

The following illustrations of adult T cell leukemia demonstrate the similarity between cases seen in the United States and those from Japan. In this case, the HTLV-I serology was positive. (Courtesy of Dr. E. Yanagihara, Honolulu, HI.)

A. PERIPHERAL BLOOD

A peripheral blood smear shows small lymphocytes with extraordinary variation in nuclear configuration with deep indentation and cloverleaf patterns. The cytoplasm is slightly azurophilic and vacuolated. Small nucleoli are noted. Wright's stain. X1000.

B. PERIPHERAL BLOOD

Occasional large blasts are present in this peripheral blood smear, although their percentage is usually low. There are finely acidophilic nuclear chromatin and small nucleoli. The cytoplasm is azurophilic and contains multiple small vacuoles. Wright's stain. X1000.

C. PERIPHERAL BLOOD

A cytospin preparation of peripheral blood reveals marked accentuation of the nuclear configurational changes with indentation and lobulation. Wright's stain. X1000.

D. PERIPHERAL BLOOD

A plastic-embedded section of buffy coat shows only limited nuclear invagination, illustrating that the degree of indentation and lobulation varies considerably with the conditions of the preparation. X1000.

E. LYMPH NODE

In this illustration, there is diffuse involvement without any follicular nodulation. Sinuses are dilated and often contain loosely scattered neoplastic cells. The capsule is not involved. H&E. X32.

F. LYMPH NODE

This section shows remarkable variation in size and nuclear configuration of neoplastic cells. This variation is more apparent than in the peripheral blood illustrations. H&E. X600.

G. LYMPH NODE

An MGP stain emphasizes the abundance of the lightly pyroninophilic character of the cytoplasm. Prominent nucleoli and one large cell are seen. MGP. X600.

PLATE III

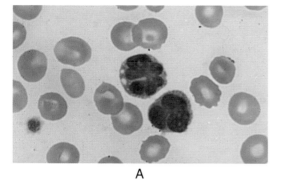

A

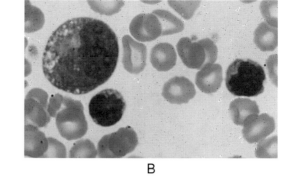

B

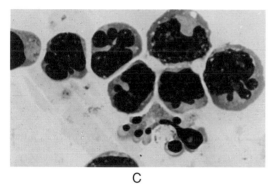

C

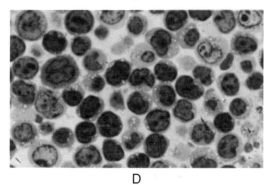

D

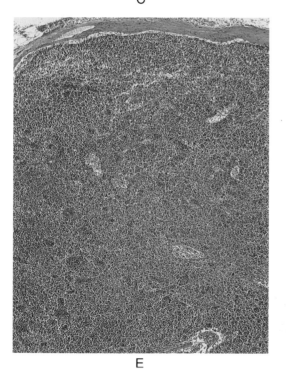

E

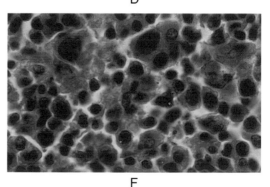

F

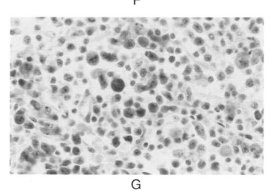

G

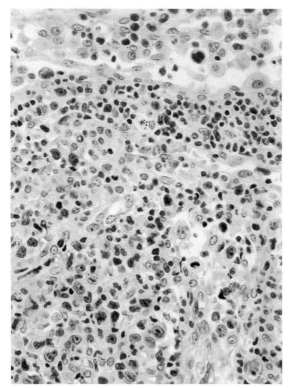

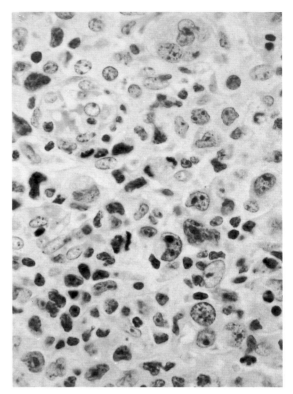

Figure 4
ADULT T CELL LEUKEMIA, LYMPH NODE
In this HTLV-I positive case from Japan, the findings are very similar to the case shown in Plate III, with a wide range in cell size and nuclear configuration. The sinuses contain numerous neoplastic cells. H&E. X400.

Figure 5
ADULT T CELL LEUKEMIA, LYMPH NODE
In this Japanese case, the range in nuclear configurational changes and cell size are apparent. X600.

in contrast to HTLV-negative peripheral T lymphomas (Lennert et al.).

Differential Diagnosis. HTLV-positive leukemia/lymphoma cases apparently cannot be distinguished from HTLV-negative cases on the basis of histopathology alone (Jaffe et al.), although the clinical features differ markedly. Cutaneous involvement is frequent in adult T cell leukemia, consisting of subcutaneous infiltrates and Pautrier abscesses, suggesting similarities to cerebriform T cell lymphoma. However, the latter disease usually has a chronic course and a chronic premycotic phase and does not have a significant association with HTLV-1.

References

Jaffe, E.S., Blattner, W.A., Blayney, D.W., et al. The pathologic spectrum of adult T-cell leukemia/lymphoma in the United States. Human T-cell leukemia/lymphoma virus-associated lymphoid malignancies. Am. J. Surg. Pathol. 8:263-275, 1984.

Knowles, D.M. Immunophenotypic and antigen receptor gene rearrangement analysis in T cell neoplasia. Am. J. Pathol. 134:761-785, 1989.

Lennert, K., Kikuchi, M., Sato, E., et al. HTLV-positive and -negative T-cell lymphomas. Morphological and immunohistochemical differences between European and HTLV-positive Japanese T-cell lymphomas. Int. J. Cancer 35:65-72, 1985.

Yanagihara, E.T., Nakamura, J., Kimura, L., and Oishi, N. Retrovirus-associated adult T-cell leukemia-lymphoma: an epidemiologic study of five cases among Hawaii-born offspring of migrant Japanese. Hematol. Oncol. 7:181-188, 1989.

SMALL T CELL NEOPLASMS INCLUDING CHRONIC LYMPHOCYTIC LEUKEMIA, T CELL TYPE

SYNONYMS AND RELATED TERMS: Chronic lymphocytic leukemia T. Rappaport: lymphocytic, well-differentiated.

Definition. Small T cell neoplasms as a group are heterogeneous as are the small B cell processes, and include what are now referred to as chronic lymphocytic leukemia T. The defining characteristic of this group is a great predominance of small lymphocytes in the neoplastic infiltrate that have membrane characteristics of T cells. Chronic lymphocytic leukemia T is rare, with an expected incidence in chronic lymphocytic leukemia populations of approximately 2 percent.

Clinical Features. The most completely defined variants of small T cell neoplasms include two morphologic variants of chronic lymphocytic leukemia, each with different clinical and pathologic features.

Prolymphocytic Leukemia of T Cell Type

The average age of onset in T prolymphocytic leukemia is approximately 60 years, and a wide age range has been reported. Males are more frequently affected. Significant splenomegaly is the most prominent physical finding and occurs in 90 percent of the patients. Hepatomegaly is described in 50 percent of the patients, and peripheral lymphadenopathy is noted in 17 to 80 percent. Skin infiltration has occasionally been reported.

Traditional therapy for chronic lymphocytic leukemia is inadequate for this aggressive disease. Splenic radiotherapy has been used with limited success,

and recent reports using aggressive regimens have been somewhat promising. The median survival is less than 6 months.

Chronic Lymphocytic Leukemia T With Azurophilic Granules

SYNONYMS AND RELATED TERMS: Chronic lymphocytosis with neutropenia; chronic lymphocytic leukemia T "cytoplasmic"; large granular lymphocyte syndrome.

Clinical Features. This variant is characteristic and distinct from the other subtypes of chronic lymphocytic leukemia. The median age at diagnosis is the mid-fifties, with a wide age distribution. Although splenomegaly may be prominent, hepatomegaly, lymphadenopathy, and skin infiltration are relatively uncommon. Lymphocytosis in excess of 100,000/µL has been described, but the majority of the patients have lymphocyte counts lower than 50,000/µL. Neutropenia with resultant recurrent infections may be a prominent feature of the disease. The course of this illness is indolent and protracted, with a reported individual patient survival rate of 10 or 20 years. Because of its lengthy course, some investigators have suggested that this entity is not neoplastic; however, the clonal nature of this process has been established (Berliner et al.). The majority of the patients have experienced a prolonged survival rate in the absence of a specific treatment or with minimal therapy, similar to that used in standard chronic lymphocytic leukemia.

Pathologic Features (Table 17). In addition to the usual criteria for diagnosing small cell neoplasms, the T nature of the predominant cell must be demonstrated. Some lymphocytes in chronic lymphocytic leukemia have been noted to contain

Table 17

MALIGNANT LYMPHOMA, SMALL LYMPHOCYTIC T, INCLUDING CHRONIC LYMPHOCYTIC LEUKEMIA T

PATTERN	
	• Marrow — diffuse effacement • Node — diffuse effacement, heterogeneous appearance
CYTOLOGY — NEOPLASTIC	**MARKERS — NEOPLASTIC**

• Prolymphocytic: acidophilic chromatin, prominent nucleoli
 	
• Large granular lymphocyte: Downey-like cells with prominent azurophilic granules, basophilic nuclear chromatin
	• Flow:
	    Prolymphocytic: both helper and suppressor phenotypes reported
	
	    Large granular lymphocyte: suppressor phenotype; some cases express natural killer antigen

INVOLVED SITES	**CLINICAL FEATURES**
• Marrow • Nodes • Skin	• Prolymphocytic: many patients in their sixties; splenomegaly, lymphadenopathy prominent • Large granular lymphocyte: neutropenia and infection may be prominent
REACTIVE COMPONENTS	**DIFFERENTIAL DIAGNOSIS**
• Not described	• Small B cell neoplasms

numerous cytoplasmic azurophilic granules. These granules have a distinct ultrastructural appearance and are presumably responsible for the high content of β-glucuronidase and acid phosphatase found in histochemical preparations. In some cases, lymphocytes in the nodes, marrow, and peripheral blood have been described as small with dense chromatin. In other cases, the lymphocytes have been larger, with irregular nuclei different from Sézary cells, or have been described as prolymphocytes. No distinctive pathologic features have been noted in the marrow infiltrates to separate this leukemia from other lymphocytic processes. The two subtypes of small T cell neoplasms described here show a considerable variation in cytologic features, although growth patterns and low magnification features are similar.

Immunologic Features. Patients with prolymphocytic leukemia have been described as having both helper and suppressor phenotypes, whereas the type with azurophilic granules predominantly has had a suppressor phenotype. In coculture experiments with activated B lymphocytes, a suppressor function has been demonstrated by cells from these patients.

Differential Diagnosis. Small B cell neoplasms are easily differentiated from small T cell lymphomas by the presence of proliferation centers in node sections, by the overall regularity of the lymphocytic infiltrate in small B cell lymphomas, and by the immunologic characteristics of the neoplastic cells.

Reference

Berliner, N., Duby, A.D., Linch, D.C., et al. T cell receptor gene rearrangements define a monoclonal T cell proliferation in patients with T cell lymphocytosis and cytopenia. Blood 67:914-918, 1986.

Additional References

Chan, W.C., Link, S., Mawle, A., et al. Heterogeneity of large granular lymphocyte proliferations: delineation of two major subtypes. Blood 68:1142-1153, 1986.

Costello, C., Catovsky, D., O'Brien, M., Morillo, R., and Varadi, S. Chronic T-cell leukemias. I. Morphology, cytochemistry and ultrastructure. Leuk. Res. 4:463-476, 1980.

Linch, D.C., Cawley, J.C., Worman, C.P., et al. Abnormalities of T-cell subsets in patients with neutropenia and an excess of lymphocytes in the bone marrow. Br. J. Haematol. 48:137-145, 1981.

Marks, S.M., Yanovich, S., Rosenthal, D.S., Moloney, W.C., and Schlossman, S.F. Multimarker analysis of T-cell chronic lymphocytic leukemia. Blood 51:435-438, 1978.

Pandolfi, F., De Rossi, G., Semenzato, G., et al. Immunologic evaluation of T chronic lymphocytic leukemia cells: correlations among phenotype, functional activities, and morphology. Blood 59:688-695, 1982.

Wallis, W.J., Loughran, T.P., Jr., Kadin, M.E., Clark, E.A., Starkebaum, G.A. Polyarthritis and neutropenia associated with circulating large granular lymphocytes. Ann. Intern. Med. 103:357-362, 1985.

CONVOLUTED (LYMPHOBLASTIC) T CELL LYMPHOMA

SYNONYMS AND RELATED TERMS: Working Formulation: malignant lymphoma; lymphoblastic (convoluted and nonconvoluted cell). Kiel: T lymphoblastic (convoluted cell type and others). Rappaport: lymphoblastic.

Definition. These neoplasms presumably arise from thymocytes; however, otherwise typical cases have been described without mediastinal masses. Although the marrow may be initially uninvolved, dissemination frequently occurs with progressive nodal, visceral, and marrow involvement and the development of a leukemic phase. As previously noted, the disseminated disorder closely resembles, or is equivalent to, acute lymphocytic leukemia T. Pathologic details are shown in Plates IV and V and figures 6-9.

Clinical Features. Convoluted (lymphoblastic) lymphoma comprises 1 to 2 percent of all lymphoid malignancies seen in the United States.

The disease occurs most frequently in teenagers or young adults, although a wide age distribution has been reported. Males are affected two to four times more frequently than females. Most patients first seek medical attention because of symptoms or signs related to the presence of a mediastinal mass (plate IV-A–C; fig. 6) or pleural or pericardial effusion. Symptoms may be dramatic, with compromise of vital intrathoracic structures.

Since this disease spreads rapidly and predictably to the bone marrow, another common mode of presentation is overt leukemia with a high white blood cell count (approximately 100,000/μL), anemia, and thrombocytopenia. Peripheral lymphadenopathy is expected in 70 percent of the cases and may lead to the initial presentation (plates IV-D, V-A). One-third of the patients present with a central nervous system disease such as leukemic meningitis (plate V-B,C) or a mass lesion in the cerebrum. The central nervous system disease may occasionally be asymptomatic, with the diagnosis made at the time of a lumbar puncture. The lung, kidney, liver, spleen, testis (plate V-D), breast, and skin may all be involved. Because the tumor disseminates so predictably and rapidly, widely disseminated disease must be presumed, and patients must be treated accordingly.

After traditional therapy for aggressive adult lymphoma, most patients experience dramatic and rapid tumor regression. Although relapse occurred predictably, the average survival for patients in the 1970s was approximately 1 year. With current regimens similar to those used for childhood leukemia and lymphoma and with the

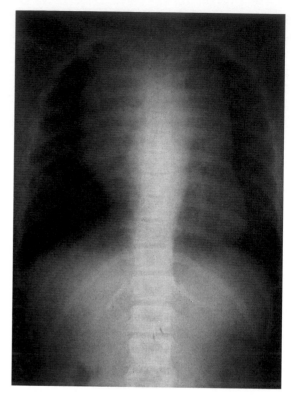

Figure 6
CONVOLUTED (LYMPHOBLASTIC) T LYMPHOMA,
CHEST X RAY
This anterior mediastinal mass was demonstrated in a 7 year old male presenting with a pleural effusion.

inclusion of early prophylactic cranial irradiation and intrathecal chemotherapy, several investigators have reported long-term, disease-free survival in approximately 50 percent of the adult and 60 percent of the pediatric patients.

Pathologic Features (Table 18). Lukes and associates have defined the following features necessary for diagnosis: an infiltrative growth pattern (plates IV-B, V-A) of noncohesive cells showing nuclear convolutions either with scalloped nuclear borders or fine linear subdivisions apparent on focusing; dispersed nuclear chromatin;

Table 18

T CELL LYMPHOMA, CONVOLUTED LYMPHOCYTE OR LYMPHOBLASTIC TYPE
(Thymic Lymphoma)

PATTERN

- Diffuse infiltrate of paracortex of nodes
- Numerous macrophages containing nuclear debris ("starry sky")
- Infiltrative destructive mediastinal mass

CYTOLOGY — NEOPLASTIC	MARKERS — NEOPLASTIC
- Cells are small to medium sized with delicate nuclear chromatin, inconspicuous nucleoli, and scant cytoplasm. Convolutions vary in depth and are seen as scalloping in some cells but on focusing, are apparent in most cells as fine branching lines. - Numerous mitoses - MGP weak or absent	- Uniformly mark as T cells; most mark as common thymocytes - CD7, CD2 positive - TdT (+) - Complement receptors present - Punctate focal acid phosphatase positivity

INVOLVED SITES	CLINICAL FEATURES
- Cervical nodes - Thymus and mediastinum - Marrow, partial, or diffuse involvement - Pleura, pericardium - Central nervous system - Gonads, particularly at relapse	- Young males with rapidly developing mediastinal mass, respiratory embarrassment, pleural or pericardial effusion - Overlaps with acute lymphocytic leukemia T, often presenting with leukemic phase and bone marrow involvement

REACTIVE COMPONENTS	DIFFERENTIAL DIAGNOSIS
- Few reactive lymphocytes - Eosinophils may be present - Macrophages with nuclear debris	- Malignant lymphoma, follicular center cell, small noncleaved cell - Leukemic infiltrate - Thymoma

55

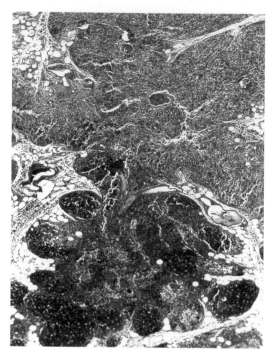

Figure 7
(Figures 7 and 8 and plate IV-A
are from the same patient)
CONVOLUTED (LYMPHOBLASTIC)
T LYMPHOMA, THYMIC MASS
This low magnification photomicrograph shows partial involvement of the thymus. Residual thymus is detected at the lower portion of the illustration and the tumorous mass at the top. H&E. X24.

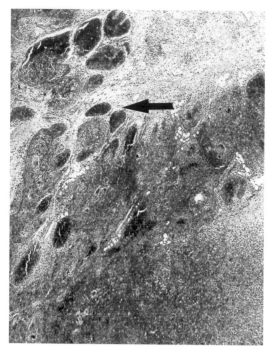

Figure 8
CONVOLUTED (LYMPHOBLASTIC)
T LYMPHOMA, THYMIC MASS
Another section demonstrates the virtual efface-ment of the thymic architecture. Only a few islands of residual thymus (arrow) are recognized within the tumor. H&E. X24.

inconspicuous nucleoli; scant cytoplasm; a high mitotic rate (plate IV-C,D); the forma-tion of E-rosettes by neoplastic-appearing cells in cytospins (plate V-B); and a strong focal acid phosphatase positivity (plate V-C). Many of these cases are first seen by pathologists as pleural effusions or periph-eral lymphadenopathy. The origin of these neoplasms from the thymus has been doc-umented in a few cases (figs. 7, 8). Re-lapse often involves the testis (plate V-D) or central nervous system (plate V-B,C).

By electron microscopy, neoplastic cells in these tumors have moderate nuclear irreg-ularity, scant rough endoplasmic reticulum (fig. 9), and closely resemble the neoplas-tic cells in acute lymphocytic leukemia T.

Immunologic Features. The T cell nature of these neoplasms is readily es-tablished. Many of these tumors are distin-guished by the simultaneous presence of E receptors, complement receptors, and acid phosphatase positivity—features also found on fetal thymocytes of 10 to 15 weeks gestation (Stein et al.). The ab-sence of sheep erythrocyte receptors on thymocytes before the tenth week of ges-tation led to an interesting postulate that

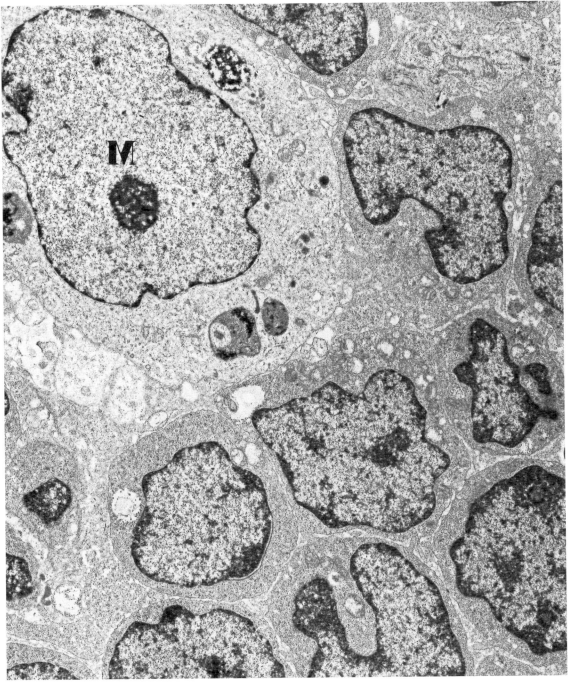

Figure 9
CONVOLUTED (LYMPHOBLASTIC) T LYMPHOMA, LYMPH NODE
Electron microscopy demonstrates cells with nuclear irregularity, distinctive finely dispersed chromatin, a sparse rough endoplasmic reticulum, and relatively inapparent nucleoli. A macrophage (M) contains phagocytosed debris. X9800.

PLATE IV

A. CONVOLUTED (LYMPHOBLASTIC) T LYMPHOMA
(Plate IV-A and figures 7 and 8 are from the same patient)
This gross photograph shows (on cut surface) a fleshy, relatively homogeneous tumor mass.

B. CONVOLUTED (LYMPHOBLASTIC) T LYMPHOMA, MEDIASTINAL MASS
(Plate IV-B,C and plate V-B,C are from the same patient)
The typical growth pattern is illustrated in this low magnification photomicrograph. At the edge of the dense cellular mass, there is infiltration of the surrounding tissue by radiating bands, with extension of lymphoma cells between individual fat cells. X32.

C. CONVOLUTED (LYMPHOBLASTIC) T LYMPHOMA, MEDIASTINAL MASS
At higher magnification, tingible body phagocytes with abundant nuclear debris may be found scattered in a primitive-appearing cellular proliferation. Tumor cells vary in size and have scanty or inapparent cytoplasm with noncohesive borders. Nuclear chromatin is light staining and nucleoli are inconspicuous. The nuclear borders are often irregular and indented; numerous fine, linear subdivisions impart the convoluted appearance of the nuclei. Mitoses are numerous. H&E. X600.

D. CONVOLUTED (LYMPHOBLASTIC) T LYMPHOMA, LYMPH NODE
This plastic-embedded section shows the range in size of the tumor cells. Nuclear chromatin is uniformly delicate, with small nucleoli and inapparent cytoplasm. Convolutions are seen in both the small and large cells. X600.

PLATE IV

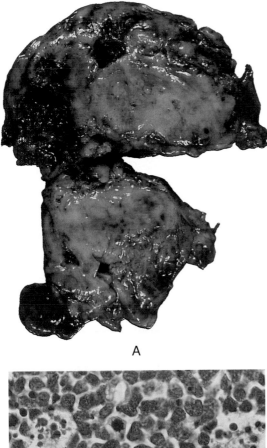

A

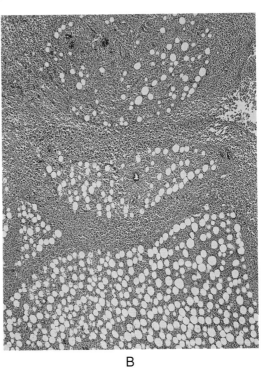

B

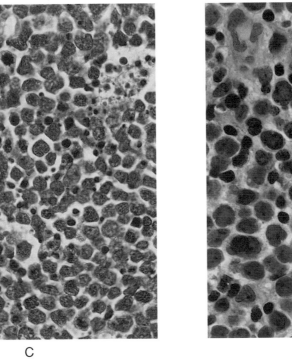

C

D

PLATE V

A. CONVOLUTED (LYMPHOBLASTIC) T LYMPHOMA, LYMPH NODE
This illustration shows the distinctive infiltrative pattern characteristic of nodal involvement by convoluted (lymphoblastic) T lymphoma. Sinuses are often preserved, and there may be residual follicular centers. Massive involvement of the hilar and perinodal soft tissue is present. X100.

B. CONVOLUTED (LYMPHOBLASTIC) T LYMPHOMA, CEREBROSPINAL FLUID, SHEEP E-ROSETTE PREPARATION, CYTOSPIN
(Plate V-B,C and plate IV-B,C are from the same patient)
Massive involvement of the cerebrospinal fluid may be seen in these patients. Only a few rosette-forming cells are found in this preparation; the range in cell size and nuclear configuration of these primitive-appearing cells is noted. Giemsa. X1000.

C. CONVOLUTED (LYMPHOBLASTIC) T LYMPHOMA, CEREBROSPINAL FLUID, CYTOSPIN
The distinct acid phosphatase punctate positivity characteristic of these tumor cells is noted in most cells. Acid phosphatase. X1000.

D. CONVOLUTED (LYMPHOBLASTIC) T LYMPHOMA, TESTICULAR RELAPSE
This neoplasm frequently relapses in the testis. The convoluted T cells infiltrate and expand the interstitial tissue. X100.

PLATE V

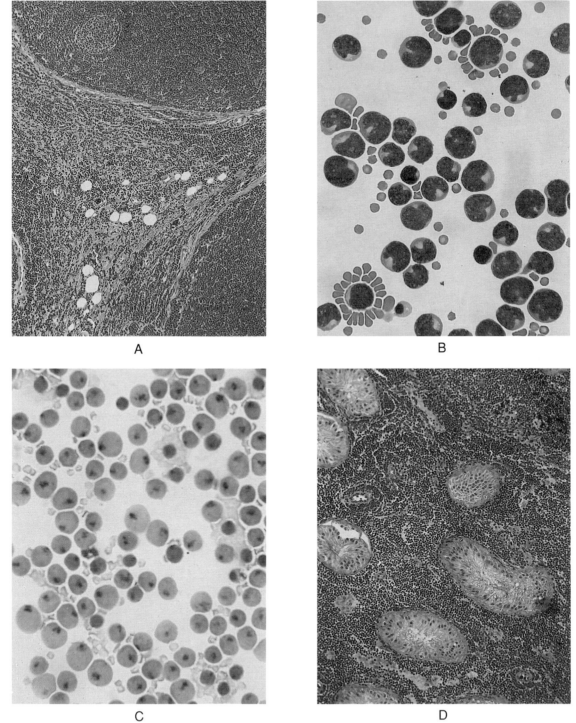

A

B

C

D

some E-rosette–negative, complement-positive neoplasms might be derived from thymocytes (Stein et al.).

Studies of these lymphomas with monoclonal antibodies have revealed considerable group variation, with most resembling common or stage II thymocytes (Bernard et al.; Weiss et al.). Approximately a third of the cases had tumor cells with surface antigens differing from the three major thymocyte populations. Cases identified as acute lymphocytic leukemia T have a phenotype similar to convoluted (lymphoblastic) T lymphomas, with a tendency toward a more immature phenotype (Weiss et al.). Rearrangements of the T β-receptor have been described.

Convoluted (lymphoblastic) lymphomas may be readily distinguished from other high grade lymphomas and myeloid leukemia by multiparameter studies. Intranuclear terminal deoxynucleotidal transferase is apparent in most convoluted (lymphoblastic) lymphoma, and CD7 is also consistently expressed as a surface antigenic marker in these malignancies. The small subset of TdT-positive acute myeloid leukemias usually expresses myeloid-associated antigens CD13 and/or CD33. TdT is not found in other T or B lymphomas (Knowles), except in possibly rare high grade B lymphomas with blastic morphology. Small noncleaved cell lymphomas (e.g., Burkitt's lymphoma) are usually TdT negative.

Differential Diagnosis. *Follicular center cell lymphomas, small noncleaved cell type.* Both small noncleaved cell and convoluted (lymphoblastic) T lymphomas have infiltrative growth patterns and morphologic evidence (numerous mitoses and macrophages) of a high growth fraction. MGP or Giemsa stains in small non-cleaved cell lymphomas show definite cytoplasmic positivity. Furthermore, nucleoli are usually inconspicuous in convoluted (lymphoblastic) T lymphomas, whereas nuclear subdivisions are readily apparent in well-fixed material. These tumors are easily shown to have B features by any type of immunologic analysis.

Thymomas. Epithelial cells are recognizable in PAS-stained preparations and very easily detected with PIP. The clinical course is different in these two processes.

Leukemia. Infiltrates of the myeloid type generally have more cytoplasm, a more open nuclear chromatin, and completely different cytochemical and immunologic patterns. Rare cases of leukemia show TdT positivity and have CD7 reactivity. These cases usually express CD13 and/or CD33 antigens.

References

Bernard, A., Boumsell, L., Reinherz, E.L., et al. Cell surface characterization of malignant T cells from lymphoblastic lymphoma using monoclonal antibodies. Blood 57:1105-1110, 1981.

Knowles, D.M. Immunophenotypic and antigen receptor gene rearrangement analysis in T cell neoplasia. Am. J. Pathol. 134:761-785, 1989.

Lukes, R.J., Parker, J.W., Taylor, C.R., et al. Immunologic approach to non-Hodgkin's lymphoma and related leukemias. Semin. Hematol. 15:322-351, 1978.

Stein, H., Petersen, N., Gaedicke, G., Lennert, K., and Landbeck, G. Lymphoblastic lymphoma of convoluted or acid phosphatase type—a tumor of T precursor cells. Int. J. Cancer 17:292-295, 1976.

Weiss, L.M., Bindl, J.M., Picozzi, V.J., Link, M.P., and Warnke, R.A. Lymphoblastic lymphoma: an immunophenotype study of 26 cases with comparison to T cell acute lymphoblastic leukemia. Blood 67:474-478, 1986.

Additional References

Barcos, M.P. and Lukes, R.J. Malignant Lymphoma of Convoluted Lymphocytes: A New Entity of Possible T-Cell Type, pp. 147-178. In: Conflicts in Childhood Cancer: An Evaluation of Current Management, Vol. 4. Sinks, L.F. and Godden, J.E. (Eds.). New York: Alan R. Liss, Inc., 1975.

Catovsky D., Bernasconi C., Verdonck P.J., et al. The association of eosinophilia with lymphoblastic leukaemia or lymphoma. Br. J. Haematol. 45:523-534, 1980.

Coleman, C.N., Cohen, J.R., Burke, J.S., and Rosenberg, S.A. Lymphoblastic lymphoma in adults. Blood 57:679-684, 1981.

Foon, K.A. and Todd, R.F., III. Immunologic classification of leukemia and lymphoma. Blood 68:1-31, 1986.

Levine, A.M., Forman, S.J., Meyer, P.R., et al. Successful therapy of convoluted T-lymphoblastic lymphoma in the adult. Blood 61:92-98, 1981.

Nathwani, B.N., Diamond, L.W., Winberg, C.D., et al. Lymphoblastic lymphoma. Cancer 48:2347-2357, 1981.

Reinherz, E.L., Nadler, L.M., Rosenthal, D.S., and Schlossman, S.F. T-cell-subset characterization of human T-CLL. Blood 53:1066-1075, 1979.

Weinstein, H.J., Vance, Z.B., Jaffe, N., et al. Improved prognosis for patients with mediastinal lymphoblastic lymphoma. Blood 53:687-694, 1979.

PERIPHERAL T CELL LYMPHOMAS, NODE BASED

SYNONYMS AND RELATED TERMS: Immunoblastic lymphoma of T cells; lymphoepithelioid lymphoma; immunoblastic lymphoma without plasmacytic differentiation; erythrophagocytic T lymphoma. Working Formulation: large cell; immunoblastic (clear cell, polymorphous, epithelioid cell component). Kiel: T-zone lymphoma; T immunoblastic. Rappaport: diffuse histiocytic. Various T lymphomas in Japan have been termed pleomorphic, large lymphoid, T cell lymphoma with hyperglobulinemia and monomorphic medium sized type, IBL-like T cell lymphoma.

Definition. Several T cell lymphomas mark immunologically as effector T cell types but have a wide variety of histologic and cytologic expressions. The following list includes most of the described types. (1) Peripheral T cell lymphomas refers to a heterogeneous group of proliferations. This term has some usefulness in broadly categorizing T lymphomas but is clearly not very specific. (2) T cell immunoblastic lymphoma identifies proliferations with features presumed to reflect varying degrees of lymphocyte transformation and changing cell kinetics (Lukes and Collins; Schneider et al.). (3) T-zone lymphoma represents an expansion of the paracortical T zone of lymph nodes by an abnormal T cell proliferation surrounding and widely separating reactive follicles (Lennert). (4) Lymphoepithelioid lymphocytic lymphoma (Lennert) has a distinctive proliferation of small to medium sized abnormal lymphocytes with peculiarly twisted nuclei and scanty cytoplasm. This lymphoma has a remarkable association with epithelioid cells and a marked tendency to become aggressive clinically with evolution to immunoblastic lymphoma T. (5) IBL-like T cell lymphoma of the Japanese (Watanabe) appears to be distinctive because of discrete foci of large, pale cytoplasmic cells that resemble transformed lymphocytes, accompanied by a proliferation of branching small vessels, and a prominent reactive plasma cell population. (6) Anaplastic T cell lymphoma (Stein et al.) relates to the Ki-1 positive lymphomas that are predominantly of the T cell type, and that exhibit lymph node sinus involvement and aggressive clinical disease. A parallel anaplastic B cell type also occurs but is less common.

The term peripheral T cell lymphoma appears to include all of these diverse types. An effective subclassification of the lymphomas of the peripheral T cell compartment having both clinical and immunologic relevance is needed. The recently proposed classification summarized below is likely to be refined as the various T cell lymphomas are defined more precisely immunologically.

A working classification of peripheral T lymphomas has been proposed based on the results of a histologic and immunohistochemical study of a large number of cases from China, England, Germany, and Japan (Suchi et al.). The low-grade group includes chronic lymphocytic leukemia and prolymphocytic leukemia, small cerebriform cell (mycosis fungoides, Sézary syndrome), lymphoepithelioid (Lennert's lymphoma), angioimmunoblastic (AILD, LgX), T zone, and pleomorphic small cell (HTLV1±). The high-grade group includes pleomorphic, medium and large cells (HTLV1±), immunoblastic (HTLV1±), and large cell anaplastic (Ki-1+). Pathologic details are shown in Plates VI-X.

Clinical Features. Peripheral T cell lymphomas account for approximately 3 to 4 percent of the lymphocytic malignancies in the United States. The disease is most common in adults in their fifties, with a wide age distribution reported. Males and females are probably equally affected. Occasional patients have had histories of prior abnormal immune disease of some type. The most common mode of presentation in this disease is peripheral lymphadenopathy. Retroperitoneal and, less frequently, mediastinal adenopathy are reported in 50 to 80 percent of the patients. "B" symptoms occur in approximately 60 percent of the patients.

Staging evaluation reveals extensive disease, with most patients at stage III or IV. The liver, lung, and bone marrow are common sites of extranodal spread. Mild anemia is expected in the majority of the cases, with absolute lymphocytopenia in approximately half. Serum protein electrophoresis reveals diffuse polyclonal hypergammaglobulinemia in 40 to 50 percent of the cases.

After multiagent chemotherapy, the complete remission rate has been quite low; median survivals have been reported in the range of 9 to 12 months. A minor subset of patients with a more favorable response to therapy has been noted.

Pathologic Features (Tables 19, 20). The criteria for diagnosis in most series have included diffuse growth patterns, a pleomorphic population of small and transformed lymphocytes, variable numbers of reactive histiocytes, and the identification of neoplastic-appearing cells in nonimmune sheep E-rosettes or with monoclonal antibodies (plate VI-A–C). In many reports, the larger cells have exhibited water-clear cytoplasm (plate VII-C), nuclear irregularity with multilobation (plate VIII-A–C), prominent nucleoli, and a resemblance to mononuclear Reed-Sternberg cells (plate VIII-A–C). T lymphomas composed exclusively of small transformed T cells have not been recognized in the West, although Japanese cases of these types have been described (Watanabe). These lymphomas are rather heterogeneous histologically due to a variation in size of the predominant cell from patient to patient.

Several variations on the above histopathologic picture have been described. A few cases have been more homogeneous in appearance and have contained predominantly small or large cells (plate VII-B–C). Lennert's lymphoma, or lymphoepithelioid cell lymphoma, is a peripheral T cell lymphoma in which large numbers of benign-appearing epithelioid histiocytes are distributed throughout the lymphomatous process (Table 21). As in other peripheral T cell lymphomas, postcapillary venules proliferate, and the infiltrate usually consists of mixtures of small lymphoid cells and transformed cells (plate IX). The T-zone lymphoma described by Lennert demonstrates (at low magnification) benign-appearing lymphoid follicles surrounded by a neoplastic infiltrate that expands the interfollicular areas of the

Table 19

T CELL LYMPHOMA, IMMUNOBLASTIC TYPES
(Immunoblastic Lymphoma T, Peripheral T, T Zone)

PATTERN	
	• Diffuse — uniform appearance throughout; some variation in frequency of intermediate and larger cells (T immunoblasts) • Follicular centers usually absent • In T-zone lymphoma, follicular centers are present in association with expansion of T zone

CYTOLOGY — NEOPLASTIC	MARKERS — NEOPLASTIC
• Mixed infiltrate of small, intermediate, and large lymphocytes; abundant water-clear cytoplasm • Small lymphocytes have irregular twisted nuclear morphology with inapparent cytoplasm • May have predominance of large cells with indented to polypoid nuclei, conspicuous nucleoli • MGP positivity in transformed cells	• Flow: great majority of cells (small and large) mark as T cells, usually T helper; polytypic B cells. Most cases lack one or more pan T antigens; have anomalous T subset expression • FSIP, PIP: most small and large cells mark as T cells, usually as T helper cells • TdT, CD1 negative • CD15 (Leu-M1) may be positive in large cells

INVOLVED SITES	CLINICAL FEATURES
• Superficial or abdominal nodes • Spleen • Marrow • Skin • Lung	• Adults, usually present with regional or generalized adenopathy • Often stage III or IV • Hyperglobulinemia, usually polytypic

REACTIVE COMPONENTS	DIFFERENTIAL DIAGNOSIS
• Scattered epithelioid macrophages often prominent; dispersed and not in distinct clusters as in lymphoepithelioid lymphomas • Eosinophils in some cases • Plasma cells frequent in those cases with polytypic hyperglobulinemia	• Malignant lymphoma, immunoblastic lymphoma B • Malignant lymphoma, follicular center cell, large noncleaved cell • Hodgkin's disease, mixed cellularity

Table 20

ANAPLASTIC LARGE CELL LYMPHOMA
(Ki-1 Positive)

DEFINITION	PATTERN
• Malignant lymphomas with Ki-1 positivity appear to be heterogeneous clinically, pathologically, and immunologically	• Preferential paracortical involvement • Sinus involvement; follicular centers often spared • Foci of necrosis may be present
CYTOLOGY — NEOPLASTIC	**MARKERS — NEOPLASTIC**
• Large cells with pleomorphic nuclei, clumped heterochromatin, one or more nucleoli, abundant cytoplasm (often vacuolated); giant forms present • Intermediate sized cells may have basophilic cytoplasm	• Almost 60 percent of Ki-1 (+) malignant lymphomas have T cell features • ~ 20 percent Ki-1 (+) malignant lymphomas have B cell features; remainder do not mark or express both B and T cell antigens • Histiocytic markers negative
INVOLVED SITES	**CLINICAL FEATURES**
• Lymph nodes, cervical, and groin area • Skin and subcutaneous tissue	• Young adults to older patients often with asymptomatic adenopathy • Regressing skin lesions and adenopathy described in children
REACTIVE COMPONENTS	**DIFFERENTIAL DIAGNOSIS**
• Eosinophils, neutrophils, and plasma cells may be present	• Ki-1 marks Reed-Sternberg cells, various T cell lymphomas including immunoblastic lymphoma T and lymphoepithelioid lymphoma, B cell malignant lymphoma, lymphomatoid papulosis, many cases of angioimmunoblastic lymphadenopathy with dysproteinemia • Often confused with carcinomas and melanomas because of sinus growth pattern • Microvillous lymphomas

Table 21

T CELL LYMPHOMA, LYMPHOEPITHELIOID LYMPHOCYTIC TYPE
(Includes Lennert's Lymphoma)

PATTERN	
	• Diffuse effacement of node or tonsil • Evenly distributed clusters of epithelioid macrophages • Vessels not prominent • Focal or multifocal immunoblastic proliferation
CYTOLOGY — NEOPLASTIC	**MARKERS — NEOPLASTIC**
• Small cells predominate; twisted, irregular nuclei • Large cells, oval or slight nuclei irregularity	• Flow: small and large cells mark as T helper • FSIP: most cells mark as T helper • PIP: small and large lymphocytes mark as T cells
INVOLVED SITES	**CLINICAL FEATURES**
• Cervical nodes • Tonsils • Skin, occasionally • Splenic white pulp	• Adult males predominate • Cervical adenopathy ± tonsillar involvement • Frequent evolution to immunoblastic lymphoma T
REACTIVE COMPONENTS	**DIFFERENTIAL DIAGNOSIS**
• B cells, eosinophils infrequent • Plasma cells uncommon • Epithelioid macrophages in small clusters	• Abnormal immune reactions • Hodgkin's disease, L&H diffuse • Malignant lymphoma, immunoblastic lymphoma T (peripheral T cell lymphoma) • Immunoblastic lymphadenopathy with clusters of histiocytes

node (plate VII-A). The interfollicular infiltrate is otherwise similar to that seen in other peripheral T cell lymphomas. Pinkus and associates described an apparently distinct variant of peripheral T cell lymphomas in which most of the neoplastic cells were large with multilobated nuclei (plate VIII-A–C). Skin involvement was present in three of the four cases presented. Watanabe described a variant of peripheral T cell lymphoma that histopathologically resembled immunoblastic lymphadenopathy and clinically was associated with hypergammaglobulinemia (plate VIII-D,E). Weiss and associates demonstrated clonal rearrangements of T β-receptor genes in three of five cases of angioimmunoblastic lymphadenopathy, which provided additional evidence for the close association of these two entities. Ki-1 marks Reed-Sternberg cells, the predominant cells in lymphomatoid papulosis, and neoplastic cells in a variety of T, B, and null-cell malignant lymphomas. A special type of large cell lymphoma, designated as anaplastic large cell lymphoma, has a distinctive appearance and strong Ki-1 positivity (plate X).

The marrow lesions in peripheral T cell lymphomas are distinctive and closely resemble the pathologic changes in the nodes (plate VI-D). By electron microscopy, some of the small cell processes have very irregular cells, similar to cerebriform cells. Usually a mixture of small and large lymphocytes are present, and electron microscopy emphasizes the nuclear lobation found to be a feature of these cases.

Immunologic Features. Peripheral T cell lymphomas are identified primarily by immunologic studies in association with sections showing a pleomorphic, diffuse lymphoma (Knowles; Picker et al.). The larger cells in these lymphomas tend to form fragile, easily disrupted E-rosettes, and may be difficult to detect in flow studies or frozen section immunoperoxidase. Peripheral T cell lymphomas are consistently TdT and CD1-antigen negative. Approximately 75 percent of the cases lack one or more pan-T antigens and approximately 20 percent may lack three pan-T antigens. PIP shows that the majority of neoplastic cells, including the large cell component, mark as T cells (plate VI-C). Lymphocytes with SIg are present in low numbers, and no evidence of monoclonality of SIg should be present.

Most cases express the helper subset with CD4 positivity and CD8 negativity but anomalous T subset expression is common (Knowles). In some cases, the large cells of peripheral T cell lymphoma are CD15 (Leu-M1) positive.

Differential Diagnosis. *Malignant lymphoma, immunoblastic lymphoma B.* Immunoblastic lymphoma B has distinct plasmacytic differentiation of the neoplastic cells and usually monotypic CIg. In general, the cytoplasm of B immunoblasts is more amphophilic than that of T immunoblasts, which tend to have clear cytoplasm. MGP and Giemsa stains are usually strongly positive in immunoblastic lymphoma B, but MGP and Giemsa positivities are not reliable for differentiation of these neoplasms. Numerous macrophages may be present in both neoplasms.

Malignant lymphoma, follicular center cell, large noncleaved cell. In some cases, this neoplasm is readily identified by the presence of neoplastic follicular nodulation or the admixture of cleaved follicular center cells with large noncleaved cells. However, immunologic procedures (FSIP or

PIP) are often required for the diagnosis of follicular center cell lymphoma, large noncleaved cell type. This neoplasm may have large numbers of reactive T cells. Thus, flow studies may be misleading if the reactive T cells are preferentially put into cell suspension.

Hodgkin's disease, mixed cellularity. Differentiation of Hodgkin's disease from peripheral T cell lymphomas may be very difficult; in fact, some cases of Hodgkin's disease apparently have T features. The growth pattern is distinctive in most peripheral T cell lymphomas, with a homogeneous effacement of architecture and an even appearance from area to area, in contrast to the more nodular appearance in many cases of Hodgkin's disease. Cells resembling Reed-Sternberg cells may be present in peripheral T cell lymphomas, and the current differentiation with PIP is difficult because these cells may be CD15 (Leu-M1) positive.

References

Knowles, D.M. Immunophenotypic and antigen receptor gene rearrangement analysis in T cell neoplasia. Am. J. Pathol. 134:761-785, 1989.

Lennert, K. Malignant Lymphomas Other Than Hodgkin's Disease: Histology, Cytology, Ultrastructure, Immunology. New York: Springer-Verlag, 1978.

Lukes, R.J. and Collins, R.D. New approaches to the classification of the lymphomata. Br. J. Cancer 31(Suppl.):1-28, 1975.

Picker, L.J., Weiss, L.M., Medeiros, L.J., Wood, G.S., and Warnke, R.A. Immunophenotypic criteria for the diagnosis of non-Hodgkin's lymphoma. Am. J. Pathol. 128:181-201, 1987.

Pinkus, G.S., Said, J.W., and Hargreaves, H. Malignant lymphoma, T-cell type. A distinct morphologic variant with large multilobated nuclei, with a report of four cases. Am. J. Clin. Pathol. 72:540-550, 1979.

Schneider, D.R., Taylor, C.R., Parker, J.W., et al. Immunoblastic sarcoma of T- and B-cell types. Hum. Pathol. 16:885-900, 1985.

Stein, H., Mason, D.Y., Gerdes, J., et al. The expression of the Hodgkin's disease associated antigen Ki-1 in reactive and neoplastic lymphoid tissue: evidence that Reed-Sternberg cells and histiocytic malignancies are derived from activated lymphoid cells. Blood 66:848-858, 1985.

Suchi, T., Lennert K., Tu, L.Y., et al. Histopathology and immunohistochemistry of peripheral T cell lymphomas: a proposal for their classification. J. Clin. Pathol. 40:995-1015, 1987.

Watanabe, S. Pathology of peripheral T-cell lymphomas and leukemias. Hematol. Oncol. 4:45-58, 1986.

Weiss, L.M., Crabtree, G.S., Rouse, R.V., and Warnke, R.A. Morphologic and immunologic characterization of 50 peripheral T-cell lymphomas. Am. J. Pathol. 118:316-324, 1985.

Additional References

Bertness, V., Kirsch, I., Hollis, G., Johnson, B., and Bunn, P.A., Jr. T-cell receptor gene rearrangements as clinical markers of human T-cell lymphomas. N. Engl. J. Med. 313:534-538, 1985.

Borowitz, M.J., Reichert, T.A., Brynes, R.K., et al. The phenotypic diversity of peripheral T-cell lymphomas. Hum. Pathol. 17:567-574, 1986.

Collins, R.D. T-neoplasms. Their significance in relation to the classification system of lymphoid neoplasms. Am. J. Surg. Pathol. 6:745-754,1982.

Cossman, J. Diffuse Aggressive Non-Hodgkin's Lymphomas, pp. 203-217. In: Major Problems in Pathology, Vol. 16. Surgical Pathology of the Lymph Nodes and Related Organs. Jaffe, E.S. and Bennington, J.L. (Eds.). Philadelphia: W.B. Saunders Company, 1985.

Greer, J.P., York, J.C., Cousar, J.B., et al. Peripheral T-cell lymphoma: a clinicopathologic study of 42 cases. J. Clin. Oncol. 2:788-798, 1984.

Horning, S.J., Weiss, L.M., Crabtree, G.S., and Warnke, R.A. Clinical and phenotypic diversity of T cell lymphomas. Blood 67:1578-1582, 1986.

Knowles, D.M., Jr., Pelicci, P.G., and Dalla-Favera, R. T-cell receptor beta chain gene rearrangements: genetic markers of T-cell lineage and clonality. Hum. Pathol. 17:546-551, 1986.

Levine, A.M., Taylor, C.R., Schneider, D.R., et al. Immunoblastic sarcoma of T-cell versus B-cell origin. I. Clinical features. Blood 58:52-61, 1981.

Lukes, R.J., Parker, J.W., Taylor, C.R., et al. Immunologic approach to non-Hodgkin lymphomas and related leukemias. Analysis of the results of multiparameter studies of 425 cases. Semin. Hematol. 15:322-351, 1978.

Palutke, M., Tabaczka, P., Weise, R.W., et al. T-cell lymphomas of large cell type: a variety of malignant lymphoma. Histiocytic and mixed lymphocytic histiocytic. Cancer 46:87-101, 1980.

PLATE VI

A. IMMUNOBLASTIC LYMPHOMA T, LYMPH NODE

In this illustration, there is diffuse effacement of the architecture without apparent follicular centers or capsular involvement by a fairly homogeneous infiltrate. PAS. X10.

B. IMMUNOBLASTIC LYMPHOMA T, LYMPH NODE

A high magnification photomicrograph shows a mixture of small and large cytoplasmic lymphocytes with numerous interspersed macrophages having distinct PAS positivity. Thin strands of connective tissue traverse the infiltrate. Macrophages in T cell neoplasms are likely to be interspersed throughout the process, as shown here (for exception see the lymphoepithelioid lymphoma in plate IX). PAS. X320.

C. IMMUNOBLASTIC LYMPHOMA T, LYMPH NODE, PIP, WITH CD45RO (UCHL-1)

A diffuse population of small and medium sized pale cytoplasmic lymphocytes with irregular nuclear shapes expand the paracortex. The cell membranes of most lymphocytes stain with this pan-T cell antibody. X160.

D. IMMUNOBLASTIC LYMPHOMA T, MARROW

Large, irregular dense foci of tumor are shown. The distribution of lymphomatous involvement of the marrow in relation to bony trabeculae in this disease is variable. PAS. X90.

PLATE VI

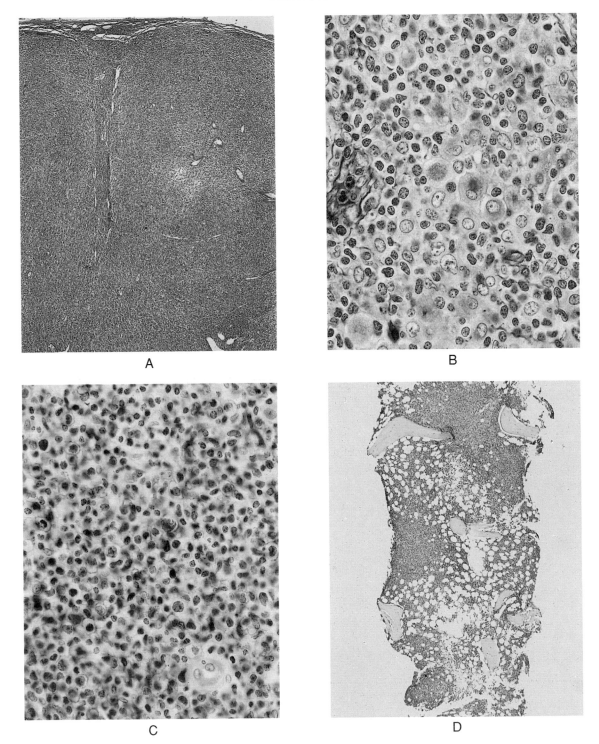

A

B

C

D

PLATE VII

A. T-ZONE LYMPHOMA, LYMPH NODE

This photograph illustrates the T-zone lymphoma described by Lennert and associates. One of the widely separated residual germinal centers is shown at the top with a tumorous infiltrate in the T zone of the node. The tumor cells were small to medium sized with relatively little nuclear irregularity. X100. (Courtesy of Prof. K. Lennert, Kiel, West Germany.)

B. IMMUNOBLASTIC LYMPHOMA T, LYMPH NODE
(Plate VII-B–E are from the same patient)

The monomorphous type is demonstrated in this illustration. A proliferation of large cells replaces most of the lymph node. There is a small amount of residual uninvolved lymph node containing a rare reactive follicle. The capsule is broadly thickened. X50.

C. IMMUNOBLASTIC LYMPHOMA T, LYMPH NODE

The pale cytoplasmic character of the monomorphous proliferation is evident at this magnification. Cellular borders appear interlocking, fine, and acidophilic. Nuclei are round to oval, have one to three nucleoli, and resemble the nuclei of in vitro transformed T lymphocytes. X600.

D. IMMUNOBLASTIC LYMPHOMA T, LYMPH NODE

The lightly pyroninophilic character of the cytoplasm is apparent in this MGP stain. MGP. X600.

E. IMMUNOBLASTIC LYMPHOMA T, LYMPH NODE

This Giemsa stain shows the pale amphophilic appearance of the cytoplasm. The stains from Plate VII-D and E are in striking contrast to the intensity of staining in immunoblastic lymphoma B. Giemsa. X600.

PLATE VII

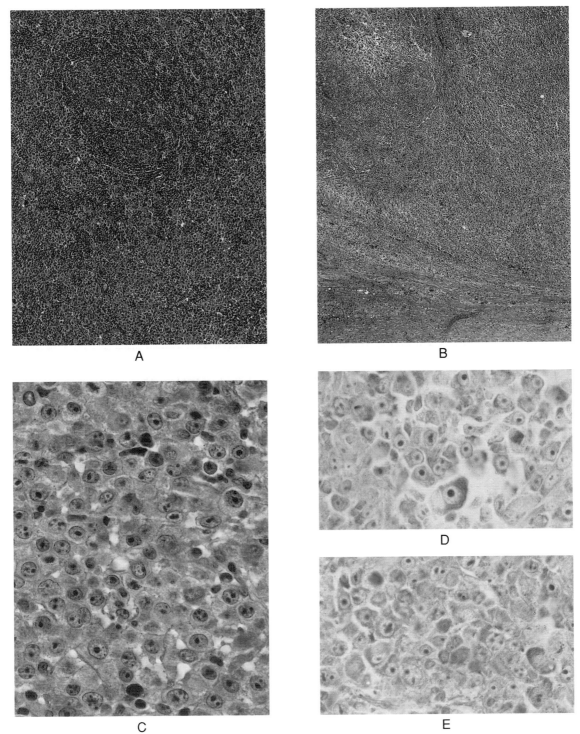

A

B

C

D

E

PLATE VIII

A. IMMUNOBLASTIC LYMPHOMA T, PLEOMORPHIC VARIANT, LYMPH NODE
(Plate VIII-A–C are from the same patient)

This photograph illustrates a pleomorphic variant described by Pinkus and associates. The neoplastic infiltrate occurs in ill-defined aggregates of large pale cytoplasmic cells distributed in the T zone. X80. (Courtesy of Dr. G. Pinkus, Boston, MA.)

B. IMMUNOBLASTIC LYMPHOMA T, PLEOMORPHIC VARIANT, LYMPH NODE

The infiltrate consists of large pale cytoplasmic cells with variable nuclear configuration along with a multinucleated cell resembling a Reed-Sternberg variant. H&E. X600. (Courtesy of Dr. G. Pinkus, Boston, MA.)

C. IMMUNOBLASTIC LYMPHOMA T, PLEOMORPHIC VARIANT, LYMPH NODE

This high magnification photomicrograph illustrates further nuclear irregularity in both the medium and large cells. X600. (Courtesy of Dr. G. Pinkus, Boston, MA.)

D. IBL-LIKE T CELL LYMPHOMA OF JAPAN, LYMPH NODE
(Plate VIII-D and E are from the same patient)

The lymph node architecture is replaced by a mixed cellular proliferation. There is a prominent, branching, medium-sized vascular proliferation with thickened walls and hyperplastic endothelium resembling postcapillary venules. Pale cytoplasmic large cells dominate the proliferation, and a plasma cell component is concentrated about the vessels. X100. (Courtesy of Dr. S. Watanabe, Tokyo, Japan.)

E. IBL-LIKE T CELL LYMPHOMA OF JAPAN, LYMPH NODE

The pale cytoplasmic cells resemble other transformed lymphocytes (T immunoblasts). Small round lymphocytes are scattered throughout, whereas cells with amphophilic plasmacytoid cytoplasm are found near the vessels. X400. (Courtesy of Dr. S. Watanabe, Tokyo, Japan.)

PLATE VIII

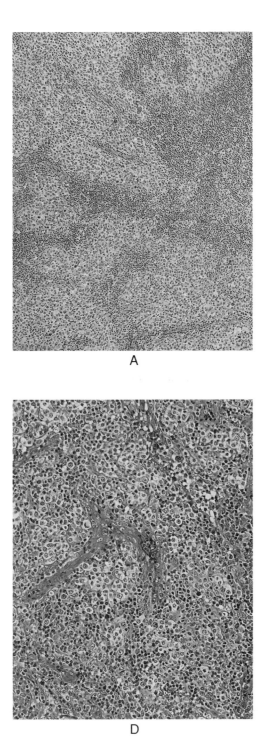

A

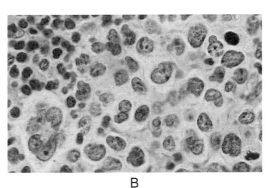

B

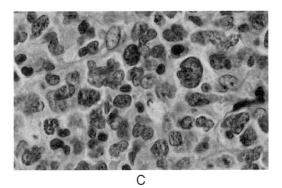

C

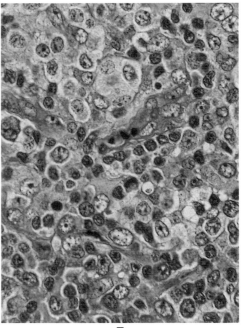

D

E

PLATE IX

A. LYMPHOEPITHELIOID LYMPHOMA, LYMPH NODE
This low magnification photomicrograph illustrates the characteristic appearance of this lymphoma in which clusters of pale cytoplasmic (epithelioid) cells are scattered in a diffuse lymphocytic population. H&E. X10.

B. LYMPHOEPITHELIOID LYMPHOMA, LYMPH NODE
(Plate IX-B–D are from the same patient)
This photograph shows the typical combination of epithelioid clusters and lymphocytes. Multiple biopsies in this patient illustrate the variation in size and character of the neoplastic cells. In this initial biopsy, there are several clusters of epithelioid cells associated with small to medium sized abnormal lymphocytes. The small lymphocytes were mostly located around vessels. X400.

C. LYMPHOEPITHELIOID LYMPHOMA, LYMPH NODE
WITH EVOLUTION TO IMMUNOBLASTIC LYMPHOMA T
In a second biopsy performed several weeks later, medium sized pale lymphocytes are now apparent, and no epithelioid clusters are found. A moderate number of eosinophils are noted. A few larger cells resembling immunoblasts are scattered throughout. X400.

D. LYMPHOEPITHELIOID LYMPHOMA
WITH EVOLUTION TO IMMUNOBLASTIC LYMPHOMA T, ABDOMINAL WALL MASS
In the third biopsy performed several months later, the lymphocytes are large and the immunoblasts are numerous. Medium sized cytoplasmic lymphocytes with cohesive cell borders are interspersed with the immunoblasts. Transformation to immunoblastic lymphoma T in lymphoepithelioid lymphomas is common. X400.

PLATE IX

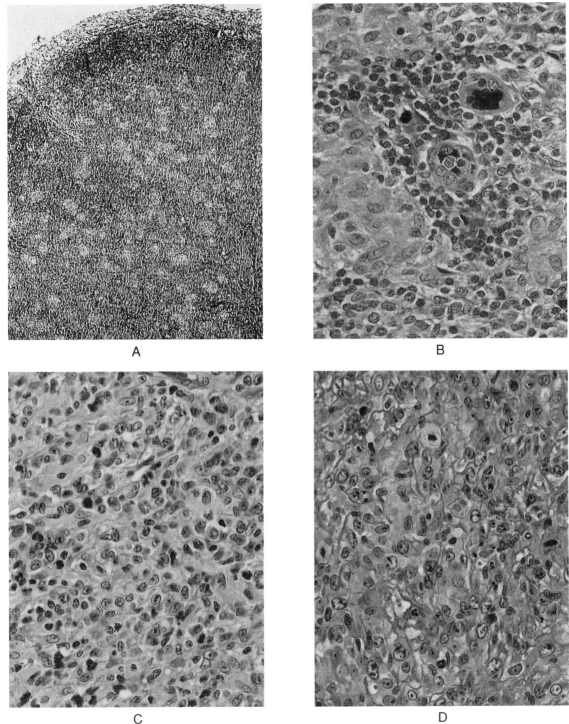

A

B

C

D

PLATE X

A. Ki-1 POSITIVE MALIGNANT LYMPHOMA, LYMPH NODE
The architecture is distorted by a prominent infiltrate of large pale cytoplasmic cells. X25. (Courtesy of Prof. K. Lennert, Kiel, West Germany.)

B. Ki-1 POSITIVE MALIGNANT LYMPHOMA, LYMPH NODE
Within the infiltrate, noncohesive large hyperlobated anaplastic cells are often found in sinuses. X250. (Courtesy of Prof. K. Lennert, Kiel, West Germany.)

C. Ki-1 POSITIVE MALIGNANT LYMPHOMA, LYMPH NODE
(Plate X-C–E are from the same patient)
This case demonstrates obvious sinus involvement typical of this type of lymphoma. PAS. X25. (Prof. K. Lennert kindly confirmed that this case was a Ki-1 positive anaplastic lymphoma.)

D. Ki-1 POSITIVE MALIGNANT LYMPHOMA, LYMPH NODE, PIP, WITH CYTOKERATIN
These large anaplastic cells have abundant cytoplasm that is often amphophilic and strongly pyroninophilic. The sinus growth pattern strongly suggested metastatic carcinoma, a possibility that was not excluded by electron microscopy. However, PIP stains for cytokeratin were negative. X100.

E. Ki-1 POSITIVE MALIGNANT LYMPHOMA, LYMPH NODE, PIP, WITH CD30 (Ber H2)
Ber H2 antibody (Ki-1 equivalent for paraffin sections) reveals numerous positive granules in the cytoplasm. Most Ki-1 positive lymphomas show membrane and/or Golgi positivity. Neoplastic cells contained IgM; a light chain was not detected. No marking was evident with T cell antibodies. Most Ki-1 positive lymphomas mark as T cell processes. X100.

PLATE X

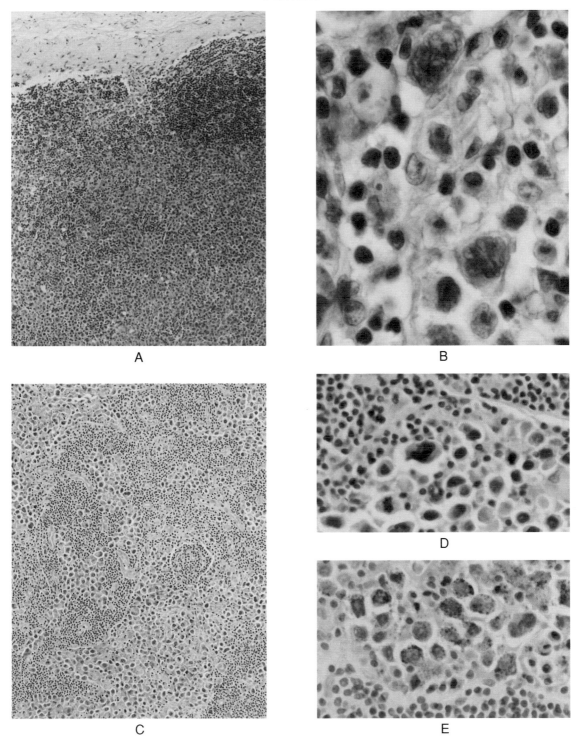

A

B

C

D

E

Said, J.W. and Pinkus, G.S. Immunoblastic sarcoma of the T cell type. Am. J. Pathol. 101:515-525, 1980.

Waldmann, T.A., Davis, M.M., Bongiovanni, K.F., and Korsmeyer, S.J. Rearrangements of genes for the antigen receptor on T cells as markers of lineage and clonality in human lymphoid neoplasms. N. Engl. J. Med. 313:776-783, 1985.

Waldron, J.A., Leech, J.H., Glick, A.D., Flexner, J.M., and Collins, R.D. Malignant lymphoma of peripheral T-lymphocyte origin: immunologic, pathologic, and clinical features in six patients. Cancer 40:1604-1617, 1977.

Weis, J.W., Winter, M.W., Phyliky, R.L., and Banks, P.M. Peripheral T-cell lymphomas: histologic, immunohistologic, and clinical characterization. Mayo Clin. Proc. 61:411-426, 1986.

CEREBRIFORM T CELL LYMPHOMAS

SYNONYMS AND RELATED TERMS: Mycosis fungoides; Sézary syndrome. Working Formulation: mycosis fungoides. Kiel: lymphocytic; mycosis fungoides; Sézary syndrome. Rappaport: mycosis fungoides.

Definition. Some of these lymphomas may be preceded by a prolonged symptomatic period in which the lymphoproliferative disorder appears indolent. A progression to an overt lymphoma may ultimately occur, with involvement of the lymph nodes, viscera, and blood. The prolonged localization of these lymphomas in the skin suggests that they arise from immunocompetent T cells specialized to provide cutaneous immunity. For pathologic details see Plates XI-XIII and figure 10.

Clinical Features. Cerebriform T cell lymphomas account for approximately 2 percent of all lymphoid malignancies in the United States. The disease occurs in middle age and affects males more commonly than females. The disease first manifests in the skin. In the mycosis fungoides variant, early skin involvement may be nonspecific, with the appearance of psoriaform or eczematoid lesions and pruritus. With time, the skin thickens, indurated plaques develop, and, later, localized or generalized tumors appear (plate XI-C,E). Visceral involvement may become apparent as lymphadenopathy and hepatosplenomegaly. In the Sézary variant, the initial disease is usually manifest as a generalized, intensely pruritic, edematous erythroderma (plate XI-D). In addition, the skin may become hyperpigmented, infiltrated, and exfoliative. Scaling and fissuring of the skin on the palms and soles is common, and dystrophy of the nail plates may be seen.

Although cerebriform T cell lymphomas have classically been viewed as restricted to the skin at presentation, recent studies indicate that the diseases in this category are widely disseminated at the time of diagnosis.

The therapy for cerebriform T cell lymphomas is encouraging in the early stages, which may last for 5 to 10 years. In spite of cosmetic improvement, however, the natural history of disease progression is not altered. Electron beam radiation may be administered safely and effectively to the entire skin and apparently induces cutaneous remission in most patients. Because most patients have extracutaneous disease at presentation, relapse is an inevitable and understandable development. In patients with advanced disease, multiagent chemotherapy produces few complete responses, with the median survival in the range of 1 to 2 years. Transformation to a high grade lymphoma may occur in the skin or extracutaneous sites and is associated with a poor prognosis. Transformation occurs in approximately 20 percent of the patients but is not uniformly present at death.

Pathologic Features (Table 22). Skin biopsies during the later stages of cerebriform T cell lymphomas show extensive

Table 22

T CELL LYMPHOMA, CEREBRIFORM LYMPHOCYTIC TYPE

PATTERN	
	• Skin — dense lymphocytic or mixed, superficial infiltrate with epidermotropism (single cells or clustered in Pautrier's abscess) • Node — may be diffuse but typically shows inter-follicular infiltrate intermixed with dermatopathic changes

CYTOLOGY — NEOPLASTIC	MARKERS — NEOPLASTIC
• Predominant cell usually small with characteristic cerebriform nuclear contour; dysplastic larger cell with condensed chromatin; rare transformed cells in early cases • Mitoses unusual; MGP usually negative • Late conversion to dominance of transformed cells or T immunoblasts	• Predominant cell usually T helper, rarely T suppressor, nonmarking or comarking as T helper and T suppressor • PIP: CD45RO (UCHL-1) (+) Transformed cells may not mark as T cells, may be CD15 (Leu-M1) (+) • PAS (+) perinuclear globules in circulating cells

INVOLVED SITES	CLINICAL FEATURES
• Skin • Superficial nodes • Circulating cells and marrow involvement often present but may be difficult to detect	• All clinical features of mycosis fungoides and Sézary syndrome may be seen • Adults may have generalized lesions (erythema, pruritus, hair loss) before diagnostic biopsy obtained • Marked erythema present in Sézary syndrome; local tumor masses • Adenopathy may develop in late phase • Transformation to high grade lymphoma occurs

REACTIVE COMPONENTS	DIFFERENTIAL DIAGNOSIS
• Reactive T and B cells, plasma cells, eosinophils, and macrophages may be present • Hypervascularity • Nodes contain dermatopathic changes with nodules of Langerhans' granule cells	• Reactive states in skin and nodes • Small B cell neoplasms of skin • Other T cell lymphomas in skin • Transformed type may be confused with Hodgkin's disease or other large cell lymphomas • Psoriaform dermatoses

lymphocytic infiltration of the dermis and, to a lesser extent, the epidermis (plate XII-A–C). The neoplastic cells are intermediate to large in size, and their nuclei have a characteristic cerebriform configuration (plates XII-B, XIII-A; fig. 10). Lymph nodes biopsied after dissemination show residual areas of dermatopathic lymphadenopathy, with involvement of T-zone areas by foci of neoplastic cells (plates XII-D, XIII-A,B). In later biopsies, nodal architecture will be effaced by a diffuse lymphomatous process that may be strikingly polymorphous (plate XIII-C). Careful cytologic examination may show scattered large Langerhans cells with folded irregular nuclei (probably residual from the dermatopathic process).

An early diagnosis of cerebriform T cell lymphomas is extremely difficult. Problems arise from the inherent complexity of the disease, inadequate sampling, and improper fixation. The lymphocytic infiltrate in the upper dermis in cerebriform T cell lymphomas should be homogeneous and dense (plate XII-A,B). With proper fixation dysplastic cells may be recognized with confidence in the skin or nodes (plate XIII-A).

The three phases of cerebriform T cell lymphomas include eczematoid, plaque, and tumor. In the eczematoid phase, there is a perivascular and periappendicular lymphocytic infiltrate with occasional eosinophils and edematous dermis. In the plaque phase, there is a mixed infiltration of the dermis with a loss of the grenz zone and infiltration of the epidermis by cerebriform cells. A cellular infiltrate consisting of prominent small to medium sized cerebriform cells with strikingly irregular nuclei is noted along with eosinophils, plasma cells, and immunoblasts. In the tumor phase, medium to large transformed lymphocytes with pale cytoplasm (T immunoblasts) are present. The tumor phase appears to represent T immunoblastic lymphoma, but residual cerebriform lymphocytes are usually found in the dermis and epidermis.

The transformation of cerebriform T cell lymphomas to a large cell lymphoma may occur in cutaneous or extracutaneous sites (plate XIII-C) and may be present at the time of the initial biopsy. In cases with sequential biopsies, original phenotypes of neoplastic T cells were usually retained. Median survival after transformation was 12 months; survival without transformation was 58 months (Salhaney et al.).

Marrow involvement in cerebriform T cell lymphomas has been significantly underestimated. With B-5 fixed marrow particle preparations, approximately 20 percent of the patients have distinct focal lesions. Leukemic phases may be very subtle. Careful examination of Wright's-stained smears may be useful (plate XI-A). Although there is a distinct PAS positivity in circulating tumor cells (plate XI-B), it is misleading to use a percentage of PAS-positive cells (i.e., 10 percent) as a diagnostic criterion of blood involvement. Other cell types may be PAS positive, many definite cases have a low percentage of positive cells in the blood, and there are always the troublesome cases counting out at 9 percent.

Immunologic Features. Neoplastic cells in the blood, node, marrow, and skin have been identified as T cells by their capacity to form E-rosettes and their reaction with anti-T monoclonal antibodies. The tumor cells in most cases express a phenotype associated with normal helper/inducer T lymphocytes and also function as helper T lymphocytes in vitro. Occasional cases mark with both CD4 and CD8 antibodies (plates XII-C, XIII-B).

Comment. These cutaneous lymphomas suggest there may be a special functional relationship between certain subpopulations of T cells and the skin. Due to the presence of cerebriform cells in the skin in a variety of benign disorders, it seems likely that some cutaneous lymphomas may evolve out of prolonged immunologic reactions taking place in the skin.

Despite the clinical and pathologic evidence suggesting a cutaneous origin for this neoplasm, proliferation kinetics suggest that the neoplastic cells migrate from the blood to the skin (Miller et al.), with a production site in the lymphatic tissue (Schwarzmeier et al.; Shackney and Skramstad). There is karyotypic evidence suggesting the origin is from a single clone rather than a multifocal process (Edelson et al.).

Many extranodal lymphomas develop after prolonged immunologic stimulation at the site of origin of the lymphoma. A similar pathogenesis for cerebriform T cell lymphoma seems likely, despite the kinetic evidence mentioned above. Widespread trafficking of the neoplastic cell should be anticipated, regardless of the source, and may account for the extension of the cutaneous involvement and the ultimate dissemination of the process.

Recognition of the early phases of cutaneous lymphomas has been difficult in part due to the presence of similar-appearing lymphoid cells in a variety of reactive dermatoses. There are indications that the disease may be recognizable in its initial stages. Thus, proper fixation of biopsies in suspected cases will certainly facilitate the recognition of the early lesions.

The relationship of mycosis cells to Langerhans granule-containing macrophages is of interest. Macrophages of this type are present in skin lesions, in nodes in dermatopathic lymphadenitis, and in nodes and marrow at the time of dissemination. Their presence in diffuse lymphomas is very suggestive of cerebriform T cell lymphomas.

Differential Diagnosis. Cerebriform T cell lymphomas should be diagnosed only when there are dense infiltrates of cerebriform cells, with both small and dysplastic forms readily demonstrated. Nodal involvement is difficult to recognize. Patients with minimal architectural distortion of the nodes and with only small aggregates of cerebriform T cells should probably not be diagnosed as having nodal involvement.

Small B cell neoplasms. Small B cell neoplasms tend to grow in the dermis, leaving a clear grenz zone, with no epidermotropism. B cell neoplasms may show neoplastic follicular nodulation and will also have immunologic features that are distinctive. The characteristic cerebriform shape of the neoplastic cell in cerebriform T cell lymphomas is easily recognized in well-prepared material.

T cell lymphomas, other than cerebriform T cell lymphomas that involve the skin, generally show pathologic changes typical of immunoblastic lymphoma T (i.e., a mixture of small lymphocytes, transformed lymphocytes, and macrophages). This involvement is often deep, with little epidermotropism.

References

Edelson, R.L., Berger, C.L., Raafat, J., and Warburton, D. Karyotype studies of cutaneous T cell lymphoma: evidence for clonal origin. J. Invest. Dermatol. 73:548-550, 1979.

Miller, R.A., Coleman, C.N., Fawcett, H.D., Hoppe, R.T., and McDougall, I.R. Sézary syndrome: a model for migration of T lymphocytes to skin. N. Engl. J. Med. 303:89-92, 1980.

Salhaney, K.E., Cousar, J.B., Greer, J.P., et al. Transformation of cutaneous T cell lymphoma to large cell lymphoma. Am. J. Pathol. 132:265-277, 1988.

PLATE XI

A. CEREBRIFORM T CELL LYMPHOMA, PERIPHERAL BLOOD
(Plate XI-A and B are from the same patient)
In the leukemic phase of this neoplasm, the tumor cells may show cytoplasmic vacuolization; fine, linear nuclear subdivisions; and distinct nuclear folding. Wright's stain. X1000.

B. CEREBRIFORM T CELL LYMPHOMA, PERIPHERAL BLOOD
The globular, block-like, and granular PAS positivity seen in the leukemic phase of cerebriform T lymphomas is illustrated. PAS. X1000.

C. CEREBRIFORM T CELL LYMPHOMA
A middle-aged black female with leonine facies had progression over several years from slight skin thickening to the nodular thickening demonstrated in this photograph.

D. CEREBRIFORM T CELL LYMPHOMA
(Plate XI-D,E, plate XII-A–D, and plate XIII-A,B are from the same patient)
This patient with erythroderma of Sézary syndrome had tumorous nodules usually seen in the tumor phase of mycosis fungoides. This photograph shows the altered color of the skin and the scaling characteristic of Sézary syndrome.

E. CEREBRIFORM T CELL LYMPHOMA
A close-up photograph reveals a skin nodule, redness of the skin, and scaling.

PLATE XI

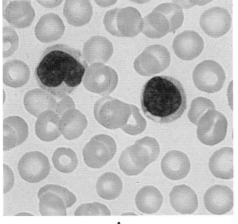

A

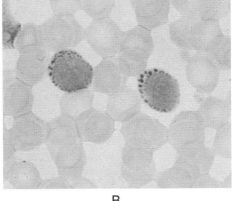

B

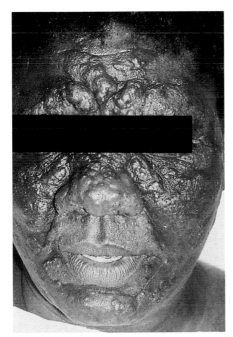

C

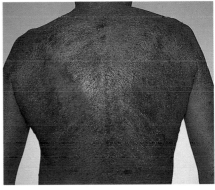

D

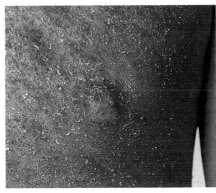

E

PLATE XII

A. CEREBRIFORM T CELL LYMPHOMA, SKIN
(Plate XII-A–D, plate XI-D,E, and plate XIII-A,B are from the same patient)

In a biopsy of an erythematous region from the case in Plate XI-E, there is extensive infiltration by tumor cells in the superficial and deep dermis with loss of the grenz zone. X100.

B. CEREBRIFORM T CELL LYMPHOMA, SKIN

This high magnification photomicrograph reveals the infiltration of the epidermis by tumor cells (epidermotropism). The cells are found as individual cells, linear aggregates, or small clusters (Pautrier's abscess). X400.

C. CEREBRIFORM T CELL LYMPHOMA, SKIN, FROZEN SECTION IMMUNOPEROXIDASE

In this case, tumor cells marked with both CD4 and CD8 antibodies. This illustration demonstrates CD8 reactivity. The positive cells extend broadly through the dermis across the grenz zone and into the epidermis in varying sized clusters. Hematoxylin. X55.

D. CEREBRIFORM T CELL LYMPHOMA, LYMPH NODE

In this illustration, there is a marked expansion of the T zone with a wide separation of the follicular centers. For high magnification appearance, see Plate XIII. X55.

PLATE XII

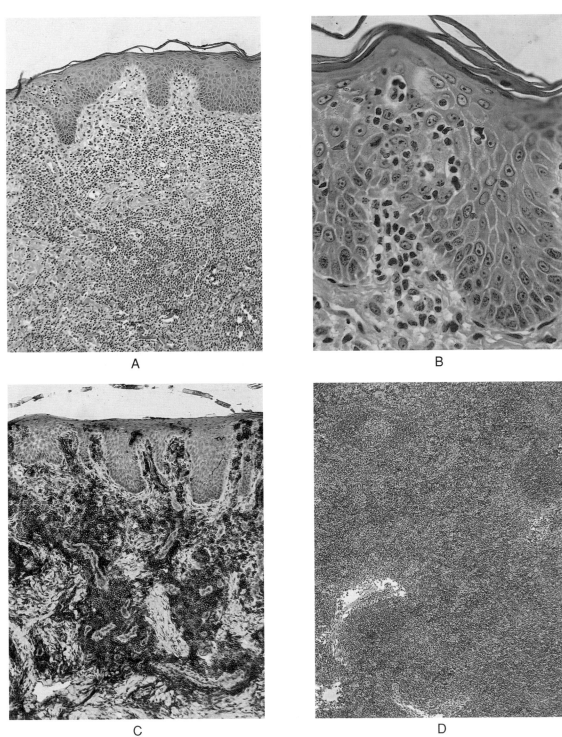

A

B

C

D

PLATE XIII

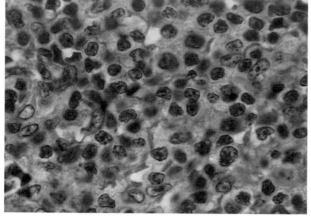

A. CEREBRIFORM T CELL LYMPHOMA, LYMPH NODE
(Plate XIII-A,B, plate XI-D,E, and
plate XII-A–D are from the same patient)

At higher magnification, the infiltration in the T-zone area shows considerable variation in the size of the neoplastic cells, with variable nuclear configuration and occasional linear subdivisions. Pale-staining cytoplasm is apparent around most of the tumor cells. Ninety percent of the cells in the peripheral blood and in the node marked with CD4 and CD8 in flow cytometry studies. X600.

B. CEREBRIFORM T CELL LYMPHOMA, LYMPH NODE, FROZEN SECTION IMMUNOPEROXIDASE, WITH CD4

With CD4 antibody, the extensive infiltration of the interfollicular area is demonstrated, while residual B areas are unstained. This tumor marked with both CD8 and CD4 antibodies. Most cases of cerebriform T cell lymphoma mark only with CD4 antibody. Hematoxylin. X55.

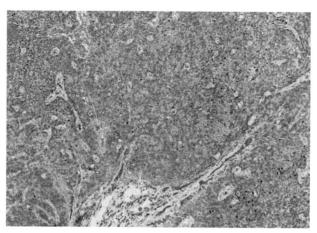

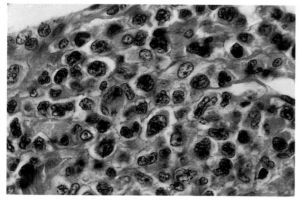

C. CEREBRIFORM T CELL LYMPHOMA WITH TRANSFORMATION, LYMPH NODE

This case of transformation shows extremely irregular tumor cells, some of which are quite large and cytoplasmic. Transformation may be identified in cerebriform T cell lymphomas when there is an interspersed component of small cells with characteristic cerebriform nuclear folding. X495.

88

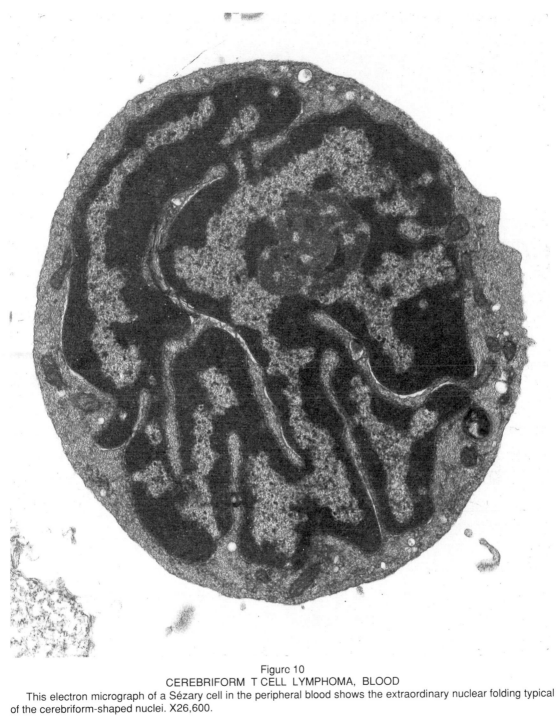

Figure 10
CEREBRIFORM T CELL LYMPHOMA, BLOOD
This electron micrograph of a Sézary cell in the peripheral blood shows the extraordinary nuclear folding typical of the cerebriform-shaped nuclei. X26,600.

Schwarzmeier, J.D., Paietta, E., Radaszkiewicz, T., Konrad, K., and Marosi, L. Proliferation kinetics of Sézary cells. Blood 57:1049-1054, 1981.

Shackney, S.E. and Skramstad, K. A dynamic interpretation of multiparameter studies in the lymphomas. Am. J. Clin. Pathol. 72(Suppl. 4):756-764, 1979.

Additional References

Broder, S., Uchiyama, T., and Waldmann, T.A. Current concepts in immunoregulatory T-cell neoplasms. Cancer Treat. Rep. 63:607-612, 1979.

Bunn, P.A., Jr., Huberman, M.S., Whang-Peng, J., et al. Prospective staging evaluation of patients with cutaneous T-cell lymphomas. Ann. Intern. Med. 93:223-230, 1980.

Foon, K.A. and Todd, R.F., III. Immunologic classification of leukemia and lymphoma. Blood 68:1-31, 1986.

Kadin, M., Nasu, K., Sako, D., Said, J., and Vonderheid, E. Lymphomatoid papulosis. A cutaneous proliferation of activated helper T cells expressing Hodgkin's disease-associated antigens. Am. J. Pathol. 119:315-325, 1985.

Knowles, D.M., Jr. and Halper, J.P. Human T-cell malignancies. Am. J. Pathol. 106:187-203, 1982.

Lutzner, M., Edelson, R., Schein, P., et al. Cutaneous T-cell lymphomas: the Sézary syndrome, mycosis fungoides, and related disorders. Ann. Intern. Med. 83:534-552, 1975.

Meijer, C.J., van der Loo, E.M., van Vloten, W.A., et al. Early diagnosis of mycosis fungoides and Sézary's syndrome by morphometric analysis of lymphoid cells in the skin. Cancer 45:2864-2871, 1980.

Nasu, K., Said, J., Vonderheid, E., et al. Immunopathology of cutaneous T-cell lymphomas. Am. J. Pathol. 119:436-447, 1985.

Ralfkiaer, E., Stein, H., Wantzin, G.L., et al. Lymphomatoid papulosis. Characterization of skin infiltrates by monoclonal antibodies. Am. J. Clin. Pathol. 84:587-593, 1985.

——————— , Wantzin, G.L., Mason, D.Y., et al. Phenotypic characterization of lymphocyte subsets in mycosis fungoides: comparison with large plaque parapsoriasis and benign chronic dermatoses. Am. J. Clin. Pathol. 84:610-619, 1985.

Rappaport, H. and Thomas, L.B. Mycosis fungoides: the pathology of extracutaneous involvement. Cancer 34:1198-1229, 1974.

Sausville, E.A., Worsham, G.F., Matthews, M.J., et al. Histologic assessment of lymph nodes in mycosis fungoides/Sézary syndrome (cutaneous T-cell lymphoma). Hum. Pathol. 16:1098-1109, 1985.

Scheffer, E., Meijer, C.J., and van Vloten, W.A. Dermatopathic lymphadenopathy and lymph node involvement in mycosis fungoides. Cancer 45:137-148, 1980.

Weinman, V.F. and Ackerman, A.B. Lymphomatoid papulosis. Am. J. Dermatopathol. 3:129-163, 1981.

Weiss, L.M., Hu, E., Wood, G.S., et al. Clonal rearrangements of T-cell receptor genes in mycosis fungoides and dermatopathic lymphadenopathy. N. Engl. J. Med. 313:539-544, 1985.

Whang-Peng, J., Bunn, P.A., Jr., Knutsen, T., et al. Clinical implications of cytogenetic studies in cutaneous T-cell lymphoma (CTCL). Cancer 50:1539-1553, 1982.

Willemze, R., Scheffer, E., and Meijer, C.J. Immunohistochemical studies using monoclonal antibodies on lymph nodes from patients with mycosis fungoides and Sézary's syndrome. Am. J. Pathol. 120:46-54, 1985.

PERIPHERAL EXTRANODAL T CELL LYMPHOMAS, MANY WITH ANGIOCENTRIC FEATURES

Ulcerative destructive lesions of the upper aerodigestive tract and face, clinically known as lethal midline granuloma, may show histopathologic and clinical features of malignancy (Table 23). Such cases have been termed polymorphic reticulosis or midline malignant reticulosis. The histopathologic changes in this type of lethal midline granuloma are similar to those in lymphomatoid granulomatosis. Jaffe considers lymphomatoid granulomatosis and lethal midline granuloma to represent the same pathologic process, an angiocentric immunoproliferative lesion that may vary in clinical aggressiveness (Lipford et al.). Benign lymphocytic vasculitides are at one end of the spectrum, and angiocentric lymphomas are at the other. In many but not all cases of such angiocentric lesions in the nose and lung, there is evidence of T cell neoplasia from aberrant T antigen expression or gene rearrangement. However, angiocentricity is not confined to T cell processes because some B cell lymphomas also exhibit vascular invasion or intravascular growth. In

Table 23

PERIPHERAL EXTRANODAL T CELL LYMPHOMAS, MANY WITH ANGIOCENTRIC FEATURES

DEFINITION	PATTERN
• Lymphomatoid granulomatosis: initially thought to be reactive but now most cases are assumed to be lymphomas • Polymorphic reticulosis (malignant midline reticulosis): a condition very similar to lymphomatoid granulomatosis in pathology, differing only in location • Angiocentric lymphoma: overtly lymphomatous clinically and pathologically; grows in and around vessels	• Generally polymorphous, with small and large cells • Definite tendency to grow partially or principally in vessels • May show extensive necrosis
CYTOLOGY	**MARKERS**
• All of these processes contain cellular infiltrates that show a wide range of size, nuclear configuration; giant cells may be present	• Lymphomatoid granulomatosis: usually has T phenotype • Polymorphic reticulosis: a few cases have shown T phenotype • Angiocentric lymphoma: the few cases studied have had a T-helper phenotype
INVOLVED SITES	**CLINICAL FEATURES**
• Lymphomatoid granulomatosis: lung and skin • Polymorphic reticulosis: nasal cavities; lymph node, liver, lung, and skin involvement late • Angiocentric lymphoma: nasal cavities, lung, skin, central nervous system	• Lymphomatoid granulomatosis: lung or skin lesions in adult • Polymorphic reticulosis: destructive facial lesion of midline in adult • Angiocentric lymphoma: clinically similar to other angiocentric processes but more likely to have disseminated disease
REACTIVE COMPONENTS	**DIFFERENTIAL DIAGNOSIS**
• Small lymphocytes, eosinophils, plasma cells, histiocytes • Minimal reactive component in angiocentric lymphoma	• Diagnosis often difficult because of confusion with benign processes, extensive necrosis, small biopsies, and rarity of disease • Some B cell lymphomas may show vascular invasion

angiocentric T cell lymphomas, the neoplastic character of the infiltrate is usually obvious because of cytologic atypia in both the small or large cell components. In all of these diseases, histologic progression to immunoblastic processes has been described, and T phenotypes have been identified in both lymphocytic and immunoblastic components (Chan et al.; Chott et al.). In terms of pathogenesis, Epstein-Barr virus DNA has been detected in nasal T cell lymphomas (Harabuchi et al.).

References

Chan, J.K., Ng, C.S., Lau, W.H., and Lo, S.T. Most nasal/nasopharyngeal lymphomas are peripheral T-cell neoplasms. Am. J. Surg. Pathol. 11:418-429, 1987.

Chott, A., Rappersberger, K., Schlossarek, W., and Radaszkiewicz, T. Peripheral T cell lymphoma presenting primarily as lethal midline granuloma. Hum. Pathol. 19:1093-1101, 1988.

Harabuchi, Y., Yamanaka, N., Kataura, A., et al. Epstein-Barr virus in nasal T-cell lymphomas in patients with lethal midline granuloma. Lancet 335:128-130, 1990.

Jaffe, E.S. Post-Thymic Lymphoid Neoplasia, pp. 218-248. In: Major Problems in Pathology, Vol. 16. Surgical Pathology of the Lymph Nodes and Related Organs. Jaffe, E.S. and Bennington, J.L. (Eds.). Philadelphia: W.B. Saunders Company, 1985.

Lipford, E.H., Jr., Margolick, J.B., Longo, D.L., Fauci, A.S., and Jaffe, E.S. Angiocentric immunoproliferative lesions: a clinicopathologic spectrum of post-thymic T-cell proliferations. Blood 72:1674-1681, 1988.

Additional References

Colby, T.V. and Carrington, C.B. Pulmonary lymphomas: current concepts. Hum. Pathol. 14:884-887, 1983.

Ho, F.C., Choy, D., Loke, S.L., et al. Polymorphic reticulosis and conventional lymphomas of the nose and upper aerodigestive tract: a clinicopathologic study of 70 cases, and immunophenotypic studies of 16 cases. Hum. Pathol. 21:1041-1050, 1990.

Ratech, H., Burke, J.S., Blayney, D.W., Sheibani, K., and Rappaport, H. A clinicopathologic study of malignant lymphomas of the nose, paranasal sinuses, and hard palate, including cases of lethal midline granuloma. Cancer 64:2525-2531, 1989.

B CELL NEOPLASMS

B cell neoplasms occur far more frequently than T cell neoplasms in the United States and Europe, particularly B cell neoplasms arising in extramarrow sites. B cell neoplasms have been recognized in all of the B cell domains and are also frequent in tissues normally containing few lymphocytes, such as the thyroid, skin, and stomach.

Recognition of B cell neoplasms has been greatly facilitated by their frequent production of monoclonal immunoglobulins detected in serum and urine, by the relative ease with which plasmacytic and follicular center cell neoplasms are diagnosed on morphologic grounds alone, by the ability to establish the monotypic nature of cytoplasmic or surface immunoglobulin in cell suspensions of tissue or blood, and by the application of immunoperoxidase methods for detecting cytoplasmic immunoglobulin in paraffin-embedded sections. Application of these methods over the last 10 years has led to a reasonable definition of the scope of B cell neoplasms in terms of morphology and clinical expression, which contrasts with the current incomplete definition of T cell processes. By defining several important clinical pathologic entities as well as contributing to a more precise understanding of the biology of the B cell component of the immune system, the studies above have been of major importance for the general understanding of lymphoid neoplasms. Furthermore, analysis of B cell neoplasms has led directly to the development of the only classification systems for lymphoid neoplasms that are immunologically oriented.

Lymphomas with follicular nodulation have been recognized with reasonable precision for many years. Predictions that such lymphomas represented a specific entity were made by Gall and associates in 1940 and Wright in 1956. The studies of Rappaport and associates of nodular lymphomas were valuable in defining the histopathologic criteria for diagnosis but were misleading in concluding that any lymphoid neoplasm might have nodular or diffuse growth patterns and that the large cells in such processes were histiocytic in type. This opinion influenced American pathologists until well into the 1970s, when it became apparent from Lennert's studies and those of Lukes and Collins that neoplasms did arise from follicular centers and had specific morphologic features, including the production of neoplastic follicular centers. Due to the histologic organization of follicular centers and the replication of this appearance in follicular lymphomas, these neoplasms were predicted to have B cell features. Lymphocyte transformation was also understandable in the context of normal and neoplastic follicular structures. Studies of follicular center cell lymphomas were instrumental in showing that many large cell "histiocytic" lymphomas of Rappaport actually were neoplasms of transformed lymphocytes. Thus, analysis of these neoplasms by light microscopy and immunologic procedures has played an important role in the development of our understanding of lymphoid neoplasms. These studies helped establish a conceptual framework for relating lymphoid neoplasms to their cell of origin and to stages

93

of the cell cycle, which are the cornerstones of the Lukes-Collins and Kiel systems for the classification of lymphomas.

Analysis of B cell neoplasms has also been important in establishing that cells in various stages of the cell cycle are present in most neoplasms (Taylor), in showing that neoplasms derived from a single subpopulation might have widely divergent pathologic and clinical expression (Lukes and Collins, 1974), and in showing that transformation in the appearance of most lymphoid neoplasms is due to cell cycle-related variations in the dividing population rather than to development of a second neoplasm (van den Tweel et al.).

Initial Sites of Presentation. Most patients with B cell neoplasms present with either marrow or nodal disease. Marrow involvement is usually massive and is often associated with peripheral blood involvement and occasionally with evidence of dissemination to the nodes and spleen. Examples of B cell neoplasms associated with marrow presentation include the various acute lymphocytic leukemias of B cell type, multiple myeloma or small lymphocytic B, and plasmacytoid lymphocytic lymphomas. Superficial or internal adenopathy is also a common presentation of B cell neoplasms, particularly in older adults. These patients may have minimal evidence of marrow involvement or peripheral lymphocytosis at presentation.

Follicular center cell lymphomas or small B cell lymphomas often present in this manner. In a few cases, systemic symptoms due to the harmful effects of paraproteinemias dominate the clinical picture. Investigation of these cases usually reveals B cell neoplasms such as multiple myeloma or plasmacytoid lymphocytic-type lymphomas. Rarely, patients with B cell neoplasms have splenomegaly and pancytopenia at presentation; most of these cases have hairy cell leukemia.

Extranodal involvement by B cell lymphomas is frequent. Most lymphomas in the thyroid and bowel are B cell in type. Salivary and conjunctival growths are often B cell in type as well.

Microscopic Features. Cell cycle and differentiating modes of some B lymphocytes are recognizable morphologically. Small B cells, transformed B cells, and plasma cells may be separated cytologically from one another, whereas pre-B cells are identifiable only by immunologic procedures. In addition, small B lymphocytes cannot be differentiated with assurance on morphologic grounds from small T cells, and transformed T and B cells may not be clearly distinguished from each other cytologically.

Over 90 percent of the cells in a mixture of reacting and neoplastic cells in B cell neoplasms may be part of the neoplastic clone in pre-B cell leukemia, small B cell neoplasms, Burkitt's lymphoma, and multiple myeloma. In contrast, T cells comprise 11 to 35 percent of the cells in some follicular center cell lymphomas (cleaved cell processes growing in a follicular pattern) (Dvoretsky et al.; Leech et al.; Lennert, 1978). Macrophages are present in large numbers in rapidly dividing processes such as noncleaved follicular center cell lymphomas, particularly Burkitt's lymphoma. Eosinophils have been noted in some follicular center cell lymphomas.

Various B cell neoplasms are compared in Table 24 by the cell cycle or differentiating mode of the predominant cell. The number of cells in each mode clearly relates to the appearance of B cell neoplasms (Shackney et al.; Taylor). Some

Table 24

CELL CYCLE AND DIFFERENTIATION MODE OF THE PREDOMINANT CELL IN VARIOUS B NEOPLASMS

Large Dividing Pool, Minimal Differentiation

- Small and large noncleaved follicular center cell lymphomas, including Burkitt's and non-Burkitt's lymphoma
- Pre-B acute lymphocytic leukemia

Small Dividing Pool, Large Dormant Pool, Minimal Plasmacytic Differentiation

- Cleaved follicular center cell lymphomas
- Small B cell neoplasms, including chronic lymphocytic leukemia
- Mantle zone lymphoma
- Hairy cell leukemia
- Parafollicular B lymphoma

Small Dividing Pool, Prominent Differentiation

- Multiple myeloma
- Plasmacytoid lymphocytic lymphomas

Large Dividing Pool, Small Dormant Pool, Varying Degrees of Differentiation

- Immunoblastic lymphoma of B cells

small B cell neoplasms (i.e., chronic lymphocytic leukemia and cleaved follicular center cell lymphomas) are composed chiefly of dormant lymphocytes with a small pool of dividing cells. These neoplasms typically contain few transformed lymphocytes and very few plasma cells. On the other hand, plasmacytic differentiation is a dominant feature in multiple myeloma and plasmacytoid lymphocytic lymphoma, and is easily demonstrated in immunoblastic lymphoma B. Neoplasms with a large dividing pool and restricted differentiation (e.g., Burkitt's lymphoma) exhibit a predominance of blasts with many mitoses and few plasma cells.

Behavior. The cell cycle-related phenomena previously described are clearly important in determining the behavior and appearance of lymphoid neoplasms (Salmon and Seligmann). Patients with disease processes that have prominent differentiation, such as multiple myeloma or plasmacytoid lymphocytic-type lymphoma, may have significant effects from immunoglobulin excretion. Patients with malignancies composed predominantly of dormant lymphocytes have relatively indolent processes with slow entry of tumor cells from a small dividing pool. Immunoglobulin excess is not a problem, and these patients may show an inability to produce normal quantities of immunoglobulin. Patients with a large dividing pool, like those with Burkitt's lymphoma, often have aggressive neoplasms and minimal evidence of immunoglobulin production.

Immunologic Markers. The earliest easily identified B cell precursors in the marrow have cytoplasmic μ-chains. Peripheral cells then acquire complete surface immunoglobulin. As differentiation to plasma cells occurs, cytoplasmic immuno-globulin is detected instead. Antigens such as CD20 are seen on peripheral B cells, but precise staging of B cell development with differentiation antigens has not yet been accomplished. It should be noted that functional B cell subpopulations may exist in a manner comparable to functional T subpopulations.

Classification. B neoplasms are arranged in Table 11 on the basis of their presumed sites of origin. Some of these neoplasms are apparently restricted in origin to specific sites. For example, pre-B acute lymphocytic leukemia has been described only in the marrow, whereas follicular center cell lymphomas apparently develop only in peripheral tissues. Other neoplasms (i.e., small cell lymphoid neoplasms with or without plasmacytic differentiation) appear to arise in either the marrow or peripheral tissue; these processes have similar pathologic and clinical features regardless of their site of origin. The site and cell of origin of hairy cell leukemia is unknown.

Chromosomal abnormalities routinely detected in certain B cell lymphomas (e.g., Burkitt's lymphoma) strongly suggest that there is a relationship between human immunoglobulin genes, rearrangement of chromosomes, and the development of neoplasia (Croce and Nowell). These and similar studies clearly indicate that detection of chromosomal abnormalities will become an integral part of the diagnostic approach to many lymphoid neoplasms.

References

Croce, C.M. and Nowell, P.C. Molecular basis of human B cell neoplasia. Blood 65:1-7, 1985.

Dvoretsky, P., Wood, G.S., Levy, R., and Warnke, R.A. T-lymphocyte subsets in follicular lymphomas compared with those in non-neoplastic lymph nodes and tonsils. Hum. Pathol. 13:618-625, 1982.

Gall, E.A., Morrison, H.R., and Scott, A.T. The follicular type of malignant lymphoma: a survey of 63 cases. Ann. Intern. Med. 14:2073-2090, 1940.

Leech, J.H., Glick, A.D., Waldron, J.A., et al. Malignant lymphomas of follicular center cell origin in man. I. Immunologic studies. J. Natl. Cancer Inst. 54:11-21, 1975.

Lennert, K. Germinal centers and germinal center neoplasms. Nippon Ketsueki Gakkai Zasshi 32:495-500, 1969.

_____ . Malignant Lymphomas Other Than Hodgkin's Disease: Histology, Cytology, Ultrastructure, Immunology. New York: Springer-Verlag, 1978.

Lukes, R.J. and Collins, R.D. New observations on follicular lymphoma. Gann Monogr. Cancer Res. 15:209, 1973.

_____ and Collins, R.D. Immunologic characterization of human malignant lymphomas. Cancer 34(Suppl. 4):1488-1503, 1974.

_____ and Collins, R.D. New approaches to the classification of the lymphomata. Br. J. Cancer 2(Suppl.): 1-28, 1975.

Rappaport, H., Winter, W.J., and Hicks, E.B. Follicular lymphoma: a re-evaluation of its position in the scheme of malignant lymphoma, based on a survey of 253 cases. Cancer 9:792-821, 1956.

Salmon, S.E. and Seligmann, M. B-cell neoplasia in man. Lancet 2:1230-1233,1974.

Shackney, S.E., Skramstad, K.S., Cunningham, R.E., et al. Dual parameter flow cytometry studies in human lymphomas. J. Clin. Invest. 66:1281-1294, 1980.

Taylor, C.R. Classification of lymphoma. Arch. Pathol. Lab. Med. 102:549-554, 1978.

van den Tweel, J.G., Lukes, R.J., and Taylor, C.R. Pathophysiology of lymphocyte transformation. A study of so-called composite lymphomas. Am. J. Clin. Pathol. 71:509-520, 1979.

Wright, C.J.E. Macrofollicular lymphoma. Am. J. Pathol. 32:201-233, 1956.

Additional References

Bhan, A.K., Nadler, L.M., Stashenko, P., McCluskey, R.T., and Schlossman, S.F. Stages of B cell differentiation in human lymphoid tissue. J. Exp. Med. 154:737-749, 1981.

Kojima, M., Imai, Y., and Mori, N. A concept of follicular lymphoma—a proposal for the existence of a neoplasm originating from the germinal center. Gann Monogr. Cancer Res. 15:195, 1973.

Lennert, K. Follicular lymphomas—a tumor of the germinal centers. Gann Monogr. Cancer Res. 15:217, 1973.

ACUTE LYMPHOCYTIC LEUKEMIA, B CELL PRECURSOR, INCLUDING PRE-B AND COMMON ACUTE LYMPHOCYTIC LEUKEMIA

SYNONYMS AND RELATED TERMS: Acute lymphoblastic leukemia.

Definition. A marrow-based neoplasm involving stem cells, B cell precursor acute lymphocytic leukemia includes a group of leukemias identified by varying combinations of reactivity with B cell-associated antigen CD19, CD10 positivity, and cytoplasmic μ-chains. Most of the cases of acute lymphocytic leukemia that do not mark as T cells fall into this group. Malignant lymphomas that involve the marrow (small noncleaved/Burkitt's) are not included. For pathologic details, see Plates XIV and XV and figures 11 and 12.

Clinical Features. B cell precursor acute lymphocytic leukemia represents the most common malignant disease seen in childhood. The average age of onset is approximately 4 years (with a range of 2-10 years), with a second minor rise in incidence in the third and fourth decades. Males are affected slightly more often than females.

The most common presenting complaints include weakness and fatigue with bleeding or bruising. Fever and chills are often present and indicate infection. Bone and joint pain are also common and may lead to a gait disturbance in the pediatric population. Cranial nerve palsies or symptoms and signs of increased intracranial pressure may occur but are rarely present at initial diagnosis.

The average hemoglobin level at diagnosis is approximately 9 g/dL. Platelets are almost always reduced, most often to the range of 75-100,000/μL. The white blood cell count is commonly elevated to the range of 50-100,000/μL, although the total white blood cell count is normal or low in approximately one-third of the cases. The serum lactic dehydrogenase is commonly elevated, as is the serum uric acid level. Treatment may produce complete remission in 90 to 95 percent of the pediatric patients, and approximately 75 percent of the pediatric patients are expected to achieve a prolonged remission and possibly cure. A poorer prognosis is associated with the black race, an age range of less than 2 years or greater than 10 years, a white blood cell count in excess of 200,000/μL, and involvement of the central nervous system at diagnosis.

Pathologic Features (Table 25). The marrow infiltrates are usually massive (plate XIV-B), with a homogeneous infiltrate of primitive cells (plate XV-A–C). Some cases show massive necrosis at presentation. The marrow involved at relapse may contain focal nodules or small aggregates of tumor cells (plate XIV-C), and testicular relapse is a recognized complication (plate XIV-D).

There are no cytologic, cytochemical, or ultrastructural findings that are specific for B cell precursor acute lymphocytic leukemia (fig. 11); PAS block positivity is often present but is not specific (plate XV-D). In patients meeting the usual criteria for acute lymphocytic leukemia, the pre-B acute lymphocytic leukemia type is recognized by the demonstration in neoplastic cells of cytoplasmic μ-chains (fig. 12) and scant or absent SIg (Vogler et al., 1978, 1981).

Immunologic Features. Most cases of acute lymphocytic leukemia that do not mark as T cells probably fall into the early B cell acute leukemia group (Nadler et al.). Cells from these cases usually show Ia reactivity, and most are CD19 positive as well. CD10 positivity is present in approximately 80 percent of the cases. TdT positivity may be demonstrated in more than 90 percent of cases of acute lymphocytic leukemia. Immunoglobulin gene rearrangement has been demonstrated in most cases, reaffirming the B cell nature of these neoplasms.

Differential Diagnosis. Most cases of acute lymphocytic leukemia present in a fully developed form with extensive marrow involvement. The diffuse nature of the involvement in acute lymphocytic leukemia is a strong point against metastatic neuroblastoma.

The differentiation of acute lymphocytic leukemia from myeloid leukemias is dependent on an integrated morphologic, cytochemical, and immunologic analysis (Browman et al.). Sudan black and ANAE stains must be carefully evaluated because small percentages of tumor cells (as low as 5 to 10 percent) may mark in myeloid leukemias. Block PAS positivity is often seen in acute lymphocytic leukemia but is not diagnostic per se. Flow studies are readily available and generally provide essential diagnostic information in categorizing these leukemic processes.

References

Browman, G.P., Neame, P.B., and Soamboonsrup, P. The contribution of cytochemistry and immunophenotyping to the reproducibility of the FAB classification in acute leukemia. Blood 68:900-905, 1986.

Nadler, L.M., Korsmeyer, S.J., Anderson, K.C., et al. B cell origin of non-T cell acute lymphoblastic leukemia. A model for discrete stages of neoplastic and normal pre-B cell differentiation. J. Clin. Invest. 74:332, 1984.

Vogler, L.B., Crist, W.M., Bockman, D.E., et al. Pre-B cell leukemia. A new phenotype of childhood lymphoblastic leukemia. N. Engl. J. Med. 298:872-878, 1978.

_____ , Crist, W.M., Sarrif, A.M., et al. An analysis of clinical and laboratory features of acute lymphocytic leukemias with emphasis on 35 children with pre-B leukemia. Blood 58:135-140, 1981.

Table 25

ACUTE LYMPHOCYTIC LEUKEMIA, B CELL PRECURSOR
(Pre-B and Common)

PATTERN	
• Diffuse with scattered residual hematopoietic cells • Rarely massive necrosis	
CYTOLOGY — NEOPLASTIC	**MARKERS — NEOPLASTIC**
• 8-15 μm cell with scant cytoplasm, smooth nuclear chromatin, nucleoli not prominent	• Flow: Ia, CD19 (+) (~ 10 percent of cases) Ia, CD19, CD10 (+) (~ 30 percent of cases) Ia, CD19, CD10, CD20 (+) (~ 50 percent of cases) (some of these show cytoplasmic μ) • TdT (+), 90 percent of cases • PAS positive blocks in many cases
INVOLVED SITES	**CLINICAL FEATURES**
• Marrow • Central nervous system • Testis at relapse	• Average age of onset 4 years; male incidence is slightly greater than female incidence • Marrow failure • Bone pain • Splenomegaly, hepatomegaly, lymphadenopathy in 50-75 percent of the patients • Marrow aspiration may not be possible due to packing by tumor
REACTIVE COMPONENTS	**DIFFERENTIAL DIAGNOSIS**
• Not described	• Myeloid leukemias • Acute lymphocytic leukemia, T • Neuroblastoma, metastatic

PLATE XIV

A. NORMAL MARROW

A marrow particle preparation from a child shows the usual degrees of cellularity and the normal mixture of megakaryocytic and other hematopoietic elements. PAS. X260.

B. ACUTE LYMPHOCYTIC LEUKEMIA, B CELL PRECURSOR TYPE, MARROW

This marrow particle shows complete effacement of normal architecture by a homogeneous infiltrate of neoplastic cells. PAS. X260.

C. ACUTE LYMPHOCYTIC LEUKEMIA, B CELL PRECURSOR TYPE, FOCAL INVOLVEMENT

After treatment for acute lymphocytic leukemia, this child had a marrow particle in which most of the marrow appears normal, although slightly more cellular than usual. A focus of leukemic involvement is present at the top central portion of the illustration. PAS. X260.

D. ACUTE LYMPHOCYTIC LEUKEMIA, B CELL PRECURSOR TYPE, TESTIS

Extensive infiltration of the testis is demonstrated. There are scattered normal tubular structures. PAS. X160.

PLATE XIV

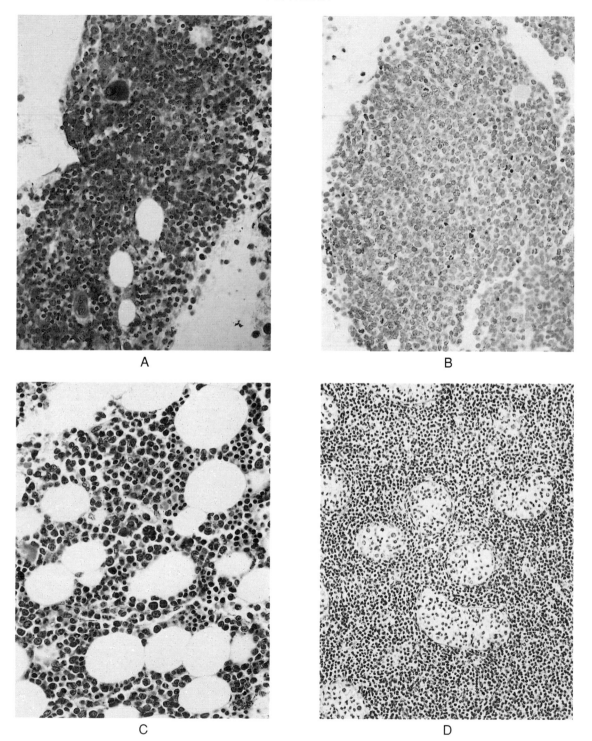

PLATE XV
ACUTE LYMPHOCYTIC LEUKEMIA, B CELL PRECURSOR TYPE, MARROW

A. These FAB L-1 tumor cells are small and have condensed chromatin, sparse cytoplasm, and irregular nuclei. Wright's stain. X650.

B. In FAB L-2 blasts, there is more variation in cell size, with some cells having distinct cytoplasm. The chromatin is slightly more dispersed than in the L-1 form. Wright's stain. X650.

C. These tumor cells show the hand mirror appearance occasionally seen in acute lymphocytic leukemia B, as well as in other lymphoid neoplasms. The chromatin is slightly more dispersed than in typical cases. Wright's stain. X650.

D. In this PAS stain, the tumor cells show a nonstaining cytoplasmic background with granular and block positivity. A granulocyte shows more diffuse positivity. PAS. X650.

PLATE XV

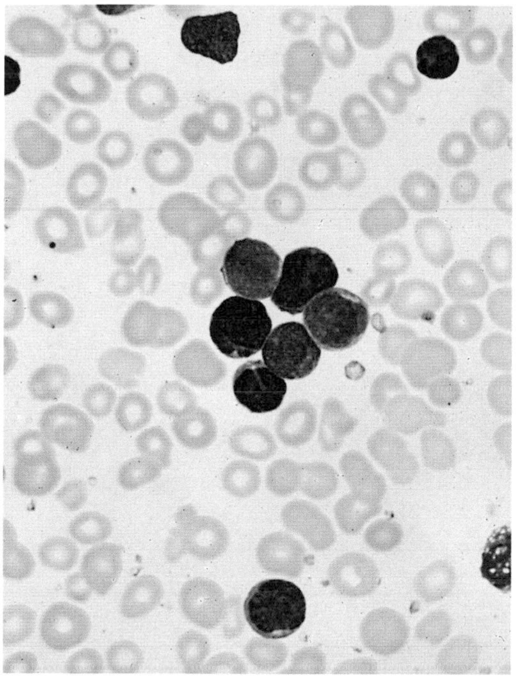

A

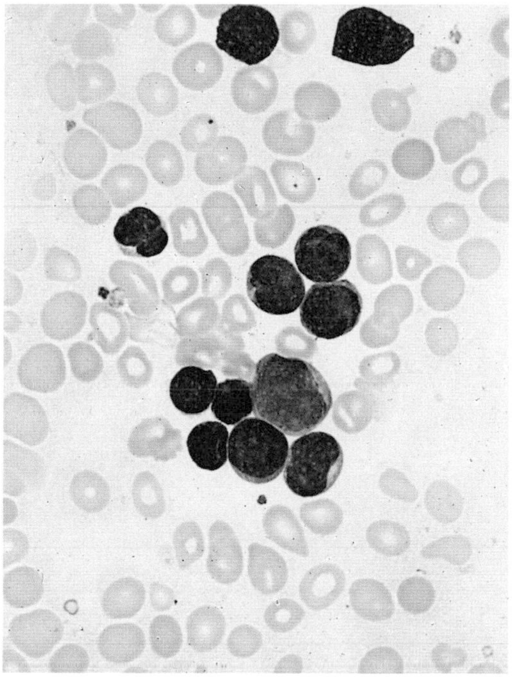

B

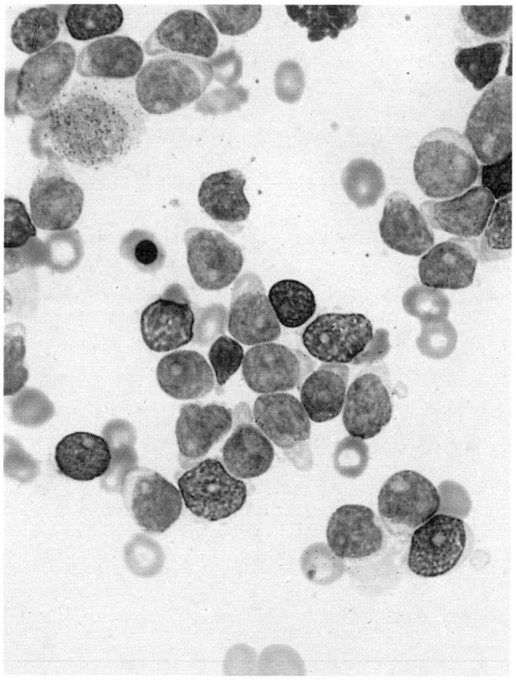

C

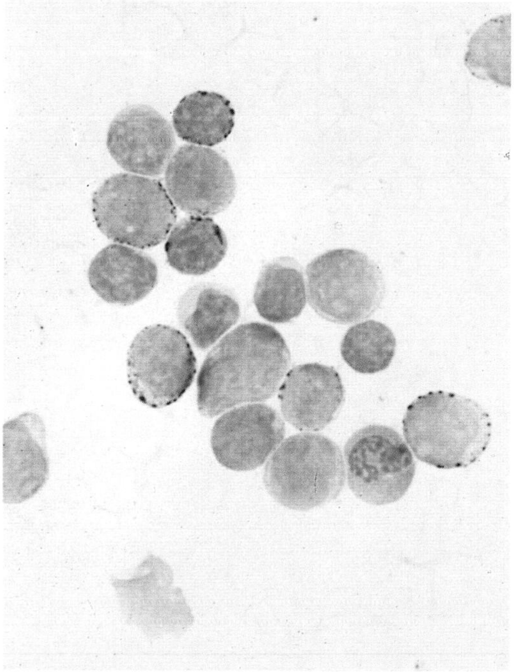

D

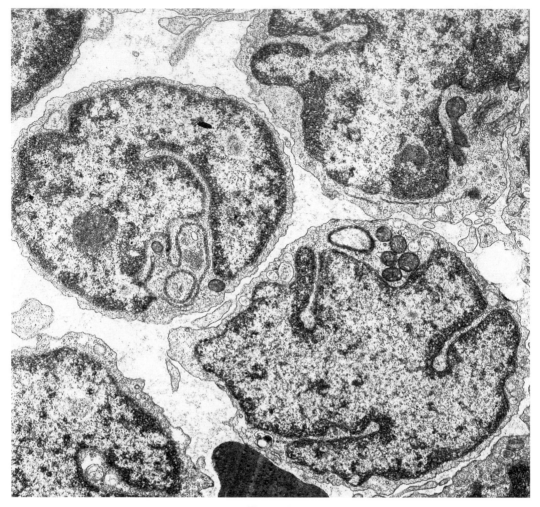

Figure 11
ACUTE LYMPHOCYTIC LEUKEMIA, B CELL PRECURSOR TYPE, MARROW
Electron microscopy usually shows small cells with marginated chromatin, sparse cytoplasm, and heavy nuclear folding with nuclear bridges. Larger cells may be seen in acute lymphocytic leukemia in which nuclear chromatin is more dispersed, and cytoplasmic polysomes and glycogen lakes are demonstrated. X17,400. (Fig. 1 from Glick, A.D., Vestal, B.K., Flexner, J.M., and Collins, R.D. Ultrastructural study of acute lymphocytic leukemia: comparison with immunologic studies. Blood 52:311-322, 1978.)

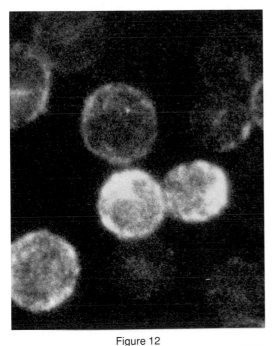

Figure 12
ACUTE LYMPHOCYTIC LEUKEMIA PRE B, MARROW
These are leukemia cells stained with fluorochrome conjugated anti-μ antisera after fixation in 95 percent ethanol and 5 percent acetic acid, as visualized under ultraviolet light microscopy. Note the concentration of staining in the region of the nuclear notch. X1200. (Courtesy of Dr. L. Vogler, Atlanta, GA.)

Additional References

Aur, R.J., Simone, J.V., Verzosa, M.S., et al. Childhood acute lymphocytic leukemia: study VIII. Cancer 42: 2123-2134, 1978.

Foon, K.A. and Todd, R.F., III. Immunologic classification of leukemia and lymphoma. Blood 68:1-31, 1986.

Gee, T.S., Haghbin, M., Dowling, M.D., et al. Acute lymphoblastic leukemia in adults and children. Differences in response with similar therapeutic regimens. Cancer 37:1256-1264, 1976.

Greaves, M.F., Janossy, G., Peto, J., and Kay, H. Immunologically defined subclasses of acute lymphoblastic leukaemia in children: their relationship to presentation features and prognosis. Br. J. Haematol. 48:179-197, 1981.

Ortega, J.A., Nesbit, M.E., Jr., Donaldson, M.H., et al. L-asparaginase, vincristine, and prednisone for induction of first remission in acute lymphocytic leukemia. Cancer Res. 37:535-540, 1977.

Pinkel, D., Simone, J., Hustu, H.O., and Aur, R.J. Nine years' experience with "total therapy" of childhood acute lymphocytic leukemia. Pediatrics 50:246-251, 1972.

ACUTE UNDEFINED LEUKEMIA

SYNONYMS AND RELATED TERMS: Acute undifferentiated leukemia; stem cell leukemia.

Definition. These acute leukemias are neoplasms of undefined cells but presumably arise from stem cells that are capable of producing any hematopoietic cell line. The meaning of the term acute undifferentiated leukemia has changed significantly in the past decade. Previously, this term signified acute stem cell leukemia or acute lymphocytic leukemia. With the use of newer immunologic techniques, however, the phenotype of many of these cases has been defined.

Clinical Features. The clinical characteristics of true undifferentiated leukemia, after exclusion of all lymphoid or myeloid cases, are not yet well understood.

Pathologic Features. The marrow contains sheets of primitive cells that do not mark cytochemically. No distinctive cytoplasmic features are seen by electron microscopy (fig. 13).

Immunologic Features. Neoplastic cells do not mark as T or B cells.

ACUTE LYMPHOCYTIC LEUKEMIA, B CELL

SYNONYMS AND RELATED TERMS: Acute lymphocytic leukemia, L-3 type.

Definition. B cell acute lymphocytic leukemia is a marrow-based neoplasm of B cell precursors. Small noncleaved cell lymphomas of Burkitt's type should not be included because they are lymphomatous with a leukemic phase.

Clinical Features. B cell acute lymphocytic leukemia represents the least common and most fulminant form of acute lymphocytic leukemia. Males are more

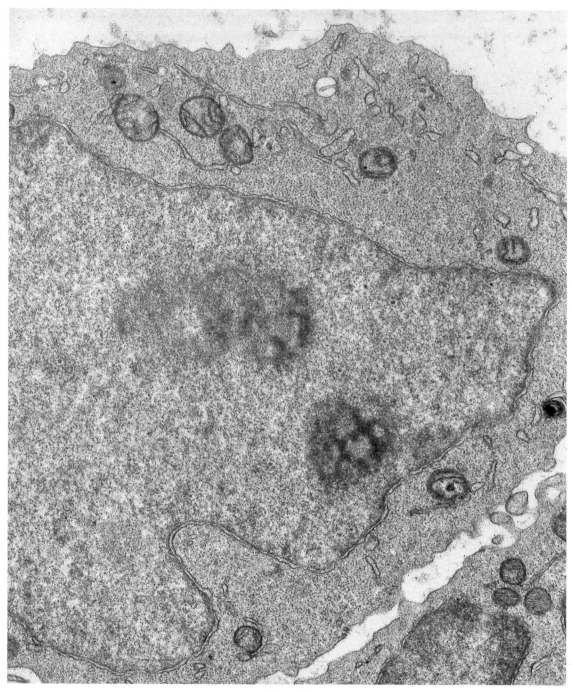

Figure 13
ACUTE UNDEFINED LEUKEMIA, MARROW
Electron microscopy shows no distinctive cytoplasmic characteristics and a slightly indented nucleus. X23,300.

commonly affected. The median age is approximately 13 years, which is older than that reported for common acute lymphocytic leukemia of childhood.

Many cases designated in the literature as B cell acute lymphocytic leukemia may represent small noncleaved cell follicular center cell lymphoma of Burkitt's type with extensive marrow involvement and a leukemic phase (Flandrin et al.; Greaves et al.). Patients may initially complain of symptoms or signs related to bone marrow infiltration and failure. Systemic symptoms are commonly noted.

Prominent findings on physical examination include lymphadenopathy, hepatosplenomegaly, and bone disease. Neurologic abnormalities related to central nervous system infiltration may also occur at presentation. Abdominal masses are frequent.

The majority of patients have leukocytosis at presentation in the range of 20 to 30,000/μL. Circulating tumor cells account for 1 to 80 percent of the differential count. Anemia, thrombocytopenia, and extensive infiltration of the marrow are expected. Elevations of uric acid levels and serum lactic dehydrogenase are commonly seen.

Although a complete remission may be obtained with combination chemotherapy, the majority of patients experience rapid relapse of disease. The median survival rate is less than 6 months from the time of diagnosis.

Pathologic Features. In sections and smears, B cell acute lymphocytic leukemia appears similar to other forms of acute lymphocytic leukemia.

Immunologic Features. In patients who have the usual marrow features of acute lymphocytic leukemia, neoplastic cells are shown to have distinct SIg, with a single light chain. The heavy chain is usually IgM.

Differential Diagnosis. B cell acute lymphocytic leukemia is often confused in the literature with malignant lymphomas of Burkitt's type presenting with extensive marrow involvement. Most patients with Burkitt's lymphoma have a primary lesion in the bowel and may be separated from those with B cell acute lymphocytic leukemia. No explanation is available for the high frequency of B cell precursor acute lymphocytic leukemia and the rarity of B cell acute lymphocytic leukemia.

References

Flandrin, G., Brouet, J.C., Daniel, M.T., and Preud'homme, J.L. Acute leukemia with Burkitt's tumor cells. Blood 45:183-188, 1975.

Greaves, M.F., Janossy, G., Peto, J., and Kay, H. Immunologically defined subclasses of acute lymphoblastic leukaemia in children: their relationship to presentation features and prognosis. Br. J. Haematol. 48:179-197, 1981.

Additional References

Raman, S., Saeed, S.M., and Kini, K.R. Acute Burkitt's leukemia. Henry Ford Hosp. Med. J. 30:37-41, 1982.

Rowley, J.D., Varlakojis, D., Kaneko, Y., and Cimino, M. A Burkitt-lymphoma variant translocation (2p-; 8q+) in a patient with ALL, L3 (Burkitt type). Hum. Genet. 58:166-167, 1981.

Stevens, D.A., O'Conor, G.T., Levine, P.H., and Rosen, R.B. Acute leukemia with "Burkitt's lymphoma cells" and Burkitt's lymphoma. Ann. Intern. Med. 76:967-973, 1972.

PROLYMPHOCYTIC LEUKEMIA

Definition. Initially described as a rare variant of chronic lymphocytic leukemia (Galton et al.), prolymphocytic leukemia is characterized by the distinctive cytologic features of its circulating neoplastic cells, and by massive splenomegaly without lymphadenopathy, marked leukocytosis, and poor response to treatment.

Clinical Features. Prolymphocytic leukemia occurs approximately one-tenth as often as chronic lymphocytic leukemia, affects slightly older patients (median age of onset 70 years vs. 64 years for chronic lymphocytic leukemia), and is slightly more common in men. Presenting symptoms include weight loss, weakness, fatigue, and abdominal discomfort due to splenomegaly. Most patients are stage III or IV at presentation. Over 75 percent have white blood cell counts greater than 100,000/μL and most have a normocytic normochromic anemia. Median survival of patients with prolymphocytic leukemia is 3 years.

Pathologic Features. The most distinctive feature of prolymphocytic leukemia, and essentially the defining characteristic, is the appearance of most cells in the peripheral blood. Tumor cells in prolymphocytic leukemia are 10-15 μm in diameter, have single nucleoli with a dense peripheral rim of chromatin, and round to slightly indented nuclei (fig. 14). The cytoplasm tends to be pale blue and free of granules or vacuoles. Sections of marrow show diffuse or nodular patterns of marrow infiltration (Nieto et al.; Stone). Node biopsies in a few cases as well as spleen infiltrates have shown follicular patterns (Bearman et al.).

Immunologic Features. Most cases of prolymphocytic leukemia have a B phenotype, with the remainder marking as T cells. A high density of surface immunoglobulin is characteristic, usually IgM with or without IgD. Approximately half of the cases show CD5 reactivity, in contrast to the higher percentage of CD5 reactivity in B-chronic lymphocytic leukemia. Prolymphocytic cells apparently do not form

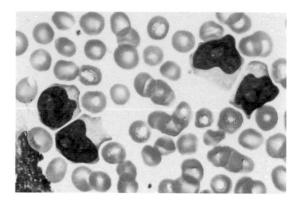

Figure 14
PROLYMPHOCYTIC LEUKEMIA
This blood smear is from a 91 year old male with massive splenomegaly and no lymphadenopathy. At the time of this peripheral blood examination, the leukocyte count was 71,000/μL and subsequently rose to 248,000/μL. The cells in this illustration have abundant basophilic cytoplasm, somewhat coarse nuclear chromatin, and single prominent nucleoli with perinucleolar chromatin condensation. These cells typed as monotypic B cells and had dense surface immunoglobulin. (Courtesy of Dr. Richard Brunning, Minneapolis, MN.)

rosettes with mouse red blood cells as in chronic lymphocytic leukemia (Melo et al., 1986a).

Karyotypic Features. Not enough cases with classic features have been studied to determine if there is a specific karyotypic abnormality in prolymphocytic leukemia.

Differential Diagnosis. The clinical and pathologic features of prolymphocytic leukemia distinguish it from some or most cases of chronic lymphocytic leukemia in blast transformation, although overlap cases have been reported (Kjeldsberg and Marty; Melo et al., 1986b,c). Enno and colleagues believed that blast transformation of chronic lymphocytic leukemia could be recognized by demonstrating a prior history of chronic lymphocytic leukemia, the coexistence of small lymphocytes and blasts in peripheral blood, and that the blasts retained the immunologic features of chronic lymphocytic leukemia cells (scant SIg, mouse rosette positivity).

Prolymphocytic leukemia may be more difficult to separate from transformation of a follicular lymphoma with extensive peripheral blood involvement. In fact, the presence in tissue sections in a few cases of follicular nodulation (Bearman) and the high density of SIg are both features of follicular lymphomas. In the initial publication on prolymphocytic leukemia, Galton and colleagues stated that the white blood cell count is rarely elevated in lymphoma, and used this criterion to separate follicular lymphoma with a leukemic phase ("lymphosarcoma cell leukemia") from prolymphocytic leukemia. However, this may be unreliable.

References

Bearman, R.M., Pangalis, G.A., and Rappaport, H. Prolymphocytic leukemia. Clinical, histopathological, and cytochemical observations. Cancer 42:2360-2372, 1978.

Enno, A., Catovsky, D., O'Brien, M., Cherchi, M., Kumaran, T.O., and Galton, D.A.G. 'Prolymphocytoid' transformation of chronic lymphocytic leukaemia. Br. J. Haematol. 41:9-18, 1979.

Galton, D.A.G., Goldman, J.M., Wiltshaw, E., Catovsky, D., Henry, K., and Goldenberg, G.J. Prolymphocytic leukaemia. Br. J. Haematol. 27:7-23, 1974.

Kjeldsberg, C.R. and Marty, J. Prolymphocytic transformation of chronic lymphocytic leukemia. Cancer 48:2447-2457, 1981.

Melo, J.V., Catovsky, D., and Galton, D.A.G. The relationship between chronic lymphocytic leukaemia and prolymphocytic leukaemia. I. Clinical and laboratory features of 300 patients and characterization of an intermediate group. Br. J. Haematol. 63:377-387, 1986a.

_____ , Catovsky, D., and Galton, D.A.G. The relationship between chronic lymphocytic leukaemia and prolymphocytic leukaemia. II. Patterns of evolution of 'prolymphocytoid' transformation. Br. J. Haematol. 64:77-86, 1986b.

_____ , Wardle, J., Chetty, M., et al. The relationship between chronic lymphocytic leukaemia and prolymphocytic leukaemia. III. Evaluation of cell size by morphology and volume measurements. Br. J. Haematol. 64:469-478, 1986c.

Nieto, L.H., Lampert, I.A., and Catovsky, D. Bone marrow histological patterns in B-cell and T-cell prolymphocytic leukemia. Hematol. Pathol. 3:79-84, 1989.

Stone, R.M. Prolymphocytic leukemia. Hematol. Oncol. Clin. North Am. 4:457-471, 1990.

SMALL B CELL NEOPLASMS, INCLUDING CHRONIC LYMPHOCYTIC LEUKEMIA, B TYPE

SYNONYMS AND RELATED TERMS: Working Formulation: small lymphocytic consistent with chronic lymphocytic leukemia. Kiel: lymphocytic; chronic lymphocytic leukemia B. Rappaport: lymphocytic, well differentiated.

Definition. Small B cell neoplasms are a heterogeneous group of diseases in which there is accumulation of small lymphocytes that mark as B cells immunologically. Patients with extensive marrow and peripheral blood involvement are often diagnosed as having chronic lymphocytic leukemia B. Some patients with tumors of similar cytologic and immunologic phenotype may have predominantly nodal involvement. These are frequent neoplasms and are generally indolent, low-grade processes. Plasmacytic differentiation is not observed. For pathologic details, see Plate XVI and figures 15-18.

Clinical Features. Lymphoid neoplasms of small B lymphocytes, including those cases with marrow involvement and lymphocytosis designated as chronic lymphocytic leukemia, comprise approximately 9 percent of all of the lymphoid malignancies in the United States.

This is a disease of older individuals, with median age of onset in the sixties; the disease is distinctly uncommon before the age of 50. Males are affected twice as often as females.

Approximately 25 percent of the patients are first diagnosed by incidental detection of lymphadenopathy or hepato-splenomegaly on routine physical examination or lymphocytosis on routine blood work. Other common presentations include recurrent infection, fatigue, and loss of sense of well-being.

Common sites of initial involvement include the bone marrow (70 percent incidence in patients with lymphoma of small B lymphocytes; 100 percent incidence in patients with chronic lymphocytic leukemia), as well as generalized lymphadenopathy. Over 90 percent of these patients are demonstrated to have stage III or IV disease at initial diagnosis; stage I disease is rare.

The Rai staging system used in this disease correlates well with expected survival as follows: Rai stage 0 is defined as lymphocytosis in blood and marrow; stage I is lymphocytosis and lymphadenopathy; stage II is lymphocytosis with hepatomegaly and splenomegaly; stage III is lymphocytosis with anemia; and stage IV is lymphocytosis with thrombocytopenia. Rai stage 0 is associated with a survival rate similar to that of the normal population, whereas Rai stage IV indicates a median survival of approximately 2 years. The disease may remain relatively stable and quiescent for years or may evolve more rapidly. Complications are related to progressive organ infiltration and dysfunction and to the development of immunologic abnormalities. Approximately 50 percent of the patients with chronic lymphocytic leukemia are hypogammaglobulinemic at diagnosis. Approximately 50 percent of the patients die from infection, presumably due to hypogammaglobulinemia. Coombs' positive hemolytic anemia is described in 10 to 20 percent of the patients, and immune thrombo-cytopenic purpura is seen in 5 to 10 percent.

Because the disease is indolent in natural history and because no currently employed regimen has been shown to be curative, aggressive multiagent chemotherapy is contraindicated. The average survival of patients with this disease, managed conservatively, is approximately 7 to 10 years.

Pathologic Features (Table 26). Marrow sections and smears usually show dense, homogeneous infiltrates of small lymphocytes with similar-appearing cells in varying numbers in the peripheral blood (figs. 15, 16). Blasts usually number less than 5 percent in the blood and are infrequently seen in the marrow. Plasma cells are very rare. Node sections show a diffuse growth of small lymphocytes, usually with complete obliteration of nodal architecture (figs. 17, 18). Many cases show pale-staining mounds or "proliferation centers" (fig. 17) in which there is an increased number of mitoses and transformed lymphocytes. Scattered follicular centers are occasionally seen.

Immunologic Features. The SIg on the predominant cells is monotypic and quantitatively homogeneous from cell to cell. The great majority of cases have SIgM or SIgM + SIgD and a single light chain type. In approximately half of the cases, the amount of fluorescence is scant and very difficult to detect. These cases generally fit into the chronic lymphocytic leukemia group. The remainder have more surface fluorescence but less than in follicular center cell lymphomas.

Other immunologic features characteristic of these cells are the absence of nuclear TdT, reactivity with B cell antigens (i.e., those defined by CD19, CD20), CD5,

Table 26

B CELL LYMPHOMA, SMALL LYMPHOCYTIC
(Includes Chronic Lymphocytic Leukemia B)

PATTERN
Node • Diffuse, very homogeneous • Diffuse, with pseudofollicles (mounds), also known as proliferation centers • Residual follicular centers at times • Capsule may be infiltrated • Sinuses often obscured Marrow • Diffuse • Focal

CYTOLOGY — NEOPLASTIC	MARKERS — NEOPLASTIC
• Small round lymphocytes, scant cytoplasm, dense chromatin • Transformed cells in proliferation centers • Mitoses in proliferation centers • MGP: Weak positivity in transformed cells; small lymphocytes negative • Giemsa: Scant cytoplasm demonstrated in small cells; transformed cells have basophilic cytoplasm	• Flow: Monotypic SIg in 90 percent of the cases (usually IgM/IgM-D) CD5 (+) CD10 (−) CD19 (+) CD20 (+) • FSIP: CD5 (+), most cases • Trisomy 12 reported in 50 percent of the chronic lymphocytic leukemia cases

INVOLVED SITES	CLINICAL FEATURES
• Superficial nodes • Marrow, extranodal • Spleen • Extranodal sites usually involved	• Older adults, slight male preponderance • Usually present with widespread disease ± leukemic phase (chronic lymphocytic leukemia B) • Lymphocytosis may be extreme (chronic lymphocytic leukemia B) • Change to immunoblastic lymphoma B (Richter's syndrome) in <1 percent of the cases

REACTIVE COMPONENTS	DIFFERENTIAL DIAGNOSIS
• Eosinophils, plasma cells rare • Mast cells common • T cells usually <10 percent • Macrophages unusual • Few vessels • Scant sclerosis	• Malignant lymphoma, follicular center cell, small cleaved cell • Plasmacytoid lymphocytic lymphoma • Small T cell neoplasms • Hairy cell leukemia • Hodgkin's disease, L&H diffuse

111

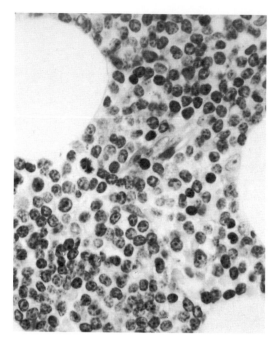

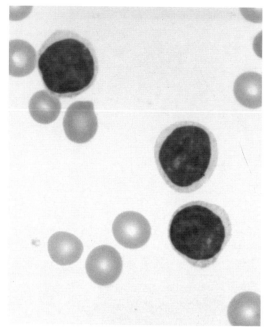

Figure 15
SMALL B CELL LYMPHOID
NEOPLASMS, MARROW
In this figure, there is effacement of architecture
with no visible hematopoietic elements. Marrow sections may show residual marrow fat, as in this case, or
sheet-like growths of small lymphocytes. H&E. X700.

Figure 16
SMALL B CELL LYMPHOID NEOPLASMS,
PERIPHERAL BLOOD
Small lymphocytes with scant cytoplasm, compact
basophilic nuclear chromatin, and homogeneous appearance are usually seen in this process. Wright's
stain. X1500.

HLA-DR antigens, and the presence of receptors for mouse erythrocytes and Epstein-
Barr virus. B cell proliferations shown to be
CD5 positive are generally neoplastic. Unlike normal B cells, these cells cannot usually be stimulated by pokeweed mitogen or
antigen to differentiate to plasma cells,
although sometimes they may be induced
to differentiate by phorbol esters (Totterman
et al.) and other mitogens (Fu et al.; Robert).

Comment. These B cell neoplasms
usually contain very few T cells and are
composed almost exclusively of small B
lymphocytes with rare blasts. By definition,
there is no detectable plasmacytic differentiation, and consequently, paraproteinemia is rare. Presumably, the small B lymphocytic pool accumulates by slow entry
from a minor population of dividing cells.
The small lymphocytes in these neoplasms may correspond to memory cells.
Small B cell neoplasms appear to arise in
both marrow and extramarrow sites. In either case, the precise relationship of this
heterogeneous group of neoplasms to
marrow stem cells or to the follicular center
cell apparatus is uncertain. It is of interest
that transformation of small B cell neoplasms to immunoblastic lymphoma B
does occur, albeit rarely, indicating the potential for plasmacytic differentiation in this
cell line (York et al.).

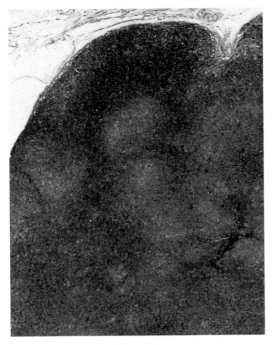

Figure 17
SMALL B CELL LYMPHOID NEOPLASMS, NODE
  There is diffuse effacement of architecture with interspersed pale growth centers or "mounds." This type of growth pattern is often seen in small cell lymphoid neoplasms and in plasmacytoid lymphocytic lymphomas. H&E. X25.

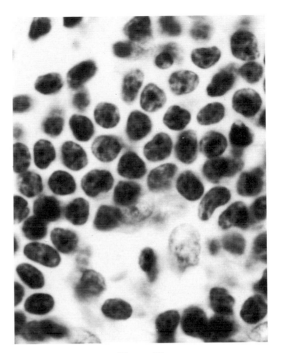

Figure 18
SMALL B CELL LYMPHOID NEOPLASMS, NODE
  At higher magnification, a monotonous infiltration of small lymphocytes with scant cytoplasm is demonstrated. A macrophage is noted at the bottom. H&E. X1500.

Transformation of Small Cell Lymphoid Neoplasms to Large Cell Lymphomas (Richter's Syndrome and Immunoblastic Lymphoma B). Transformation occurs in 3 to 10 percent of the patients with chronic lymphocytic leukemia and has been noted from 11 to 240 months after the initial diagnosis, with a mean of 63 months. Most patients developed fever, weight loss, or increasing peripheral adenopathy. Sixty-seven percent of the patients had an abdominal mass with pain. One-half of the patients had an elevated peripheral leukocyte count equal to or higher than at initial presentation, and one-third showed a significantly reduced leukocyte count at transformation. Serum proteins studied in 11 cases demonstrated hypogammaglobulinemia in six cases, hypergammaglobulinemia in two cases, and a monotypic IgM in three cases. Survival was poor regardless of therapy, ranging from 0 to 10 months, with a mean survival of 3 months. The site of transformation was usually an extranodal abdominal site, including the spleen, liver, bowel, or kidney; abdominal nodes were occasionally involved. Transformation involved the marrow in 50 percent and nodes in 30 percent of the patients. Over 50 percent of the patients showed focal persistence of the small B cell neoplasm in

113

PLATE XVI

A. SMALL B CELL NEOPLASMS
ASSOCIATED WITH HODGKIN'S DISEASE, NODE
(Plate XVI-A and B are from the same patient)

This low magnification view shows the border zone between the diffuse infiltrate of small lymphocytes and an area with more polymorphous appearance in which larger cells are apparent. H&E. X40.

B. SMALL B CELL NEOPLASMS
ASSOCIATED WITH HODGKIN'S DISEASE

At a higher magnification, monomorphous aggregates of small lymphocytes are seen along with scattered large cells, several of which are acceptable as Reed-Sternberg cells. H&E. X300.

C. SMALL B CELL NEOPLASMS
EVOLVING TO IMMUNOBLASTIC LYMPHOMA B, NODE
(Plate XVI-C and D are from the same patient)

There is diffuse effacement of nodal architecture with some infiltration into the adjacent fat in this illustration. X40.

D. SMALL B CELL NEOPLASMS
EVOLVING TO IMMUNOBLASTIC LYMPHOMA B, NODE

A higher magnification shows clusters of large transformed lymphocytes with amphophilic cytoplasm. Paraffin immunoperoxidase showed a monotypic κ-light chain bearing population. Giemsa. X300.

PLATE XVI

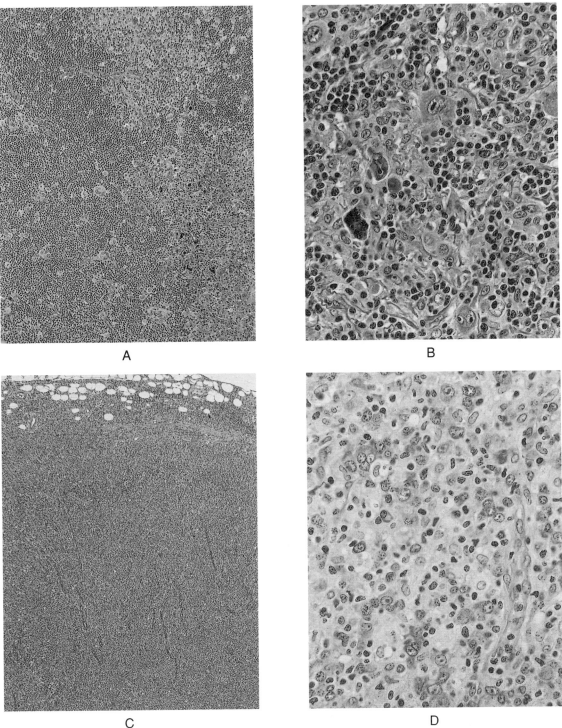

A

B

C

D

the site of transformation or in a separate location.

Two morphologic patterns of transformation were described in the involved tissues. Approximately 40 percent of the cases demonstrated a diffuse, fairly uniform infiltration of large transformed lymphocytes. These cells had large nuclei, peripherally dispersed chromatin, one or two prominent nucleoli, and a moderate amount of eosinophilic cytoplasm. "Prolymphocytoid" is the term often applied to the peripheral blood manifestation of this form. The remaining cases demonstrated a pleomorphic infiltrate with a predominance of large transformed lymphocytes. These transformed cells were intermixed with small lymphocytes, bizarre giant cells, and multinucleated cells resembling Reed-Sternberg cells (plate XVI-A,B). A few reports identified transformed lymphocytes with plasmacytic differentiation or immunoblasts (plate XVI-C,D).

Nine cases studied immunologically at the time of transformation showed monotypic B cell markers. Two cases with immunologic studies at initial presentation were restudied at transformation and showed identical immunologic markers (Frenkel et al.; Laurent et al.).

Differential Diagnosis. *Malignant lymphoma, follicular center cell, small cleaved cell type.* Neoplastic follicular nodulation is a characteristic feature of this neoplasm, in contrast to pseudofollicles or proliferation centers. Lymphocytes are generally irregular. In flow studies or FSIP, 10 to 30 percent T cells are present chiefly in the interfollicular areas. CD5 is negative. In PIP, CDw75 (LN-1) positivity is characteristic.

Plasmacytoid lymphocytic lymphoma. Pseudofollicles may be present in plasmacytoid lymphocytic lymphoma, as in malignant lymphoma, small B cell type. In the former, however, there are varying degrees of amphophilic cytoplasm that are distinctly plasmacytic in some cases. Giemsa and MGP stains are clearly positive. On PIP, CIg is monotypic.

Small T cell lymphoma. This neoplasm produces a diffuse infiltrative growth pattern and has irregular to knobby nuclear profiles. Small to large giant cells are present (as in adult T cell leukemia). Immunologic differences may be brought out in flow, FSIP, or PIP studies. In the latter, the pan-T marker CD45RO (UCHL-1) would show almost universal marking in small T cell lymphomas.

Hairy cell leukemia. Involvement of the marrow in hairy cell leukemia may be diffuse but is often focal and may be relatively subtle, in contrast to the usual appearance in small B cell neoplasms. Hairy cell nuclei show fine nuclear chromatin with indentations, whereas nuclei in small B cell neoplasms tend to be round with denser nuclear chromatin. The cytoplasm in hairy cell leukemia is prominent and pale with cohesive cell borders; tartrate-resistant acid phosphatase (TRAP) positivity is usually demonstrable. On flow and FSIP studies, there is CD5 negativity in hairy cell leukemia.

Hodgkin's disease, lymphocytic and/or histiocytic (L&H) diffuse. This neoplasm shows an infiltration of small lymphocytes with varying nuclear configurations associated with the L&H variants of Reed-Sternberg cells, whereas in small B cell lymphomas, the large cell component is mainly in the proliferation centers. L&H variants are CD20 (L26) positive and may be much more apparent in PIP preparations than in H&E sections.

References

Frenkel, E.P., Ligler, F.S., Graham, M.S., et al. Acute lymphocytic leukemic transformatin of chronic lymphocytic leukemia: substantiation by flow cytometry. Am. J. Hematol. 10:391-398, 1981.

Fu, S.M., Chiorazzi, N., Kunkel, H.G., Halper, J.P., and Harris, S.R. Induction of in vitro differentiation and immunoglobulin synthesis of human leukemic B lymphocytes. J. Exp. Med. 148:1570-1578, 1978.

Laurent, G., Gourdin, M.F., Flandrin, G., et al. Acute blast crisis in a patient with chronic lymphocytic leukemia. Acta Haematol. (Basel) 65:60-66, 1981.

Robert, K.H. Induction of monoclonal antibody synthesis in malignant human B cells by polyclonal B cell activators. Relationship between B cell subsets and prognosis. Immunol. Rev. 48:123-143, 1979.

Totterman, T.H., Nilsson, K., and Sundström, C. Phorbol ester-induced differentiation of chronic lymphocytic leukaemia cells. Nature 288:176-178, 1980.

York, J.C., Glick, A.D., Cousar, J.B., and Collins, R.D. Changes in the appearance of hematopoietic and lymphoid neoplasms. Hum. Pathol. 15:11-38, 1984.

Additional References

Han, T., Ozer, H., Bloom, M., Sagawa, K., and Minowada, J. The presence of monoclonal cytoplasmic immunoglobulins in leukemic B cells from patients with chronic lymphocytic leukemia. Blood 59:435-438, 1982.

Harris, N.L. and Bhan, A.K. B-cell neoplasms of the lymphocytic, lymphoplasmacytoid, and plasma cell types. Hum. Pathol. 16:829-837, 1985.

Kosiner, B., Kempin, S., Passe, S., et al. Characterization of B-cell leukemias. Blood 56:815-823, 1980.

Rai, K.R., Sawitsky, A., Cronkite, E.P., et al. Clinical staging of chronic lymphocytic leukemia. Blood 46:219-234, 1975.

Rundles, R.W. and Moore, J.O. Chronic lymphocytic leukemia. Cancer 42(Suppl. 2):941-945, 1978.

Stein, H. and Mason, D.Y. Immunological Analysis of Tissue Sections in Diagnosis of Lymphoma, pp. 127-169. In: Recent Advances in Haematology, Vol. 4. Hoffbrand, A.V. (Ed.). Edinburgh: Churchill Livingstone, 1985.

Swerdlow, S.H., Murray, L.J., Habeshaw, J.A., and Stansfeld, A.G. Lymphocytic lymphoma/B-chronic lymphocytic leukaemia—an immunohistopathological study of peripheral B lymphocyte neoplasia. Br. J. Cancer 50:587-599, 1984.

PLASMACYTOID LYMPHOCYTIC LYMPHOMA, INCLUDING WALDENSTRÖM'S MACROGLOBULINEMIA

SYNONYMS AND RELATED TERMS: Working Formulation: small lymphocytic, plasmacytoid. Kiel: lymphoplasmacytic/lymphoplasmacytoid. Rappaport: lymphocytic, well-differentiated with plasmacytoid features.

Definition. Plasmacytoid lymphocytic lymphoma appears to arise from marrow or extramarrow sites. Some of the neoplasms in this group are widespread at presentation, with affected tissues infiltrated by small lymphocytes, plasmacytoid lymphocytes, and plasma cells. Immunoblasts vary in frequency. A monoclonal gammopathy is usually detectable; patients with monoclonal IgM are considered to have Waldenström's macroglobulinemia. However, some patients with plasmacytoid lymphocytic morphology may have a monotypic IgG or IgA spike, or their cells may be nonsecretory.

The cell of origin in marrow-based processes is probably a marrow B precursor. In extramarrow sites, the cell of origin has not been identified but may arise from postfollicular center B cells. For pathologic details, see Plates XVII-XX and figures 19 and 20.

Clinical Features. Plasmacytoid lymphocytic lymphoma is a disease of the elderly, usually occurring in the sixth or seventh decades of life, although younger patients have been reported. This group comprises approximately 7 percent of all of the lymphoid malignancies in the United States. There is a slight male preponderance. IgM paraprotein produced in Waldenström's macroglobulinemia causes the hyperviscosity syndrome, which is expressed by mucosal bleeding and purpura,

117

epistaxis, and various neurological complaints including vertigo, peripheral neuropathy, and ataxia. Occasionally, patients have syncopal episodes, congestive heart failure, digital gangrene, or Raynaud's phenomenon.

On physical examination, patients may demonstrate mucous membrane bleeding and dilation of retinal veins with associated retinal hemorrhage on fundoscopic examination. Abnormal bleeding is common and has been shown in some cases to be caused by a functional coagulation factor deficiency due to the presence of a paraprotein. Aside from symptoms related to increased viscosity, patients may present with complaints similar to those seen in other lymphomatous processes. Hepatomegaly is seen in approximately 50 percent of all of the cases, lymphadenopathy in an equal proportion, and splenomegaly in approximately 30 percent of the cases. Bone lesions are quite uncommon in this disease, with osteolytic bone abnormalities reported in 7 percent of the cases. Likewise, renal failure is only rarely seen, although Bence-Jones proteinuria has been reported in 10 to 30 percent of the patients. Plasmacytoid lymphocytic lymphoma may present with isolated lung, skin, or conjunctival masses (plate XX-A–D).

Therapeutic options include plasmapheresis and chemotherapy. Plasmapheresis effectively removes circulating IgM paraprotein because approximately 80 percent of IgM is found in the intravascular compartment. Plasmapheresis offers immediate relief of the symptoms and signs related to hyperviscosity but does not reduce the tumor burden, in contrast to chemotherapy. When oral daily chlorambucil and intermittent corticosteroids are administered, the average life expectancy in responding patients is 4 years; nonresponders live an average of 2 years.

Plasmacytoid lymphocytic lymphoma has also been described without an IgM paraproteinemia. In these cases, IgG or IgA paraprotein is produced, or no paraprotein may be detectable. The clinical hyperviscosity syndrome is not found in this subset of patients. The median age is 60 years, with a range of 30 to 80 years. The presenting symptoms include anemia, fever, night sweats, lymphadenopathy, and extranodal mass lesions. Approximately half of these patients have organomegaly and/or lymphadenopathy at diagnosis. Most patients are anemic and have marrow involvement. This variant is relatively indolent in natural history. With a relatively nonaggressive single agent or combination chemotherapy, the expected survival is 3 to 7 years.

Pathologic Features (Table 27). Histopathologic changes are similar to those in small B cell neoplasms but with several important differences. Architectural distortion in nodes may be massive or slight (plate XVII-A). In plasmacytoid lymphocytic lymphoma, follicular structures and sinuses are partially preserved. In marrow particles, infiltrates are often nodular (plate XIX-A).

Plasmacytic differentiation may be subtle or overt in the form of Russell bodies (plates XVII-B,C; XVIII-A,B). In either case, plasmacytic differentiation is most apparent in PAS, Giemsa, and MGP preparations (plates XVIII-D–F; XIX-B). The amount of plasmacytic differentiation may vary dramatically from one site to another in simultaneous biopsies. Plasma cells may aggregate in small or large foci, often near the sinuses of nodes. Plasmacytic

Table 27

PLASMACYTOID LYMPHOCYTIC LYMPHOMA

PATTERN	
	• Diffuse lymphocytic process • Partial retention of nodal architecture with retention of sinuses and follicles on occasion • Pale foci containing transformed lymphocytes and mitoses (pseudofollicles) similar to those in small B cell neoplasms • Bone marrow involvement is focal, patchy, or diffuse
CYTOLOGY — NEOPLASTIC	**MARKERS — NEOPLASTIC**

• Predominantly small round lymphocytic population, varying numbers of plasmacytoid cells
 	
• Plasmacytic differentiation varies, may not be apparent in H&E stain; in imprints, cytoplasm is blue with May Gruenwald Giemsa, basophilic in Giemsa, and pyroninophilic in MGP stains
	• Flow, FSIP, PIP: Monotypic Ig demonstrated in most cases
	    CD45 (+)
	    CD20, L26 (+)
	    CD19 (+)
	    CDw75 (−)
	
	• PAS (+) intranuclear inclusions (Dutcher bodies)
	
	• Heavy chains usually IgM; IgG, IgA less frequent

INVOLVED SITES	**CLINICAL FEATURES**
• Lymph nodes, spleen, and bone marrow • Various other sites including lung, conjunctiva, gastrointestinal tract	• Lymphadenopathy • Hyperviscosity syndrome of Waldenström in 50 percent of the cases • Monoclonal hyperglobulinemia, usually IgM • Monoclonal Ig spike frequently not present • Leukemic expression occasionally • Stages III and IV usual, may be localized • Evolution to malignant lymphoma, immunoblastic lymphoma B in approximately 25 percent of the cases
REACTIVE COMPONENTS	**DIFFERENTIAL DIAGNOSIS**
• Benign follicles often present • Small T cells present in variable numbers • Mast cells frequent	• Small B/T cell neoplasms • Mantle zone lymphoma • Malignant lymphoma, follicular center cell, small cleaved cell, diffuse • Chronic lymphadenitis

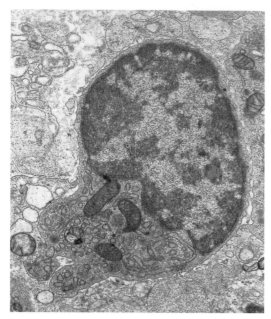

Figure 19
PLASMACYTOID LYMPHOCYTIC LYMPHOMA,
ULTRASTRUCTURE OF
PLASMACYTOID LYMPHOCYTE
Note the small lymphocytic nucleus, abundant cytoplasm, and rough endoplasmic reticulum in this figure. X13,300. (Fig. 10-7A from Vogler, L.B., Glick, A.D., and Collins, R.D. B Cell Neoplasms: Correlation of Recent Developments with the Biology of Normal B Lymphocytes, pp. 197-223. In: Progress in Clinical Pathology, Vol. IX. Stefanini, M., Gorstein, F., and Fink, L. [Eds.]. Orlando: Grune and Stratton, 1983.)

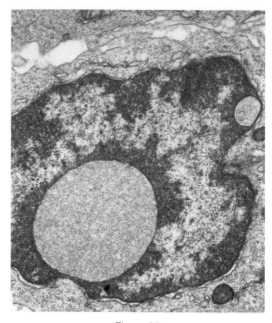

Figure 20
PLASMACYTOID LYMPHOCYTIC LYMPHOMA
This electron micrograph shows a cytoplasmic projection into the nucleus, a feature that is often seen in plasmacytoid lymphocytic lymphoma. X18,900. (Fig.10-7B from Vogler, L.B., Glick, A.D., and Collins, R.D. B Cell Neoplasms: Correlation of Recent Developments with the Biology of Normal B Lymphocytes, pp. 197-223. In: Progress in Clinical Pathology, Vol. IX. Stefanini, M., Gorstein, F., and Fink, L. [Eds.]. Orlando: Grune and Stratton, 1983.)

differentiation is readily apparent in electron micrographs (fig. 19). Tumorous plasma cells may be strongly PAS positive, particularly in IgA- or IgM-producing neoplasms. "Intranuclear" inclusions (Dutcher bodies) are cytoplasmic projections (plates XVIII-C–F; XIX-B; fig. 20) and are most easily recognized in PAS stains; however, they may react negatively with immunoperoxidase using anti-immunoglobulin antisera. Marrow smears, touch imprints, or peripheral smears show a mixture of lymphocytes, plasma cells, and apparent intermediates (plate XVII-D,E).

Although most cases of plasmacytoid lymphocytic lymphoma contain homogeneous-appearing populations of small lymphocytes and plasma cells, some cases have more variation in cell size (plate XVIII-A). Immunoblasts, some of which may be plasmacytoid, vary in frequency (plate XVIII-B). The diagnosis of immunoblastic lymphoma B should be made only when there are monomorphous aggregates or nodules of immunoblasts (plate XIX-C–E).

Immunologic Features. Lymphocytic and plasmacytic components usually have an SIg with the same heavy and light chain and the same idiotype as that found in the serum. Similar membrane patterns of SIg are found on most blood lymphocytes, although the peripheral counts are usually not elevated. Monotypic CIg is readily demonstrated by PIP. Occasional patients have mixed patterns of serum and cellular immunoglobulin, indicating biclonal proliferations.

Although the neoplastic clone has been traced in multiple myeloma to the earliest B precursor, the relationship of plasmacytoid lymphocytic neoplasms to pre-B cells has not been established. Furthermore, some of these neoplasms appear to arise in peripheral tissue, presumably from a post-follicular center B cell population.

Transformation of Plasmacytoid Lymphocytic Lymphoma to Immunoblastic Lymphoma B. Transformation occasionally occurs with a mean interval of 56 months after the initial diagnosis. Patients developing immunoblastic lymphoma B may have fever, anemia, adenopathy, a soft tissue mass, or an abdominal mass (usually an enlarged spleen or liver). There is often an absolute decrease in the abnormal serum immunoglobulin. Survival data emphasize the aggressiveness of transformation, with most patients dying after 1 to 5 months.

Involvement by immunoblastic lymphoma B is almost equally divided among the nodes, marrow, lung, and soft tissue. Morphologically, the transformed process consists of a diffuse growth of large transformed lymphocytes, usually with abundant basophilic and pyroninophilic cytoplasm (plate XIX-C–E). In many cases, a pleomorphic appearance is caused by an admixture of plasma cells and small lymphocytes. Some cases contained bizarre Reed-Sternberg-like cells (McCallister et al.;

Osterberg and Rausing). Rare cases with sequential cell marker studies had identical surface immunoglobulin markers on the neoplastic immunoblasts at transformation (Leonhard et al.; Sun et al.).

Differential Diagnosis. *Small B cell lymphomas.* A growth pattern showing pseudofollicles may be similar in both of these neoplasms. Because subtle plasmacytic features are only appreciated in Giemsa and MGP stains, these must be available to differentiate the two processes. In both small B cell and plasmacytoid lymphocytic-type neoplasms, the lymphocytic components have small round nuclei with dense chromatin. The cytoplasm is generally scant in the small B cell processes and found in variable amounts in plasmacytoid lymphocytic type. In PIP studies, there is a prominent monotypic cytoplasmic immunoglobulin in plasmacytoid lymphocytic-type processes.

Small T cell neoplasms. Cells in small T neoplasms vary widely in size and may be associated with numerous T immunoblasts. Small lymphocytes vary in nuclear configuration, with abundant cytoplasm that may be clear or slightly acidophilic. Immunologic studies in this neoplasm would, of course, show T features.

Mantle zone lymphoma. In this lymphoma, there is usually a wide expansion of small lymphocytes around small or distorted benign follicular centers. Follicular centers may also persist in plasmacytoid lymphocytic-type neoplasms. Lymphocytes are small to medium in size in mantle zone lymphoma, with an irregular to elongated nuclear configuration. CIg is not demonstrable by PIP, but CD74 (LN-2) is distinctly positive in this process.

Follicular center cell, small cleaved cell type, diffuse. The node is diffusely

PLATE XVII
PLASMACYTOID LYMPHOCYTIC LYMPHOMA
(Plate XVII is from the same patient)

A. LYMPH NODE
There is effacement of architecture by a diffuse growth of small cells. In the central portion of the photograph, the nuclei appear more separated because the cells have more abundant cytoplasm. X60.

B. LYMPH NODE
A higher magnification shows that the cells in the central area of Plate XVII-A have distinct cytoplasm and appear somewhat plasmacytic. X630.

C. LYMPH NODE
A touch imprint of an affected node shows the mixture of lymphocytes, plasma cells, and plasmacytoid lymphocytic cells frequently seen in this neoplasm. The plasmacytoid lymphocyte is a small cell with clumped chromatin and limited amounts of basophilic cytoplasm. Wright's stain. X1000.

D,E. PERIPHERAL BLOOD
This composite photograph shows the appearance of circulating cells in the patient in whom the previous lymph node was biopsied. D. This illustration shows a small lymphocyte on the right and a more plasmacytoid-appearing cell on the left. Wright's stain. X1000. E. This photograph shows lymphocytic cells, some with abundant cytoplasm. Wright's stain. X1000.

PLATE XVII

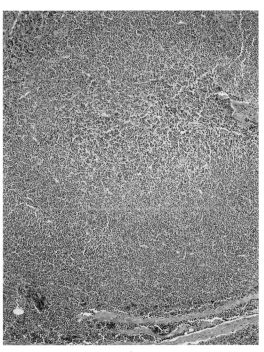

A

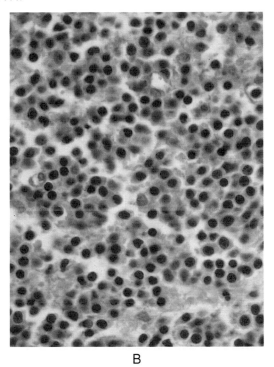

B

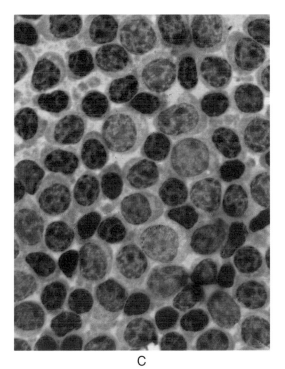

C

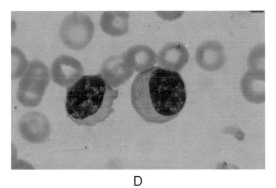

D

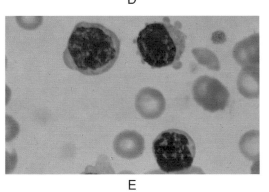

E

PLATE XVIII

A. PLASMACYTOID LYMPHOCYTIC LYMPHOMA, LYMPH NODE
This high magnification photograph shows a mixture of plasmacytoid lymphocytes and a scattering of immunoblasts. More immunoblasts are present in the polymorphous lymphoplasmacytic lymphoma described by Lennert (see plate XVIII-B). X1000.

B. POLYMORPHOUS LYMPHOPLASMACYTIC LYMPHOMA OF LENNERT, LYMPH NODE
This photomicrograph shows the increased number of immunoblasts seen in polymorphous lymphoplasmacytic lymphoma. In contrast, the immunoblastic lymphoma shown in Plate XIX-D and E demonstrate a monomorphous population of immunoblasts. Giemsa. X600.

C,D. PLASMACYTOID LYMPHOCYTIC LYMPHOMA
Dutcher bodies, characteristic of plasmacytoid lymphocytic lymphoma, are illustrated in this split photomicrograph. In H&E stains, Dutcher bodies are usually indistinct, pale-pink, globular structures; in PAS-stained tissue sections, they appear intensely positive if the globulin is IgM or IgA. On electron microscopy, these structures appear to be situated between the two nuclear membranes and thus are not really intranuclear. C. There are several intranuclear-appearing acidophilic globular structures of varying size surrounded by clear, unstained halos. These Dutcher bodies are unusually prominent for an H&E stain, possibly as a result of the effectiveness of the B-5 fixation. The subtle plasmacytoid character of the lymphocytic population is apparent. X800. D. Numerous intensely positive PAS intranuclear globular structures surrounded by a clear halo are found scattered in a lymphocytic population. PAS. X800.

E. PLASMACYTOID LYMPHOCYTIC LYMPHOMA, LYMPH NODE
(Plate XVIII-E and F are from the same patient)
This photograph shows the striking PAS positivity of the cytoplasmic inclusions. PAS. X400.

F. PLASMACYTOID LYMPHOCYTIC LYMPHOMA, LYMPH NODE
This photomicrograph emphasizes the pyroninophilia present in many of these neoplasms. PAS and MGP stains are often required to recognize this type of plasmacytic differentiation. MGP. X400.

PLATE XVIII

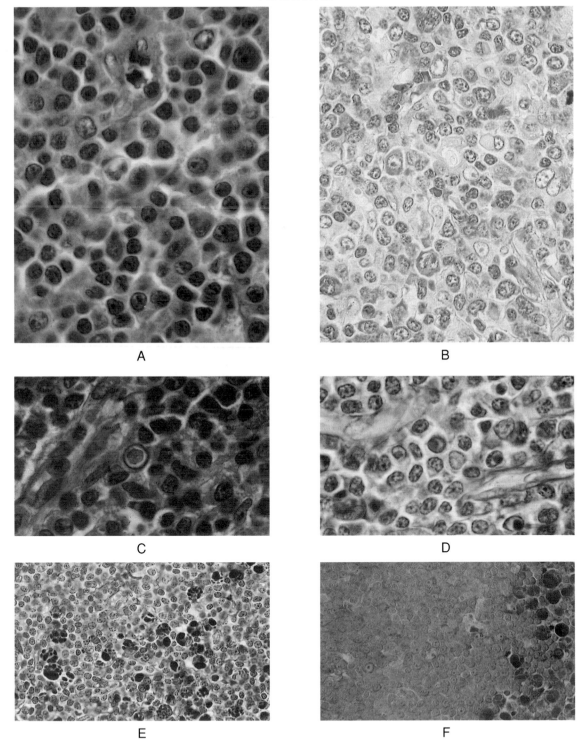

A

B

C

D

E

F

PLATE XIX

A. PLASMACYTOID LYMPHOCYTIC LYMPHOMA, MARROW
(Plate XIX-A and B are from the same patient)

Marrow involvement often takes the form of ill-defined nodular aggregates of lymphocytes and plasma cells. The cytoplasm of plasma cells may be PAS positive, as in this case. PAS. X160.

B. PLASMACYTOID LYMPHOCYTIC LYMPHOMA, MARROW

At higher magnification, the mix of lymphocytes and PAS-positive plasma cells is shown. There is a Dutcher body in the center of the picture. PAS. X650.

C. PLASMACYTOID LYMPHOCYTIC LYMPHOMA EVOLVING TO IMMUNOBLASTIC LYMPHOMA B, STOMACH
(Plate XIX-C–E are from the same patient)

This gross photograph shows an ulcerated nodular lesion in the stomach of a patient with a long history of plasmacytoid lymphocytic lymphoma with an IgM spike and hyperviscosity.

D. PLASMACYTOID LYMPHOCYTIC LYMPHOMA EVOLVING TO IMMUNOBLASTIC LYMPHOMA B, LYMPH NODE

An adjacent node shows diffuse effacement by immunoblastic cells with distinct plasmacytoid differentiation. H&E. X400.

E. PLASMACYTOID LYMPHOCYTIC LYMPHOMA EVOLVING TO IMMUNOBLASTIC LYMPHOMA B, LYMPH NODE

This high magnification photomicrograph shows that the large cells have distinct pyroninophilia and large nuclei with prominent nucleoli. MGP. X600.

PLATE XIX

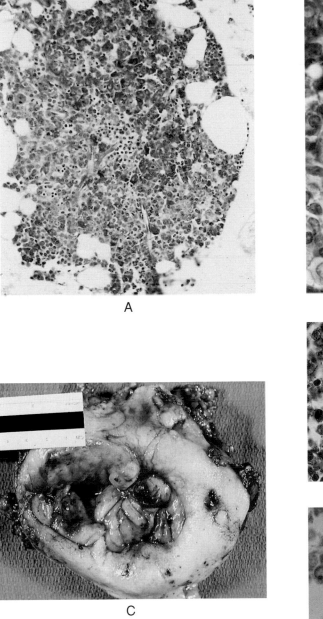

A

C

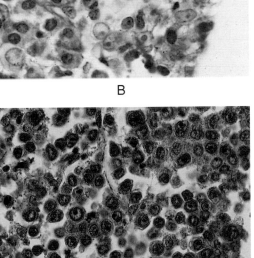

B

D

E

PLATE XX
PLASMACYTOID LYMPHOCYTIC LYMPHOMA
(Plate XX-B–D are from the same patient)

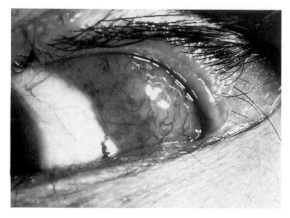

A. This man in his fifties developed a conjunctival mass. This type of lesion is often plasmacytoid lymphocytic lymphoma. Staging showed no evidence of systemic disease, and a paraprotein was not present.

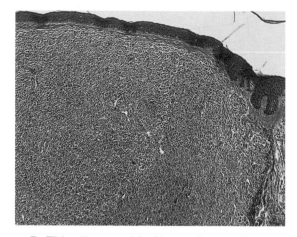

B. This 45 year old white male developed a skin nodule on his back. After biopsy, lesions recurred locally with satellite nodules. There was no apparent systemic disease. This low magnification photomicrograph shows a large nodule with a fairly monomorphic appearance of plasmacytoid lymphocytic cells. There is extension into the adjacent dermis. X50.

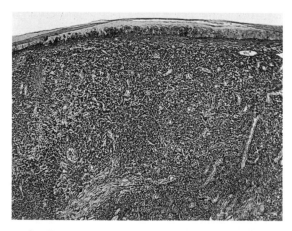

C. Paraffin immunoperoxidase staining is shown in this illustration and in Plate XX-D. This is the reaction with κ-antisera. The intense staining is an indication of monotypism.

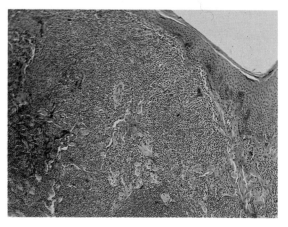

D. This illustration demonstrates the negative reaction with λ-antisera. X50.

involved and there are no growth centers; sinuses are usually not preserved. Nuclei vary in size but are in the same size range as those of the lymphocytes in the small lymphocytic B processes. Nuclear morphology is irregular with nuclear cleavage, and cytoplasmic borders are not apparent. CIg is more easily demonstrated in plasmacytoid lymphocytic type than in follicular center cell, small cleaved cell type, diffuse.

Hodgkin's disease, L&H diffuse. Nodes are diffusely involved, and reactive follicular centers are infrequent or absent. Sinuses are not apparent. Histiocytes are prominent and frequently scattered. Lymphocytes are small and often irregular or twisted in appearance with inapparent cytoplasm. The major distinguishing feature is the presence of L&H variants in this neoplasm, with these variants exhibiting CD20, CDw75 (LN-1) and EMA on PIP.

Chronic lymphadenitis. Nodes are diffusely involved, often without residual follicles, although the sinuses may remain. The cellular composition is predominantly lymphocytic. There are a few immunoblasts and benign plasma cells, and PIP is polytypic.

References

Leonhard, S.A., Muhleman, A.F., Hurtubise, P.E., and Martelo, O.J. Emergence of immunoblastic sarcoma in Waldenström's macroglobulinemia. Cancer 45:3102-3107, 1980.

McCallister, B.D., Bayrd, E.D., Harrison, E.G., and McGuckin, W.F. Primary macroglobulinemia. Am. J. Med. 43:394-434, 1967.

Osterberg, G. and Rausing, A. Reticulum cell sarcoma in Waldenström's macroglobulinemia after chlorambucil treatment. Acta Med. Scand. 188:497-504, 1970.

Sun, N.C., Fishkin, B.G., Nies, K.M., Glassy, E.F., and Carpentier, C. Lymphoplasmacytic myeloma. Cancer 43:2268-2278, 1979.

Additional References

Choi, Y.J., Yeh, G., Reiner, L., and Spielvogel, A. Immunoblastic sarcoma following Waldenström's macroglobulinemia. Am. J. Clin. Pathol. 71:121-124, 1979.

De Waele, M., Coulie, R., and Van Camp, B. Waldenström-like lymphoma with monoclonal IgG1-kappa: evidence of common clonal origin. Br. J. Haematol. 48:95-101, 1981.

Dutcher, T.F. and Fahey, J.L. The histopathology of the macroglobulinemia of Waldenström. J. Natl. Cancer Inst. 22:887-917, 1959.

Fudenberg, H.H. Waldenström's Macroglobulinemia in Cancer Chemotherapy. II. Hahnemann Symposium on Cancer Chemotherapy. Brodsky, I. and Khan, S.B. (Eds.). New York: Grune and Stratton, 1972.

Harrison, C.V. The morphology of the lymph node in the macroglobulinaemia of Waldenström. J. Clin. Pathol. 25:12-16, 1972.

Hopper, J.E. Comparative studies on monotypic IgM, lambda and IgG, kappa from an individual patient. IV. Immunofluorescent evidence for a common clonal synthesis. Blood 50:203-211, 1977.

Levine, A.M., Lichtenstein, A., Gresik, M.V., et al. Clinical and immunologic spectrum of plasmacytoid lymphocytic lymphoma without serum monoclonal IgM. Br. J. Haematol. 46:225-233, 1980.

Lukes, R.J. and Collins, R.D. Immunologic characterization of human malignant lymphomas. Cancer 34(Suppl. 4):1488-1503, 1974.

_____, Parker, J.W., Taylor, C.R., et al. Immunologic approach to non-Hodgkin's lymphomas and related leukemias. Semin. Hematol. 15:322-335, 1978.

Pettersson, D., Mellstedt, H., and Holm, G. Characterization of the monoclonal blood and bone marrow B lymphocytes in Waldenström's macroglobulinaemia. Scand. J. Immunol. 11:593-599, 1980.

Rywlin, A.M., Civantos, F., Ortega, R.S., and Dominguez, C.J. Bone marrow histology in monoclonal macroglobulinemia. Am. J. Clin. Pathol. 63:769-778, 1975.

Stein, H. and Mason, D.Y. Immunological Analysis of Tissue Sections in Diagnosis of Lymphoma, pp. 127-169. In: Recent Advances in Haematology, Vol. 4. Goldberg, A. et al. (Eds.). Edinburgh: Churchill Livingstone, 1985.

_____, Staudinger, M., Tolksdorf, G., and Lennert, K. Immunologic markers in the differential diagnosis of non-Hodgkin's lymphomas. J. Cancer Res. Clin. Oncol. 101:29-42, 1981.

Van Camp, B., Reynaert, P., and Broodtaerts, L. Studies on the origin of the precursor cells in multiple myeloma, Waldenström's macroglobulinaemia and benign monoclonal gammopathy. I. Cytoplasmic isotype and idiotype distribution in peripheral blood and bone marrow. Clin. Exp. Immunol. 44:82-89, 1981.

MULTIPLE MYELOMA

Definition. Multiple myeloma arises from the marrow. There is usually minimal significant extension to extramarrow sites, although circulating tumor cells are often demonstrable. The cell of origin is a marrow B precursor; the capacity for plasmacytic differentiation by the neoplasm is retained. For pathologic details, see Plate XXI and figures 21-24 and Spjut et al.

Clinical Features. The age-adjusted mortality rate in multiple myeloma in white males is 2.5 per 100,000 population, and the rate for females is 1.7 per 100,000. Sixty percent of the patients are males, and the disease is seen most commonly after the age of 55 years. Blacks account for 65 percent of the affected individuals in the United States.

Bone pain is the most common initial complaint, occurring in 68 percent of the patients. Bacterial infection is the cause for presentation in 12 percent of the patients. Weakness and fatigue from anemia are seen in 66 percent of the patients, and systemic symptoms such as fever and weight loss are unusual.

The most frequent finding on physical examination is pallor, reflecting the degree of anemia. Bone deformity and tenderness are commonly found, and extramedullary tumor masses are occasionally seen. At diagnosis, slight splenomegaly is reported in 5 percent of the patients, hepatomegaly in 21 percent, and lymphadenopathy in 4 percent. Nephrotic syndrome, congestive heart failure, peripheral neuropathy, and/or macroglossia may be found as a consequence of coexisting amyloidosis.

A mild anemia (mean hemoglobin of 11 g/dL) is found in 62 percent of the cases at the time of diagnosis. Leukopenia ($<4000/\mu L$) is found in 16 percent, and thrombocytopenia ($<100,000/\mu L$) is present in 13 percent. Approximately 30 percent of the patients have serum creatinine levels over 2 mg/dL at the time of diagnosis, and an equal number are hypercalcemic. Hyperuricemia is reported in 40 to 60 percent. A monoclonal serum paraprotein may be found in 75 percent of the cases, hypogammaglobulinemia in 10 percent, and normal SPEP in 15 percent. Of the patients with monoclonal heavy chain in the serum, 71 percent have IgG, 28 percent have IgA, and 1 percent have IgD. A globulin peak in the urine is demonstrated in 75 percent of the cases, consisting of κ-light chains in 58 percent. Less than 1 percent of the patients have no detectable monoclonal protein in either serum or urine.

Abnormal skeletal radiographs are expected, with combinations of osteoporosis, lytic bone lesions, and fractures seen most commonly. Normal skeletal radiographs are reported in 20 percent of the cases.

Bartl and associates have shown that there is significant variation in the morphology of the predominant cell in myeloma and that the quantity of tumor in the biopsy also provides useful prognostic information. With the use of chemotherapy and local radiotherapy to the sites of bone pain or fracture, the response rate is approximately 75 to 80 percent, with the return of more normal hematologic parameters and an increased sense of well-being. The median survival is approximately 2 to 3 years. The most common causes of death are infection and renal failure.

Pathologic Features (Table 28). The microscopic changes that are diagnostic of multiple myeloma include massive replacement of marrow by homogeneous

Table 28

MULTIPLE MYELOMA

PATTERN	
• Monomorphous nodules of myeloma cells in bone marrow associated with thinning and lysis of bony trabeculae • Diffuse and extensive at times	

CYTOLOGY — NEOPLASTIC	MARKERS — NEOPLASTIC

• Monomorphous accumulation of abnormal plasma cells
• Nuclei vary in size, but nuclear chromatin is consistent in character. Most commonly, finely granular and acidophilic with single large nucleolus. Occasionally, the chromatin is compact and basophilic, and nucleoli are small or inapparent.
• Mitoses extremely rare
• Presence of mitoses and B immunoblasts herald change in kinetics and possible emergence of immunoblastic lymphoma B/dysplastic myeloma
	• CIg: Easily demonstrated
	  Monoclonal IgG, 70 percent
	  IgA, 28 percent
	  IgD, 1 percent
	
	• SIg scant

INVOLVED SITES	CLINICAL FEATURES
• Principally bone marrow • Extramedullary sites uncommon	• Monostotic type occasionally seen with single lytic bone lesion preceding classic type by few or many years • Multiple lytic bone lesions in skull, ribs, pelvis, even long bones common; rare sclerotic bone lesions • Leukemic form with high white count rare; small numbers of myeloma cells in the blood common • Bone pain common • Myeloma kidney with obstructive protein casts and renal features common • Bence-Jones proteinuria of Ig light chains in 60 percent of the cases • Hypogammaglobulinemia in 10 percent of the cases; normal SPEP in 15 percent of the cases

REACTIVE COMPONENTS	DIFFERENTIAL DIAGNOSIS
• Small lymphocytes rare • Reactive plasma cells scant or absent • Osteoclastic proliferation	• Severe reactive plasmacytosis • Plasmacytoid lymphocytic lymphoma • Granulocytic sarcoma • Hairy cell leukemia

131

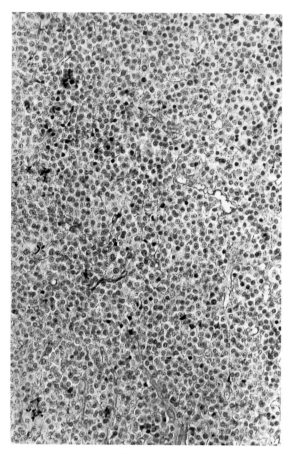

Figure 21
MULTIPLE MYELOMA, MARROW
This nodule of myeloma cells with sheet-like growth replaced marrow fat and hematopoietic tissue. Homogeneity of this process is striking; there are few vessels and little fibrosis. PAS. X100. (Fig. 1 from Canale, D. and Collins, R.D. Use of bone marrow particle sections in the diagnosis of multiple myeloma. Am. J. Clin. Pathol. 61:382-392, 1974.)

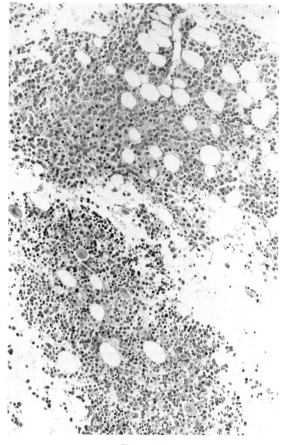

Figure 22
MULTIPLE MYELOMA, MARROW
A small nodule of myeloma cells is noted in the particle at the top of the figure, with partial replacement of fat. Adjacent marrow is infiltrated by myeloma cells and hematopoietic tissue is sharply reduced. The normal particle at the bottom contains few myeloma cells. Focal involvement of marrow particles is fairly common in multiple myeloma. PAS. X100. (Fig. 3 from Canale, D. and Collins, R.D. Use of bone marrow particle sections in the diagnosis of multiple myeloma. Am. J. Clin. Pathol. 61:382-392, 1974.)

sheets of plasma cells or the presence of homogeneous nodules of plasma cells (≥50 percent high power field in diameter in marrow particle sections). These histopathologic features (figs. 21-24) are diagnostic of multiple myeloma, because the plasma cells even in extreme reactive states are not aggregated into large

clumps and are mixed with other marrow elements. The percentage of plasma cells in the marrow aspirate does not differentiate multiple myeloma from reactive plasmacytosis, although percentages greater than 50 percent are highly suggestive of multiple myeloma. Some patients with multiple myeloma will not have discrete

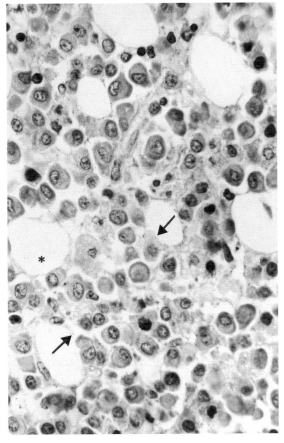

Figure 23
MULTIPLE MYELOMA, MARROW
This high magnification view shows broad infiltrate of myeloma cells (between arrows) and circumscription of fat globule (*) by myeloma infiltration. Little hematopoietic tissue is present. PAS. X400. (Fig. 4 from Canale, D. and Collins, R.D. Use of bone marrow particle sections in the diagnosis of multiple myeloma. Am. J. Clin. Pathol. 61:382-392, 1974.)

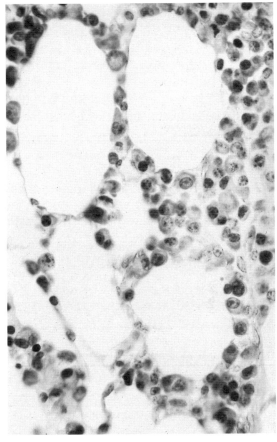

Figure 24
MULTIPLE MYELOMA, MARROW
This pattern of reduced marrow cellularity is unusual in myeloma. Groups of myeloma cells are interspersed among fat globules, and hematopoietic tissue is virtually absent. Diagnoses of myeloma may be made in such cases by demonstrating monotypic CIg with PIP. PAS. X400.

tumors of plasma cells. Diagnoses may be made in these cases by demonstrating dysplasia, plasmacytosis, and monotypic CIg with PIP.

Cytologically, neoplastic cells in multiple myeloma show some variation in cell size and nuclear size (plate XXI-A). Nucleoli are usually present and are rarely prominent. Nuclear chromatin is not basophilic or compact. Electron microscopy may reveal normal-appearing plasma cells or abnormal nuclear forms indicative of dysplasia.

Immunologic Features. Plasma cells from patients with multiple myeloma generally have the same heavy and light chains as present in the paraprotein. Patients with multiple myeloma have circulating mononuclear lymphocytoid cells on

133

PLATE XXI

A. MULTIPLE MYELOMA, MARROW
This smear demonstrates myeloma cells with large nucleoli and minimal dysplastic changes. Wright's stain. X520.

B. MULTIPLE MYELOMA, DYSPLASTIC, SOFT TISSUE
Dysplastic myeloma cells with bizarre nuclei and intranuclear inclusions are demonstrated. Only a few cells have recognizable plasmacytic features. This soft tissue mass developed in a patient several years after therapy for multiple myeloma. X900.

C. MULTIPLE MYELOMA, DYSPLASTIC, TESTIS
(Plate XXI-C and D are from the same patient)
A testicular mass developed in an elderly man 2 years after diagnosis of myeloma. Widespread dissemination occurred, and he died shortly thereafter with dysplastic myeloma.

D. MULTIPLE MYELOMA, DYSPLASTIC, TESTIS
An immunoperoxidase stain shows a monotypic light chain pattern in the testicular mass. X430.

E. MULTIPLE MYELOMA EVOLVING TO DYSPLASTIC MYELOMA/IMMUNOBLASTIC LYMPHOMA B, RIB LESION
High magnification shows some of the features that indicate a process in transition to a high-grade neoplasm of the immunoblastic lymphoma B type. A single mitosis is present in the center of the field along with large multinucleated cells. Mitoses are not found in the usual case of multiple myeloma. X600.

PLATE XXI

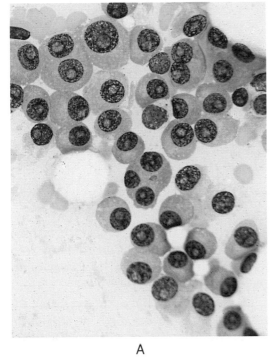

A

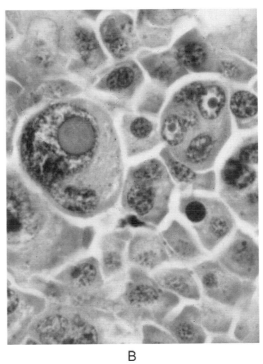

B

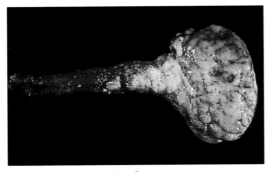

C

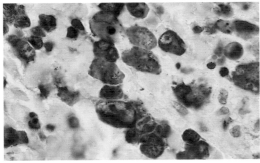

D

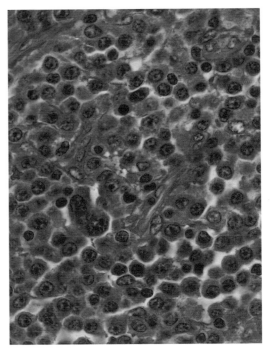

E

which there is SIg identical to the serum paraprotein (Holm et al.). The implication is that there is a circulating population of cells responsible for the spread of multiple myeloma. Studies of a few patients with multiple myeloma using antibodies against idiotypic determinants of myeloma proteins indicated that the oncogenic event in multiple myeloma occurs in the marrow at the earliest stage of B cell development (Kubagawa et al.).

Multiple myeloma has been extensively investigated via biosynthetic, biochemical, and cell-cloning techniques. Although there is usually a concordance between the immunoglobulin in plasma cells and the circulating paraproteins, there are cases in which abnormal immunoglobulin chain synthesis or defective cellular transport results in "nonsecretory" myeloma, Bence-Jones myeloma (Preud'homme et al., 1976), immunoglobulin heavy chain diseases (Preud'homme et al., 1979; Seligmann et al.), or light chain deposition disease (Preud'homme et al., 1980).

Solitary Myeloma of Bone

These patients have a single bony lesion. Criteria for diagnosis include the presence of a solitary bone tumor; a biopsy showing myeloma cell histology with monotypic CIg; a negative random bone marrow examination; the absence of anemia, hypercalcemia, or renal involvement; the absence of a serum paraprotein or presence of low serum paraprotein with disappearance after surgery or radiation therapy; and normal levels of immunoglobulins or low levels that increase to normal after surgery and/or radiation therapy.

Solitary myeloma of bone represents a distinct entity from multiple myeloma as is evidenced by the higher male predominance, earlier age of onset, higher incidence of neurologic involvement, and longer survival than with multiple myeloma. However, most patients with solitary myeloma eventually develop multiple lesions. Marrow involvement may be recognized only by demonstrating monotypic CIg with PIP.

Extramedullary Plasmacytoma

This tumor is characterized by its frequent presentation in the upper air passages, a high incidence of spread to soft tissues, dissemination to bone, and rare marrow involvement. It is extremely radiosensitive and has a better prognosis than myeloma.

Plasmacytomas have rarely been described in other areas such as the node, oral cavity, stomach, or cervix. These processes usually arise in the setting of some immunologic abnormality—angiofollicular hyperplasia for the nodes and Sjögren syndrome for the oral cavity. The neoplastic potential of these processes is uncertain, but they may remain localized for long periods.

Transformation of Multiple Myeloma to Dysplastic Myeloma (Immunoblastic Lymphoma of B Cells). Some patients with multiple myeloma enter an aggressive phase characterized by rapidly deteriorating clinical status with the growth of dysplastic plasmacytic cells in bone, soft tissue, or viscera (plate XXI-B–E). The cytoplasmic immunoglobulin in the majority of these dysplastic cases shows a persistence of the same heavy and light chains as the original paraprotein, although serum paraproteins may decrease. Transformation of multiple myeloma to a pre-B phenotype has not been reported but theoretically might occur. Transformation to a dysplastic phase has occurred 7 to 67 months after the initial diagnosis (with a mean of 28 months). Eighty-three percent of the patients developed soft tissue lesions, often in the lung or abdomen. Therapy has consisted of conservative management, multiagent chemotherapy, and chemotherapy plus radiation therapy. Survival was approximately 6 months in all of the cases.

Histologic evidence of transformation occurred most commonly in the soft tissue or lung, with marked dysplasia as well as giant and multinucleated forms of plasmacytoid cells. The overall appearance ranged from large transformed lymphocytes with plasmacytic differentiation to plasma cells with bizarre features (plate XXI-B). Scattered mature plasma cells were present in most cases. Some patients evaluated for cytoplasmic immunoglobulin at transformation with an immunoperoxidase technique have shown the same heavy and light chains as in the original serum paraprotein (Falini et al.).

Differential Diagnosis. The diagnosis of multiple myeloma should not be made simply on the basis of the percentage of plasma cells but by the demonstration of nodular aggregates of plasma cells with distinctive cytologic features.

Severe reactive plasmacytosis. Plasma cells are not found in nodules, although they may be present in the marrow in very high percentages, particularly when there is decreased hematopoiesis due to marrow injury. The plasma cells in reactive states have cartwheel chromatin and generally are not nucleolated, although they may be multinucleated. They are usually found in aggregates along vessels. The PIP is polyclonal.

Plasmacytoid lymphocytic lymphoma. In this neoplasm, the nodules in the bone marrow are dominantly lymphocytic with varying degrees of eccentric amphophilic cytoplasm. Scattered plasma cells are marked brilliantly with PAS, and mast cells are distinctly increased. On PIP, the plasmacytic elements are usually IgM positive, in contrast to IgG or IgA in multiple myeloma.

Hairy cell leukemia. The cellular proliferation is cohesive, with patchy aggregates of medium sized cells or with a diffuse effacement of architecture. Nuclei are oval or elongated with finely dispersed chromatin and inapparent nucleoli. In multiple myeloma, chromatin is denser, central nucleoli are usually present and are prominent, and growth is noncohesive. On PIP, cytoplasmic positivity is not demonstrated in hairy cell leukemias, but TRAP positivity is present.

Granulocytic sarcomas. A variety of sites including the bone may be involved. Proliferating cells have a diffuse growth pattern and eccentric acidophilic cytoplasm. Nuclei are oval with finely dispersed chromatin and central small nucleoli. On cytochemistry, there may be Sudan black and ACAE positivity.

References

Bartl, R., Frisch, B., Fateh-Moghadam, A., et al. Histologic classification and staging of multiple myeloma. Am. J. Clin. Pathol. 87:342-355, 1987.

Falini, B., De Solas, I., Levine, A.M., et al. Emergence of B-immunoblastic sarcoma in patients with multiple myeloma. Blood 59:923-933, 1982.

Holm, G., Mellstedt, H., Pettersson, D., and Biberfeld, P. Idiotypic immunoglobulin structures on blood lymphocytes in human plasma cell myeloma. Immunol. Rev. 34:139-164, 1977.

Kubagawa, H., Vogler, L.B., Conrad, M., et al. Studies on the clonal origin of multiple myeloma. Use of individually specific (idiotype) antibodies to trace the oncogenic event to its earliest point of expression in B-cell differentiation. J. Exp. Med. 150:792-807, 1979.

Preud'homme, J.L., Hurez, D., Danon, R., Brouet, J.C., and Seligmann, M. Intracytoplasmic and surface-bound immunoglobulins in "non-secretory" and Bence-Jones myeloma. Clin. Exp. Immunol. 25:428-436, 1976.

_____ , Brouet, J.C., and Seligman, M. Cellular immunoglobulins in human gamma- and alpha-heavy chain diseases. Clin. Exp. Immunol. 37:283-291, 1979.

_____ , Morel-Maroger, L., Brouet, J.C., et al. Synthesis of abnormal immunoglobulins in lymphoplasmacytic disorders with light chain deposition. Am. J. Med. 69:703-710, 1980.

Seligmann, M., Mihaesco, E., Preud'homme, J.L., Danon, F., and Brouet, J.C. Heavy chain diseases. Immunol. Rev. 48:145-167, 1979.

Spjut, H.J., Dorfman, H.D., Fechner, R.E., and Ackerman, L.V. Tumors of Bone and Cartilage. Fascicle 5, Second Series. Washington: Armed Forces Institute of Pathology, 1971.

Additional References

Bardwick, P.A., Zvaifler, N.J., Gill, G.N., et al. Plasma cell dyscrasia with polyneuropathy, organomegaly, endocrinopathy, M protein, and skin changes: the POEMS syndrome. Medicine (Baltimore) 59:311-322, 1980.

Bataille, R. and Sany, J. Solitary myeloma. Cancer 48:845-851, 1981.

Biberfeld, P., Mellstedt, H., and Pettersson, D. Ultrastructural and immunocytochemical characterization of circulating mononuclear cells in patients with myelomatosis. Acta Pathol. Microbiol. Scand. [A] 85:611-624, 1977.

Blattner, W.A., Blair, A., and Mason, T.J. Multiple myeloma in the United States, 1950-1975. Cancer 48:2547-2554, 1981.

Canale, D.D., Jr. and Collins, R.D. Use of bone marrow particle sections in the diagnosis of multiple myeloma. Am. J. Clin. Pathol. 61:382-392, 1974.

Corwin, J. and Lindberg, R.D. Solitary plasmacytoma of bone vs. extramedullary plasmacytoma and their relationship to multiple myeloma. Cancer 43:1007-1013, 1979.

Endo, T., Okumura, H., Kikuchi, K., et al. Immunoglobulin E (IgE) multiple myeloma. Am. J. Med. 70:1127-1132, 1981.

Hamburger, A. and Salmon, S.E. Primary bioassay of human myeloma stem cells. J. Clin. Invest. 60:846-854, 1977.

Joyner, M.V., Cassuto, J.P., Dujardin, P., et al. Non-excretory multiple myeloma. Br. J. Haematol. 43:559-566, 1979.

Kapadia, S.B. Multiple myeloma. Medicine (Baltimore) 59:380-392, 1980.

Kyle, R.A. Multiple myeloma. Mayo Clin. Proc. 50:29-40, 1975.

Mundy, G.R., Raisz, L.G., Cooper, R.A., Schechter, G.P., and Salmon, S.E. Evidence for the secretion of an osteoclast stimulating factor in myeloma. N. Engl. J. Med. 291:1041-1046, 1974.

Salmon, S.E., Hamburger, A.W., Soehnlen, B., et al. Quantitation of differential sensitivity of human tumor stem cells to anticancer agents. N. Engl. J. Med. 298:1321-1327, 1978.

Sato, I., Abo, T., Onodera, S., and Kumagai, K. Detection of monoclonal B lymphocytes in multiple myeloma by immunofluorescence tests of surface immunoglobulins. Scand. J. Haematol. 21:433-444, 1978.

Warner, T.F. and Krueger, R.G. Circulating lymphocytes and the spread of myeloma. Lancet 1:1174-1176, 1978.

Wiltshaw, E. The natural history of extramedullary plasmacytoma and its relationship to solitary myeloma of bone and myelomatosis. Medicine (Baltimore) 55:217-238, 1976.

Zarrabi, M.H., Stark, R.S., Kane, P., Dannaher, C.L., and Chandor, S. IgM myeloma, a distinct entity in the spectrum of B-cell neoplasia. Am. J. Clin. Pathol. 75:1-10, 1981.

HAIRY CELL LEUKEMIA OR LEUKEMIC RETICULOENDOTHELIOSIS

Definition. The function and site of action of the cells from which this neoplasm arises are not known, although the proliferating cells are B cells. Hairy cell leukemia affects principally the marrow and spleen, and a leukemic phase is common. For pathologic details, see Plates XXII-XXV and figures 25-29.

Clinical Features. Hairy cell leukemia comprises approximately 3 percent of the lymphoid malignancies in the United States and approximately 2 percent of all leukemias.

The disease is seen most commonly in the fifth decade, with patients ranging in age from the second to eighth decades.

Males are affected four times more frequently than females. Marrow failure is the most common mode of presentation. Granulocytopenia and infection are reported in 17 percent of the patients, thrombocytopenia and bleeding in 9 percent, and anemia with weakness and fatigue in the majority. Splenomegaly and left upper quadrant pain is the presenting complaint in approximately 15 percent of the newly diagnosed patients.

Splenomegaly occurs in 93 percent of patients and may be massive. Hepatomegaly is found in approximately 40 percent of patients, and lymphadenopathy occurs in 30 percent.

Initial hematologic observations include anemia in approximately 85 percent of the cases, granulocytopenia in approximately 50 percent, and thrombocytopenia in 80 percent of the cases. Although thrombocytopenic bleeding is common in the disease, qualitative defects in platelet function have also been described. Paraproteinemia has been described in a few patients but rarely with osteolytic lesions.

The course of this disease is variable. Some patients experience a very slow, chronic progression of disease, whereas others have a more rapid and progressive downhill course. The median survival is 5 to 6 years.

The most prominent complication is infection, which is the immediate cause of death in the majority of the patients. Bacterial, fungal, and acid-fast infections are all common because these patients have a decreased production of granulocytes and monocytes, a deficiency in antibody-mediated cytotoxicity by monocytes, and an inadequate monocyte chemotaxis. Studies of humoral immunity have revealed no major defect.

Pathologic Features (Table 29). Due to the rarity of overt leukemic phases and the usual inability to aspirate marrow, the marrow biopsy is the single most important diagnostic method. The marrow may show focal or generalized effacement of architecture (plate XXIII-A–C). In altered areas, there is decreased hematopoietic tissue, delicate PAS positive stromal framework, and infiltration by small cells with abundant eosinophilic or clear cytoplasm and ovoid folded nuclei with a bland nuclear chromatin pattern. Nucleoli are inconspicuous, and mitotic figures are rare. Nuclei of tumor cells never appear as closely packed as those of chronic lymphocytic leukemia or small cell lymphomas. Mast cells may be increased.

The spleen is usually enlarged and has a firm, homogeneous cut surface without evidence of discrete tumor masses (plate XXIV-A); infarcts may be present. Histologically, the red pulp is diffusely infiltrated, often obliterating the white pulp (plate XXV-A–C). Blood-filled "pseudosinuses" (these sinuses do not have the usual structure of splenic sinuses) lined by hairy cells are seen in most cases (plate XXV-A). There may be numerous plasma cells around the blood vessels and scattered in the cords. The liver involvement usually has a sinusal and portal distribution with slight architectural distortion (fig. 25). Pseudosinuses similar to splenic lesions may be seen in the portal areas of the liver and resemble angiomatous lesions. Lymph nodes may be focally or diffusely involved (plate XXIV-B); lymphoid follicles often are spared, despite extensive infiltration. Soft tissues in the abdomen may be heavily infiltrated.

Peripheral Blood Cytology. Hairy cells derive their name from the characteristic

Table 29

HAIRY CELL LEUKEMIA

PATTERN	
	• Focal, patchy, or diffuse marrow involvement • Spleen — red pulp infiltrate with widely separated white pulp; pseudosinuses present in spleen • Node — interfollicular infiltrate

CYTOLOGY — NEOPLASTIC	MARKERS — NEOPLASTIC

• Distinctive due to abundant pale cytoplasm, small round or indented nuclei, well demarcated cell borders
 	
• Hairy microfilaments not readily apparent in smears
 	
• Mitoses: None
 	
• MGP: Negative
	• Monotypic SIg; hairy cells have an unusual phenotype on flow:
	    CD5 (–)
	    CD10 (–)
	    Leu-M5 (+)
	    CD20, CD25 (+)
	
	• Prominent capping phenomenon on immuno-fluorescence of living cells
	
	• Tartrate-resistant acid phosphatase present in most cases
	
	• Hairy microfilaments most evident on phase microscopy of wet mounts

INVOLVED SITES	CLINICAL FEATURES
• Marrow • Spleen • Rarely lymph node or abdominal soft tissue	• Adult (M > F), pancytopenia, splenomegaly • May have few circulating cells • "Dry" marrow aspirates • Hematopoiesis often hypoplastic • Rare bone pain and lytic lesions at presentation • Transformation to high-grade neoplasm rare

REACTIVE COMPONENTS	DIFFERENTIAL DIAGNOSIS
• Hematopoietic elements may be interspersed in marrow • Scattered plasma cells • Few mast cells, eosinophils	• Small B/T cell neoplasms • Plasmacytoid lymphocytic lymphoma • Multiple myeloma • Mastocytosis

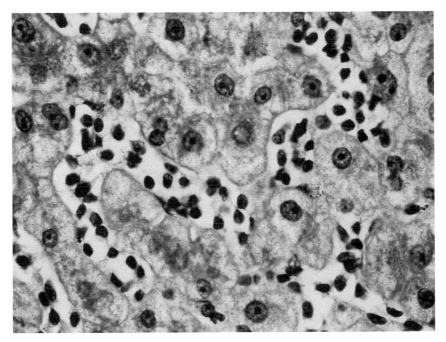

Figure 25
HAIRY CELL LEUKEMIA, LIVER
This figure shows extensive sinus infiltrate with hairy cells that appear to be percolating through the expanded sinuses. H&E. X400.

cytoplasmic projections best seen on Wright's-stained smears, wet preparations viewed with phase microscopy, and ultrastructural examination (plate XXII-A–C). Hairy cells are slightly larger than lymphocytes, and their nuclei may be round, oval, bean, or dumbbell shaped. Prominent nucleoli are rare. The nuclear chromatin pattern is bland and smudged in appearance. Occasionally, fine cytoplasmic granules are present. Rod-shaped inclusions are rarely seen and are thought to represent ribosomal lamellar complexes.

Ultrastructural Features. The nuclear profiles often display one or more indentations with a modest degree of peripheral chromatin condensation. Highly developed nucleoli are uncommon. The cytoplasmic

surface projections are characteristic (figs. 26, 27) but may not be apparent in spleen sections (fig. 28). Numerous cytoplasmic vacuoles and vesicles are present, as well as occasional membrane-bound granular structures that may represent lysosomes containing acid phosphatase activity. Glycogen is frequently present, and mitochondria are numerous. Up to 50 percent of the cases of hairy cell leukemia are said to contain distinctive ribosomal lamellar complexes in a variable number of cells per individual case. The function of these complexes is not known, and similar structures are occasionally seen in other hematologic malignancies and benign conditions.

Cytochemistry. At least seven isoenzymes of acid phosphatase are present in

PLATE XXII
HAIRY CELL LEUKEMIA, PERIPHERAL BLOOD
(Plate XXII-B and plate XXV are from the same patient)

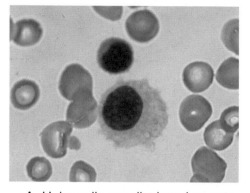

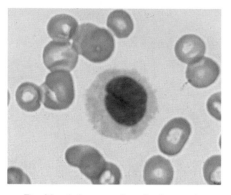

A. Hairy cells are displayed as cytoplasmic mononuclear cells in comparison with small lymphocytes. Nuclei of hairy cells are round to oval, and the nuclear chromatin is loosely aggregated and acidophilic. The cytoplasm is pale, slightly coarse, and sometimes vacuolated. The periphery of the cell is slightly irregular due to fine linear or indistinct projections. Wright's stain. X1000.

B. Nuclei may be indented, as shown in this illustration. Wright's stain. X1000.

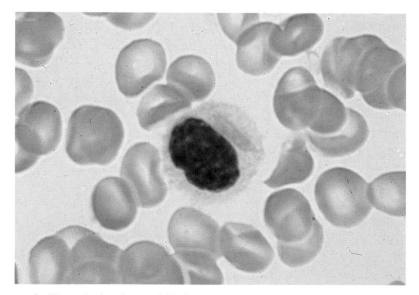

C. The tubular, basophilic structure in the cytoplasm of this hairy cell corresponds to the ribosomal-lamellar complex identified by electron microscopic examination. Wright's-Giemsa stain. X1035.

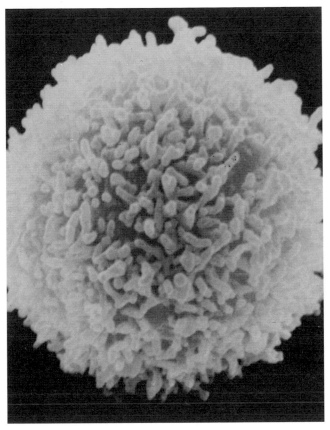

Figure 26
HAIRY CELL LEUKEMIA
This is a scanning electron micrograph of a hairy cell with a surface consisting predominantly of microvilli. Ruffles may be seen in addition to microvilli. (From Schnitzer, B. and Hammack, W.J. B-lymphocyte nature of hairy cells in hairy cell leukaemia. [Letter to the Editor.] Lancet 2:649, 1974.)

hematopoietic cells, but only isoenzyme number five is found in hairy cells. In addition, it is the only isoenzyme (except the one found in Gaucher's disease) that is resistant to L (+) tartrate (Cawley et al.). TRAP positivity is useful in recognizing hairy cell leukemia (plates XXIII-D; XXV-D). The importance of technical considerations about the methodology of the cytochemical techniques is emphasized by Yam and associates, who recommend the naphthol-ASBI phosphoric acid-fast garnet GBC method. Within a given case of hairy cell leukemia, variation in staining intensity is seen from cell to cell, and occasional cases will show little or no positivity in any cells. Most cases of hairy cell leukemia

demonstrate finely granular PAS positivity in the cytoplasm. Likewise, α-naphthyl acetate esterase positivity may be seen in a diffuse or granular pattern often localized near one pole of the cytoplasm (Variakojis et al.).

Immunologic Features. Hairy cells have been identified as B cells by their monotypic SIg with light chain restriction, by their reactivity with B cell-associated antigens including Ia and CD20, and by the clonal rearrangement of immunoglobulin genes. Hairy cells cross-react with some antibodies marking plasma cells and myeloma cells, and an antibody designated HC-2 appears to be restricted in reactivity to hairy cell leukemia cells.

PLATE XXIII
HAIRY CELL LEUKEMIA, MARROW
(Plate XXIII-B and C are from the same patient)

A. Extensive involvement of the marrow with considerable architectural distortion may be present in hairy cell leukemia. Little hematopoietic tissue is apparent in this biopsy. Contrast this appearance with the focal involvement shown in Plate XXIII-B. X75.

B. This low magnification photomicrograph shows patchy involvement of the marrow, often seen in hairy cell leukemia. There is abundant interspersed fat and hematopoietic elements; overall cellularity is not increased. X75.

C. A high magnification photomicrograph of the infiltrate in Plate XXIII-B shows a focus of hairy cell leukemia in the center of the field surrounded by normal hematopoietic elements. X1160

D. This illustration demonstrates a tartrate-resistant acid phosphatase stain on a section of a plastic-embedded trephine biopsy. Nearly every hairy cell shows a positive reaction. TRAP. X1160.

PLATE XXIII

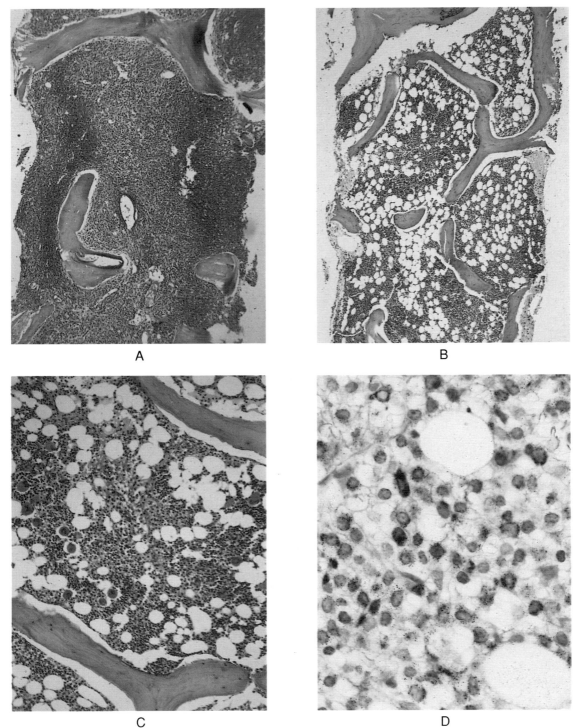

A

B

C

D

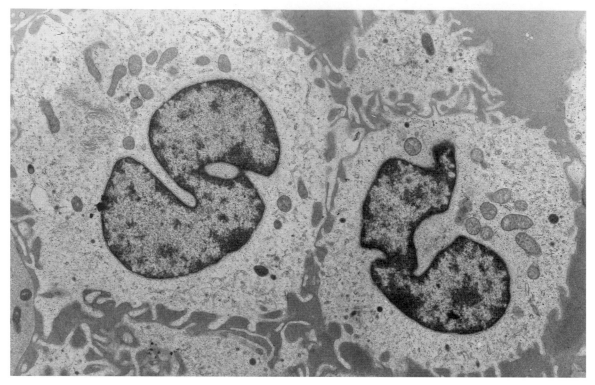

Figure 27
HAIRY CELL LEUKEMIA, BUFFY COAT PREPARATION
In this electron micrograph, the nuclei are deeply indented and irregular in shape, the chromatin is moderately condensed, and the cytoplasm is abundant. The most prominent feature of the leukemic cells is the presence of numerous delicate cytoplasmic projections. Uranyl acetate, lead citrate. X8000.

There is general agreement that the surface phenotype of hairy cells indicates they have the features of B cells late in the differentiation pathway (Anderson et al.; Robinson et al.). Normal counterparts of hairy cells have been identified in the peripheral blood as activated B cells (Posnett et al., 1982, 1984), and most reports surmise that hairy cell leukemia is a tumor of plasma cell precursors (Anderson et al.). However, immunoperoxidase and ultrastructural studies show that most immunoglobulin is on the cell surface rather than in the cytoplasm, and no clear-cut intermediates between hairy cells and plasma cells have been identified (Gooi et al.). Thus, despite careful investigations, the function, site of action, and source of hairy cells are unknown (Hooper et al.). Although the leukemic cells in hairy cell leukemia usually have a monotypic SIg (fig. 29), it is not clear whether these cells develop the capacity to excrete immunoglobulin. Finally, the possibility exists that there are functional subpopulations of hairy cells, because cases of hairy cell leukemia vary somewhat in ultrastructure and cytochemical reactions, as well as surface phenotype (Cawley et al.; Jansen et al.).

PLATE XXIV

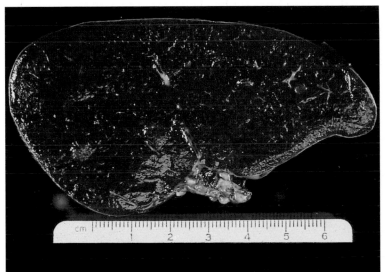

A. HAIRY CELL LEUKEMIA, SPLEEN

The spleen is usually enlarged in hairy cell leukemia, and the cut surface usually has a homogeneous appearance. Rarely, small ill-defined nodules may be detected, as in this case.

B. HAIRY CELL LEUKEMIA, NODE

Nodal involvement in hairy cell leukemia may be relatively subtle, but in this case, there is a diffuse hairy cell infiltrate that replaces the normal architecture of the lymph node. Aggregates of lymphocytes surrounded by hairy cells are apparent. H&E. X125.

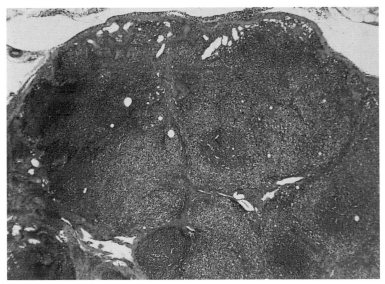

PLATE XXV
(Plate XXV and plate XXII-B are from the same patient)

A. HAIRY CELL LEUKEMIA, SPLEEN
There is marked infiltration of the cords of Billroth of the red pulp with only a small Malpighian body remaining. Several pseudosinuses are packed with masses of erythrocytes. X25.

B. HAIRY CELL LEUKEMIA, SPLEEN
The cords of Billroth are greatly broadened by an infiltration of cytoplasmic mononuclear cells, whereas the sinuses contain only a few scattered mononuclear cells. X40.

C. HAIRY CELL LEUKEMIA, SPLEEN, IMPRINT
Hairy cells in imprints usually have abundant cytoplasm (often without surface projections) and round to oval nuclei with inapparent nucleoli. Wright's stain. X1000.

D. HAIRY CELL LEUKEMIA, SPLEEN, IMPRINT
An acid phosphatase stain after tartrate treatment shows the characteristic positivity of hairy cells. TRAP. X1000.

PLATE XXV

A

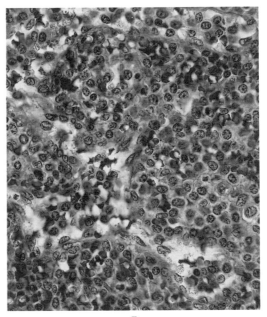

B

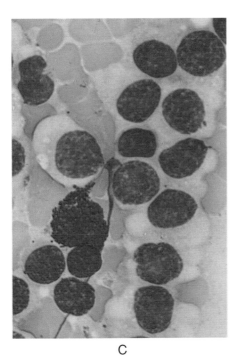

C

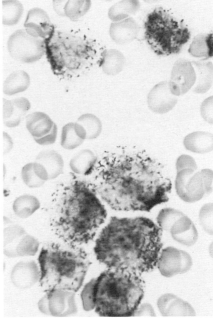

D

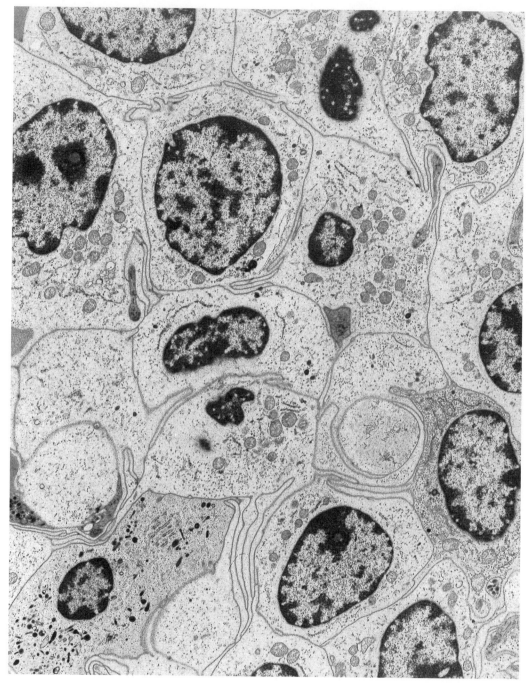

Figure 28
HAIRY CELL LEUKEMIA, SPLEEN
By electron micrography, the lymphoid-appearing cells show elaborate interdigitations of long, thin cytoplasmic projections. The cytoplasm is moderately abundant and contains small mitochondria, strands of rough endoplasmic reticulum, and rare, small electron-dense granules. Uranyl acetate, lead citrate. X6000.

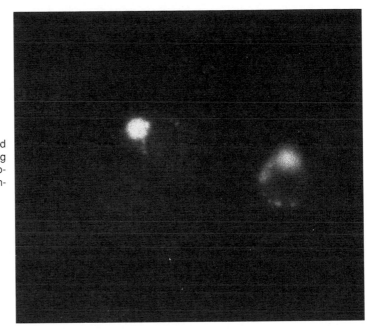

Figure 29
HAIRY CELL LEUKEMIA,
PERIPHERAL BLOOD
Hairy cells exposed to fluorescein-tagged anti-Ig antisera show an exaggerated capping phenomenon. A very large area of bright fluorescence at one pole of the cell is demonstrated. X1000.

Differential Diagnosis. *Small B/T cell neoplasms.* Growth patterns in nodes or marrow are usually diffuse. In hairy cell leukemia, involvement in the marrow may be patchy and difficult to appreciate, and nodal involvement is often around follicular centers. Hairy cells are distinctly cytoplasmic with only slight nuclear irregularity. The extent of nuclear irregularity in hairy cell leukemia is in contrast to the striking irregularity present in small T cell neoplasms. Nuclear chromatin is usually denser and nuclei are generally rounder in small B cell neoplasms. Immunologic studies uniformly show the T nature of small T cell neoplasms, and small B cell neoplasms are often CD5 positive. TRAP reactions are often positive in hairy cell leukemia.

Plasmacytoid lymphocytic lymphoma. Infiltrates in the marrow are predominantly lymphocytic, with scattered large PAS positive plasma cells. CIg is distinctly monotypic, and plasmacytic differentiation is usually readily demonstrated by MGP and PAS stains.

Multiple myeloma. The growth patterns in multiple myeloma are usually quite different, and there is massive involvement of the marrow. Myeloma cells show amphophilic cytoplasm that is distinctly MGP positive, and cytoplasmic CIg is readily demonstrated on PIP.

Mastocytosis. Infiltrates in the marrow may be focal, and involvement of the nodes may have a similar distribution to that of hairy cell leukemia. Mast cell granules are usually readily demonstrated with toluidine blue stains. TRAP reactions are positive in hairy cell leukemia. Cell suspensions show monotypic SIg in hairy cell leukemia, and there are clear-cut ultrastructural differences.

References

Anderson, K.C., Boyd, A.W., Fisher, D.C., et al. Hairy cell leukemia: a tumor of pre-plasma cells. Blood 65:620-629, 1985.

Cawley, J.C., Burns, G.F. and Hayhoe, G.J. Hairy cell leukemia. Recent Results Cancer Res. 72:1-123, 1980.

Gooi, J.H., Burns, G.F., and Cawley, J.C. Hairy-cell leukaemia. J. Clin. Pathol. 32:1244-1247, 1979.

Hooper, W.C., Buss, D.H., and Parker, C.L. Leukemic reticuloendotheliosis (hairy cell leukemia). Leuk. Res. 4:489-503, 1980.

Jansen, J., Schuit, H.R., Meijer, C.J., van Nieuwkoop, J.A., and Hijmans, W. Cell markers in hairy cell leukemia studied in cells from 51 patients. Blood 59:52-60, 1982.

Posnett, D.N., Chiorazzi, N., and Kunkel, H.G. Monoclonal antibodies with specificity for hairy cell leukemia cells. J. Clin. Invest. 70:254-261, 1982.

_____, Wang, C.Y., Chiorazzi, N., Crow, M.K., and Kunkel, H.G. An antigen characteristic of hairy cell leukemia cells is expressed on certain activated B cells. J. Immunol. 133:1635-1640, 1984.

Robinson, D.S., Posnett, D.N., Zola, H., and Catovsky, D. Normal counterparts of hairy cells and B-prolymphocytes in the peripheral blood. Leuk. Res. 9:335-348, 1985.

Variakojis, D., Vardiman, J.W., and Golomb, H.M. Cytochemistry of hairy cells. Cancer 45:72-77, 1980.

Yam, L.T., Janckila, A.J., Li, C.Y., and Tam, K.W. Cytochemistry of tartrate-resistant acid phosphatase. Leukemia 1:285-288, 1987.

Additional References

Bouza, E., Burgaleta, C., and Golde, D.W. Infections in hairy-cell leukemia. Blood 51:851-859, 1978.

Braylan, R.C., Jaffe, E.S., Triche, T.J., et al. Structural and functional properties of the "hairy" cells of leukemic reticuloendotheliosis. Cancer 41:210-227, 1978.

Burke, J.S. The value of the bone marrow biopsy in the diagnosis of hairy cell leukemia. Am. J. Clin. Pathol. 70:876-884, 1978.

Catovsky, D., Pettit, J.E., Galetto, J., Okos, A., and Galton, D.A. The B-lymphocyte nature of the hairy cells of leukaemic reticuloendotheliosis. Br. J. Haematol. 26:29-37, 1974.

_____, Pettit, J.E., Galton, D.A., Spiers, A.S.D., and Harrison, C.V. Leukaemic reticuloendotheliosis ("Hairy" cell leukaemia). Br. J. Haematol. 26:9-27, 1974.

Foon, K.A. and Todd, R.F., III. Immunologic classification of leukemia and lymphoma. Blood 68:1-31, 1986.

Fu, S.M., Winchester, R.J., Rai, K.R., and Kunkel, H.G. Hairy cell leukemia: proliferation of a cell with phagocytic and B-lymphocyte properties. Scand. J. Immunol. 3:847-851, 1974.

Golde, D.W., Saxon, A., and Stevens, R.H. Macroglobulinemia and hairy cell leukemia. N. Engl. J. Med. 296:92-93, 1977.

Golomb, H.M. Hairy cell leukemia: an unusual lymphoproliferative disease. Cancer 42(Suppl. 2):946-956, 1978.

_____. Progress report on chlorambucil therapy in postsplenectomy patients with progressive hairy cell leukemia. Blood 57:464-467, 1981.

_____, Catovsky, D., and Golde, D.W. Hairy cell leukemia. Ann. Intern. Med. 89(5 part 1):677-683, 1978.

Hsu, S.M., Yang, K., and Jaffe, E.S. Hairy cell leukemia: a B cell neoplasm with a unique antigenic phenotype. Am. J. Clin. Pathol. 80:421-428, 1983.

Katayama, I. and Finkel, H.E. Leukemic reticuloendotheliosis. Am. J. Med. 57:115-126, 1974.

_____ and Schneider, G.B. Further ultrastructural characterization of hairy cells of leukemic reticuloendotheliosis. Am. J. Pathol. 86:163-182, 1977.

Mori, N., Tsunoda, R., Kojima, M., Andres, T., and Kadin, M.E. Ultrastructural localization of immunoglobulins in hairy cell leukemia. Hum. Pathol. 15:1042-1047, 1984.

Nanba, K., Soban, E.J., Bowling, M.C., and Berard, C.W. Splenic pseudosinuses and hepatic angiomatous lesions. Am. J. Clin. Pathol. 67:415-426, 1977.

Saxon, A., Stevens, R.H., and Golde, D.W. T-lymphocyte variant of hairy-cell leukemia. Ann. Intern. Med. 88:323-326, 1978.

MANTLE ZONE LYMPHOMA

Definition. This malignant lymphoma appears to arise from the mantle zone of the secondary follicles and is remarkable for the production of wide tumorous mantle zones around small follicular centers (Pallesen et al.; Weisenburger et al., 1982). For pathologic details, see Plate XXVI.

Clinical Features. Mantle zone lymphoma has only recently been described and comprises fewer than 10 percent of all cases of well- or poorly differentiated lymphocytic lymphomas of Rappaport. The median age at onset is 56 years, with a range from 35 to 76 years. Males are affected twice as frequently as females.

Approximately 60 percent of the patients present with systemic symptoms including fever, weight loss, and night sweats. Peripheral lymphadenopathy and left upper quadrant pressure related to splenic enlargement are also prominent initial complaints. Physical examination reveals generalized lymph node enlargement in the majority of the patients (60 percent), with splenomegaly in 80 percent and hepatomegaly in 30 percent. The spleen may be massively enlarged.

On laboratory analysis, the median hemoglobin level is 12 g/dL (with a range of 8.8-14.9 g/dL), with a median white blood cell count of 6800/μL; patients with a leukemic picture in the peripheral blood have not been described. The median platelet count is reported to be 225,000/μL. Polyclonal hypergammaglobulinemia on serum protein electrophoresis has been reported in approximately 30 percent of the patients, whereas monoclonal serum paraproteins may be seen in as many as 20 percent of the patients. Coombs' positive hemolytic anemias have been reported.

Widespread disease is expected in the vast majority of the patients, and approximately 90 percent of the patients demonstrate stage III or IV disease. Bone marrow involvement has been reported in 66 percent of the patients, with liver involvement in 30 to 60 percent. Generalized lymphadenopathy is expected, involving both peripheral and retroperitoneal sites.

Nonaggressive chemotherapy produces complete remission in the majority of the cases. The median survival is in excess of 3 years in the limited number of patients reported.

Pathologic Features (Table 30). The morphology of mantle zone lymphoma is distinctive in that follicular centers may be detected in the midst of ill-defined nodules of small lymphocytes in the nodes and spleen (plate XXVI-A,C). Follicular centers are small and atrophic in some cases but are active in others. The cells in these growths closely resemble normal mantle zone lymphocytes (plate XXVI-B). Marrow involvement has been reported in 6 of 12 cases (Weisenburger et al., 1981). Other B cell lymphomas (see Differential Diagnosis) may have a growth pattern closely resembling that of mantle zone lymphoma.

Immunologic Features. Immunologic studies have confirmed the B cell nature of this process. The few cases studied have had IgM-λ as the predominant SIg in two cases and IgG + IgM-λ in one case. With PIP, there is a characteristic pattern of positive reactivity of the mantle zone lymphoma cells with CD74 (LN-2) and a negative reactivity with CDw75 (LN-1) (plate XXVI-D,E).

Differential Diagnosis. *Malignant lymphoma, follicular center cell, small cleaved cell type.* Neoplastic follicular nodules are present and contain a homogeneous population of cleaved follicular center cells, in contrast to the generally atretic or small benign reactive follicular centers surrounded by broad mantle zones in mantle zone lymphoma. On PIP, CDw75 positivity is present in the neoplastic cells in small cleaved cell-type lymphomas, whereas in mantle zone lymphoma, the broad mantle zone areas mark with CD74. Cytologically, the small cleaved cell is much more irregular with inapparent cytoplasm than the rounder cell that predominates in mantle zone lymphoma.

PLATE XXVI

A. MANTLE ZONE LYMPHOMA, LYMPH NODE
Benign-appearing residual follicular centers are surrounded by a dense neoplastic proliferation of small lymphoid cells in the mantle region. The sinuses are open, with follicular centers of varying size. X188.

B. NORMAL MANTLE ZONE, TONSIL
A normal mantle zone is shown in this high magnification photomicrograph. Lymphocytes are small, round, and only slightly irregular with basophilic chromatin. There are indistinct cytoplasmic borders (compare with plate XXVI-C). H&E. X800.

C. MANTLE ZONE LYMPHOMA, NODE
(Plate XXVI-C and E are from the same patient)
A high magnification photomicrograph of a typical mantle zone lymphoma shows lymphocytes of small to intermediate size with somewhat variable configuration and indistinct cytoplasmic borders. H&E. X800.

D. MANTLE ZONE LYMPHOMA, NODE, PIP, WITH CD74 (LN-2)
A characteristic pattern of positivity is shown with CD74 reactive cells surrounding a benign follicular center with scattered positive reactive cells (compare with plate XXVI-E). X320.

E. MANTLE ZONE LYMPHOMA, NODE, PIP, WITH CDw75 (LN-1)
In this illustration, a typical pattern of reactivity is observed with marked positivity in the follicular center and a negative mantle zone. X130.

PLATE XXVI

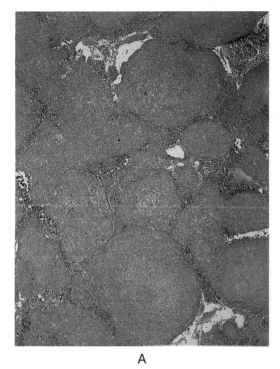

A

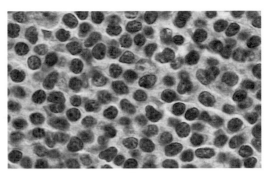

B

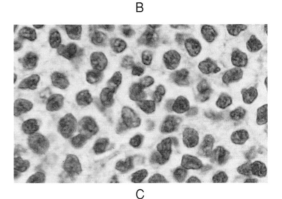

C

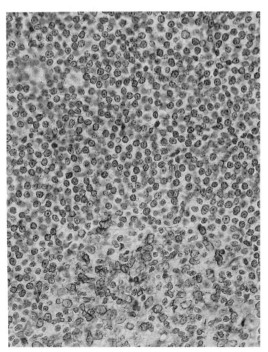

D

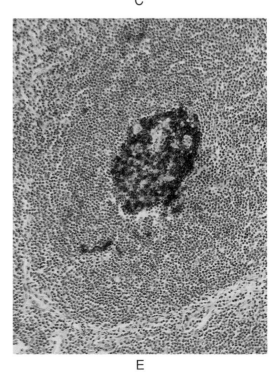

E

Table 30

MANTLE ZONE LYMPHOMA

PATTERN
• Small, almost atretic follicular centers in some cases surrounded by broad mantle zones (pattern may be mimicked by other B cell neoplasms)
• Mantle zone width uniformly greater than that of follicles
• Medullary sinuses may be dilated
• Mitoses rare

CYTOLOGY — NEOPLASTIC	MARKERS — NEOPLASTIC
• Round, slightly irregular nuclei; nuclear irregularity much less than in follicular center cell, small cleaved cell	• Flow, FSIP: Monotypic SIg (IgM ± D) CD19 (+), CD20 (+)
• Nuclear chromatin condensed; nucleoli absent	• PIP: Weak monotypic CIg some cases CDw75 (LN-1) (−) CD74 (LN-2) (+)
• Minimal cytoplasm [MGP, PAS, Giemsa (−)]	
• Rare plasma cells	

INVOLVED SITES	CLINICAL FEATURES
• Superficial nodes	• Adult males with superficial adenopathy ± splenomegaly (may be massive)
• Spleen, liver	• B symptoms, particularly weight loss, may be present; most patients have advanced stage disease
• Bone marrow, blood	• Appears to have indolent course

REACTIVE COMPONENTS	DIFFERENTIAL DIAGNOSIS
• Follicular centers polytypic	• Malignant lymphoma, follicular center cell, small cleaved cell (follicular)
	• Small B/T cell neoplasms
	• Mantle zone hyperplasia
	• Angiofollicular hyperplasia

Small B/T cell neoplasms. Follicular centers may be preserved in small B cell neoplastic processes but have no particular relationship to the proliferating cell. Mantle zone lymphoma has a pseudonodular appearance due to the presence of large numbers of mantle zone lymphocytes around small atretic follicular centers. Pseudofollicles or proliferation centers are present in small B cell neoplastic processes but not in mantle zone lymphoma. Immunologically, small T cell neoplasms mark distinctly with flow, FSIP, or PIP. Small B cell neoplasms show a monotypic SIg on flow or FSIP and are also CD5 positive.

Mantle zone hyperplasia. Mantle zone lymphoma should be diagnosed only when there is considerable distortion or effacement of nodal architecture by broad areas of proliferation around small follicular centers.

Angiofollicular hyperplasia. The follicular centers in this process are usually distinctive, with whorled lymphocytes around small vascular structures. There is usually a characteristic vascular component or numerous plasma cells. Monotypic surface immunoglobulin is not present in angiofollicular hyperplasia.

References

Pallesen, G., Madsen, M., and Pedersen, B.B. B-prolymphocytic leukaemia—a mantle zone lymphoma? Scand. J. Haematol. 22:407-416, 1979.

Weisenburger, D.D., Nathwani, B.N., Diamond, L.W., Winberg, C.D., and Rappaport, H. Malignant lymphoma, intermediate lymphocytic type. Cancer 48:1415-1425, 1981.

_____, Kim, H., and Rappaport, H. Mantle-zone lymphoma: a follicular variant of intermediate lymphocytic lymphoma. Cancer 49:1429-1438, 1982.

Additional References

Harris, N.L. and Bhan, A.K. Mantle-zone lymphoma. A pattern produced by lymphomas of more than one cell type. Am. J. Surg. Pathol. 9:872-882, 1985.

Palutke, M., Eisenberg, L., Mirchandani, I., Tabaczka, P., and Husain, M. Malignant lymphoma of small cleaved lymphocytes of the follicular mantle zone. Blood 59:317-322, 1982.

Samoszuk, M.K., Epstein, A.L., Said, J., Lukes, R.J., and Nathwani, B.N. Sensitivity and specificity of immunostaining in the diagnosis of mantle zone lymphoma. Am. J. Clin. Pathol. 85:557-563, 1986.

MARGINAL ZONE LYMPHOMA

Definition. This rare lymphoma has produced massive involvement of the spleen in the two cases we have studied (Cousar et al.). The predominant cell closely resembles the reactive marginal zone cells of the human spleen by histology and electron microscopy. The relationship of marginal zone cells to other B cell neoplasms is unclear, as is the normal function of these cells.

Clinical Features. Our patients were adults who had moderate to massive splenomegaly, as well as superficial and hilar adenopathy. The natural history for this neoplasm has not been established because of the scarcity of cases.

Pathologic Features (Table 31). Nodal and splenic involvement consists of ill-defined nodules of small lymphocytes with abundant clear cytoplasm and round nuclei (figs. 30, 31). Electron microscopy is distinctive for long serpentine patterns of rough endoplasmic reticulum (fig. 32).

Immunologic Features. Immunologic studies in our two cases showed a monotypic surface immunoglobulin with moderate to strong immunofluorescence. The SIg in both cases was IgG-κ and IgM +

Table 31

MARGINAL ZONE LYMPHOMA

PATTERN		
• Spleen — growths diffuse, extensive, may be multifocal, with minimal extension into red pulp; mitoses frequent • Lymph node — growths diffuse, usually with complete effacement of architecture; nodes often contain residual follicular centers		
CYTOLOGY — NEOPLASTIC	**MARKERS — NEOPLASTIC**	
• Approximately 12 µm, round or oblong nuclei; partially dispersed chromatin with peripheral accentuation • Cytoplasm abundant, clear, with distinct cell borders • Electron microscopy shows abundant cytoplasm, mixture of single and clustered ribosomes; abundant rough endoplasmic reticulum	• Flow: Monotypic SIg, usually IgM-κ	
INVOLVED SITES	**CLINICAL FEATURES**	
• Spleen ± liver • Lymph nodes, superficial and deep • Bone marrow	• Only a few cases reported • Adults with splenomegaly (occasionally massive) ± hepatomegaly; lymphadenopathy superficial and deep, usually generalized • Often present with abdominal pain, weight loss; have advanced stage • Bone marrow usually involved • Prognosis poor	
REACTIVE COMPONENTS	**DIFFERENTIAL DIAGNOSIS**	
• Residual follicles in nodes • Macrophages rare	• Malignant lymphoma, follicular center cell, small cleaved cell • Mantle zone lymphoma • Malignant lymphoma, parafollicular B	

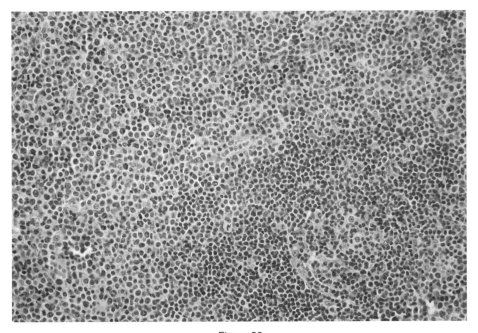

Figure 30
MARGINAL ZONE LYMPHOMA, SPLEEN
Growth pattern in this neoplasm may produce large nodules of tumor, occasionally adjacent to residual follicular centers. X100.

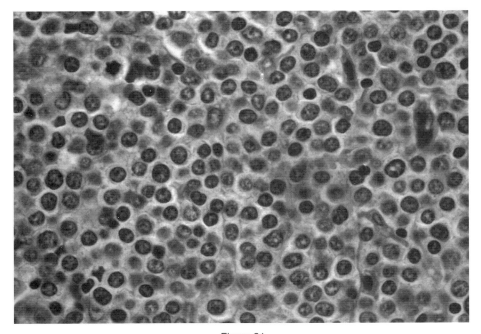

Figure 31
MARGINAL ZONE LYMPHOMA, SPLEEN
Note the small to medium sized neoplastic cells with centrally located round nuclei, partially dispersed nuclear chromatin, and moderately abundant clear cytoplasm. X650.

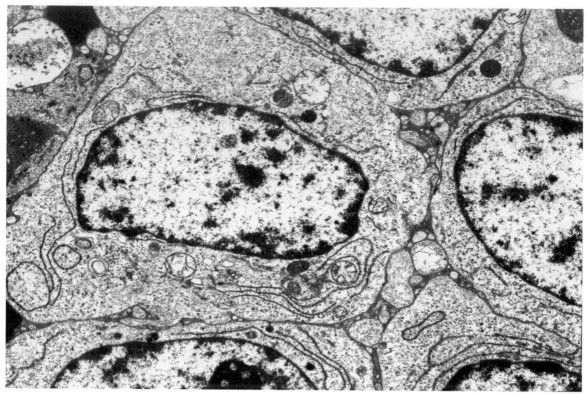

Figure 32
MARGINAL ZONE LYMPHOMA, SPLEEN
In this figure, the ultrastructure shows oblong nuclei and cytoplasm with long serpentine rough endoplasmic reticulum profiles. The centrally placed round nuclei, abundant cytoplasm, and rough endoplasmic reticulum profiles are characteristic of these cases. Uranyl acetate. X9800.

IgD-κ with 13 to 30 percent E-rosette-forming cells, respectively.

Differential Diagnosis. *Malignant lymphoma, follicular center cell, small cleaved cell type.* Neoplastic follicular nodules are usually produced, and the predominant lymphocyte is an irregular small lymphocyte. The cytoplasm is usually inapparent, and cell borders are not seen. In marginal zone lymphoma, the lymphocytic nuclei are separated by abundant cytoplasm and cell borders may be apparent.

Mantle zone lymphoma and parafollicular B cell lymphoma. Differentiation of the proliferating cell in marginal zone lymphoma from mantle zone lymphoma and parafollicular B cell malignant lymphoma is somewhat controversial and may be difficult at best. Marginal zone lymphoma is very rare and apparently involves primarily the spleen. Mantle zone lymphomas are much more common and typically show a broad zone of proliferation around small follicular centers in the nodes. Parafollicular B lymphomas show sheet-like infiltrates with hyperplastic follicular centers. The electron microscopic appearance of the marginal zone lymphoma is distinctive with long serpentine rough endoplasmic reticulum profiles. Currently, it is not known whether there are immunologic differences in these processes.

Reference

Cousar, J.B., McKee, L.C., Greco, F.A., Glick, A.D., and Collins, R.D. Report of an unusual B-cell lymphoma, probably arising from the perifollicular cells (marginal zone) of the spleen. Lab. Invest. 42:109, 1980.

PARAFOLLICULAR B CELL LYMPHOMA

SYNONYMS AND RELATED TERMS: Monocytoid B cell lymphoma.

Definition. This rare and recently recognized B cell lymphoma (Cousar et al.; Sheibani et al., 1986, 1988) resembles a distinctive B cell population that is particularly evident in reactive states such as toxoplasmic lymphadenitis. The term parafollicular B cell lymphoma emphasizes its morphologic and immunologic features and is more descriptive than the alternative monocytoid. Parafollicular B cells apparently have none of the structural, cytochemical, immunologic, or functional characteristics of monocytes; they resemble monocytes only by having abundant cytoplasm.

Clinical Features. Only a few cases have been reported. Patients have been adults with superficial adenopathy, without splenomegaly or marrow involvement. Both localized and generalized adenopathy has been described. One patient had retroperitoneal adenopathy, and one had rheumatoid arthritis. There are too few cases to predict the natural history or response to treatment. Transformation to a large cell type apparently may occur.

Pathological Features (Table 32). Nodal architecture was altered distinctively by a massive parafollicular and interfollicular infiltrate of lymphoid cells, often around hyperplastic, benign follicular centers (figs. 33-35). Neoplastic cells resemble those seen in toxoplasmic lymphadenitis (figs. 36, 37) and are larger than small lymphocytes. They have moderately abundant clear cytoplasm, round to slightly indented nuclei, and inconspicuous nucleoli (fig. 38). Plasmacytoid cells with PAS positive cytoplasmic globules may be present as well.

Parafollicular B cells by electron microscopy have abundant cytoplasm, interdigitating cytoplasmic borders, numerous granules, and glycogen. Other lymphocytes do not typically have granules or glycogen to the same extent.

Immunologic Features. The few cases reported have shown a monotypic SIg (μ, 2 cases; γ, 2 cases) and have reacted with CD20 and CD22. In one case, large plasmacytoid cells in the interfollicular infiltrate marked monotypically (weakly), with the same heavy and light chain (IgG-κ) detected on flow and FSIP in the predominant interfollicular component.

Differential Diagnosis. The differential diagnosis is the same as the one previously described for marginal zone lymphoma.

References

Cousar, J.B., McGinn, D.L., Glick, A.D., List, A.F., and Collins, R.D. Report of an unusual lymphoma arising from parafollicular B-lymphocytes (PBLs) or so-called "monocytoid" lymphocytes. Am. J. Clin. Pathol. 87:121-128, 1987.

Sheibani, K., Sohn, C.C., Burke, J.S., et al. Monocytoid B-cell lymphoma. Am. J. Pathol. 124:310-318, 1986.

_____ , Burke, J.S., Swartz, W.G., Nademanee, A., and Winberg, C.D. Monocytoid B-cell lymphoma. Clinicopathologic study of 21 cases of a unique type of low-grade lymphoma. Cancer 62:1531-1538, 1988.

Table 32

PARAFOLLICULAR B LYMPHOMA

PATTERN
• Hyperplastic, benign follicular centers, which may be obscured late in course by massive tumor growth • Massive parafollicular and interfollicular lymphocytic infiltrate extending into sinuses • No necrosis

CYTOLOGY — NEOPLASTIC	MARKERS — NEOPLASTIC

• Neoplastic cells are 2-3x size of small lympho-cytes, have small nuclei with condensed chromatin and abundant clear cytoplasm
 	
• Rare mitoses
 	
• Plasmacytoid neoplastic cells may be present, contain PAS (+) globules
	• Flow, FSIP: Monotypic SIg, few T cells
	  CD20, CD22 (+)
	  CDw75 (+)
	  CD74 (+)
	  CD19 (±)
	
	• PIP: Monotypic CIg

INVOLVED SITES	CLINICAL FEATURES
• Superficial nodes in the few reported cases Inguinal	• Only a few cases reported; probably low grade • Usually have superficial adenopathy without hepatosplenomegaly; adenopathy may be generalized • Bone marrow not involved

REACTIVE COMPONENTS	DIFFERENTIAL DIAGNOSIS
• Hyperplastic follicles	• Reactive (toxoplasmic) lymphadenitis • Malignant lymphoma, follicular center cell, small cleaved cell (follicular) • Hairy cell leukemia • Systemic mast cell disease

162

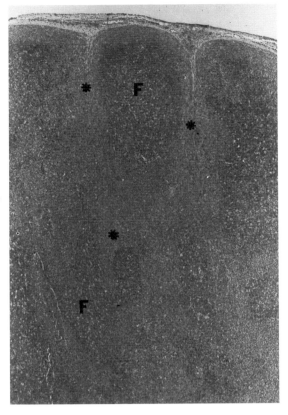

Figure 33
PARAFOLLICULAR B CELL LYMPHOMA, LYMPH NODE
In this illustration, the neoplastic infiltrate (*) is parafollicular, subcapsular, and interfollicular in distribution. Several hyperplastic follicular centers (F) are present. H&E. X20. (Fig. 1 from Cousar, J.B., McGinn, D.L., Glick, A.D., List, A.F., and Collins, R.D. Report of an unusual lymphoma arising from parafollicular B-lymphocytes (PBLs) or so-called "monocytoid" lymphocytes. Am. J. Clin. Pathol. 87:121-128, 1987.)

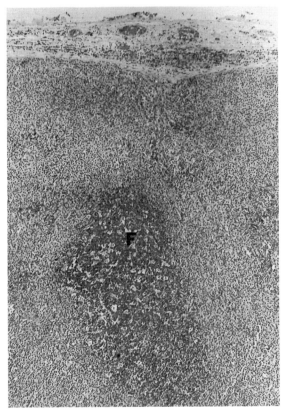

Figure 34
PARAFOLLICULAR B CELL LYMPHOMA, LYMPH NODE
Higher magnification demonstrates the parafollicular B cell lymphomatous infiltrate surrounding a hyperplastic follicle (F). H&E. X65. (Fig. 1 from Cousar, J.B., McGinn, D.L., Glick, A.D., List, A.F., and Collins, R.D. Report of an unusual lymphoma arising from parafollicular B-lymphocytes (PBLs) or so-called "monocytoid" lymphocytes. Am. J. Clin. Pathol. 87:121-128, 1987.)

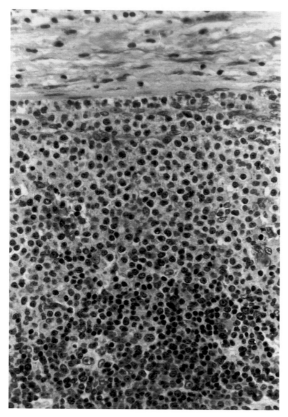

Figure 35
PARAFOLLICULAR B CELL LYMPHOMA, LYMPH NODE
Note the involvement of the subcapsular sinus by parafollicular B cells. Neoplastic cells appear to percolate through the mantle zone of a hyperplastic follicle. X260. (Fig. 2 from Cousar, J.B., McGinn, D.L., Glick, A.D., List, A.F., and Collins, R.D. Report of an unusual lymphoma arising from parafollicular B-lymphocytes (PBLs) or so-called "monocytoid" lymphocytes. Am. J. Clin. Pathol. 87:121-128, 1987.)

Figure 36
TOXOPLASMIC LYMPHADENITIS
Note the hyperplastic follicle with proliferation of parafollicular B cells (*). H&E. X160. (Fig. 3 from Cousar, J.B., McGinn, D.L., Glick, A.D., List, A.F., and Collins, R.D. Report of an unusual lymphoma arising from parafollicular B-lymphocytes (PBLs) or so-called "monocytoid" lymphocytes. Am. J. Clin. Pathol. 87:121-128, 1987.)

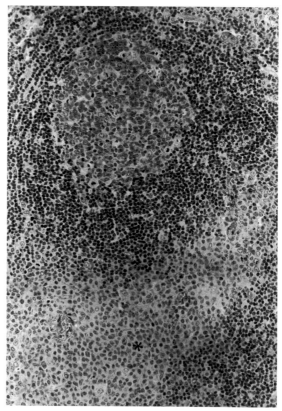

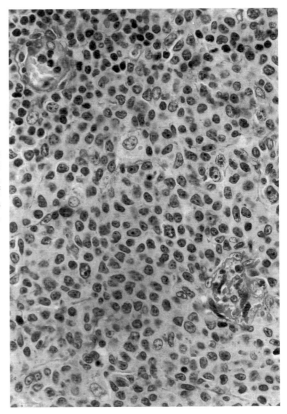

Figure 37
TOXOPLASMIC LYMPHADENITIS
Parafollicular B cells are small to medium sized, possess abundant clear cytoplasm, and contain slightly indented nuclei with indistinct nucleoli. H&E. X650. (Fig. 4 from Cousar, J.B., McGinn, D.L., Glick, A.D., List, A.F., and Collins, R.D. Report of an unusual lymphoma arising from parafollicular B-lymphocytes (PBLs) or so-called "monocytoid" lymphocytes. Am. J. Clin. Pathol. 87:121-128, 1987.)

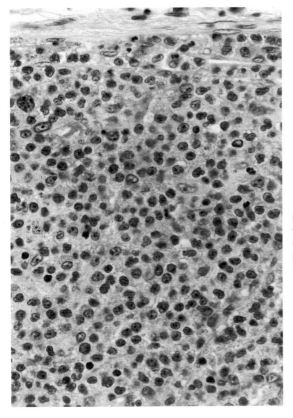

Figure 38
PARAFOLLICULAR B CELL LYMPHOMA, LYMPH NODE
These neoplastic parafollicular B cells are cytologically similar to those of toxoplasmic lymphadenitis. H&E. X650. (Fig. 4 from Cousar, J.B., McGinn, D.L., Glick, A.D., List, A.F., and Collins, R.D. Report of an unusual lymphoma arising from parafollicular B-lymphocytes (PBLs) or so-called "monocytoid" lymphocytes. Am. J. Clin. Pathol. 87:121-128, 1987.)

FOLLICULAR CENTER CELL LYMPHOMAS, INCLUDING BURKITT'S LYMPHOMA

SYNONYMS AND RELATED TERMS: Small Cleaved. Working Formulation: follicular or diffuse, small cleaved. Kiel: centrocytic; centroblastic-centrocytic. Rappaport: nodular, poorly differentiated lymphocytic; nodular, mixed lymphocytic-histiocytic; diffuse lymphocytic, poorly differentiated. **Large cleaved.** Working Formulation: follicular or diffuse, predominantly large cells. Kiel: centrocytic; centroblastic-centrocytic. Rappaport: nodular, histiocytic; diffuse mixed lymphocytic-histiocytic. **Small noncleaved** (includes Burkitt's and non-Burkitt's variants). Working Formulation: small noncleaved cell, Burkitt's, follicular areas. Kiel: malignant lymphoma lymphoblastic, Burkitt's type and other B lymphoblastic. Rappaport: undifferentiated, Burkitt's and non-Burkitt's. **Large noncleaved.** Working Formulation: follicular or diffuse, predominantly large cell or large noncleaved cell. Kiel: centroblastic. Rappaport: nodular, histiocytic; diffuse histiocytic with, without sclerosis.

Definition. Follicular center cell lymphomas comprise a complex group of malignant lymphomas usually arising from follicular (germinal) centers in the nodes, spleen, tonsil, and gut. Thus, they are of peripheral B cell origin. Follicular center cell lymphomas usually develop in superficial or retroperitoneal nodes but occasionally arise in extranodal sites such as the thyroid or stomach. The predominant cell in follicular center cell lymphomas may be of dormant (cleaved) or transformed (noncleaved) type. Overt plasmacytic differentiation is rare in either case.

Burkitt's lymphoma is a B cell neoplasm composed of small noncleaved follicular center cells. It is a distinct clinical pathologic entity and is reported in higher frequency in Africa. The Burkitt's subtype has a uniform nuclear size and configuration, whereas the non-Burkitt's subtype shows more variation in these features. Although immunologically similar, these two subtypes differ in pathogenesis and, to a certain extent, in clinical expression. For pathologic details, see Plates XXVII-XXXVI and figures 39-50.

Comment. The demonstration that lymphomas arise from follicular center cells was a key step in the modern approach to hematopathology (Lennert, 1969, 1973; Lukes and Collins). The distinctive histologic appearance of these lymphomas facilitated their initial recognition by light microscopy and subsequent evaluation by immunologic techniques. Because of their frequency and the relative precision with which they were recognized, we have a reasonable understanding of the full scope of these lymphomas and may be more thoughtful in our analysis of all lymphomas. Knowledge of the full range of the morphologic and clinical expression of follicular center cell lymphomas is the cornerstone of the practice of hematopathology.

The presumption is that B cells in follicular centers represent a single functional subpopulation that is responsible for producing, on stimulation, plasma cell precursors (fig. 39). Neoplasms of this lymphocyte subpopulation resemble their normal precursors structurally and functionally (fig. 40). The analysis of follicular center cell lymphomas has led to the following important conclusions: (1) The majority of non-Hodgkin's lymphomas are derived from follicular center cells. (2) Follicular center cell lymphomas may have a follicular or diffuse growth pattern or they may change from follicular to diffuse over time. Neoplastic follicular nodulation is a specific marker of these lymphomas; it has absolute immunologic specificity in marking a specific type of B cell process. (3) Lymphomas of varying histopathology, clinical expression, and prognosis may arise from a single functional subpopulation of

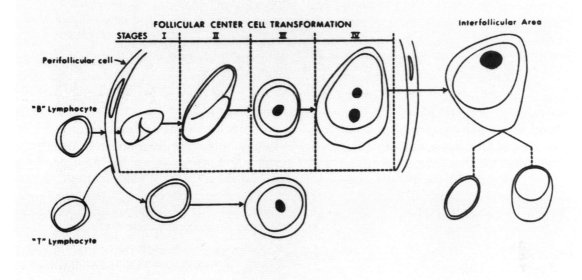

Figure 39
FOLLICULAR CENTER CELL CONCEPT
This is a schematic representation of the normal transformation of follicular center cells in comparison with the transformation of T cells. The scheme of Lukes-Collins is based on the observations of a large number of cases in which the morphological features of lymphomatous follicles seemed to fall into these four cytological groups that resemble counterparts in normal follicular centers. This proposal is at variance with the concept of Lennert, which is based mainly on experimental systems. (Fig. 2 from Lukes, R.J. and Collins, R.D. New approaches to the classification of the lymphomata. Br. J. Cancer 31[Suppl. 2]:1-28, 1975.)

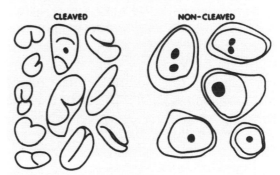

Figure 40
NORMAL FOLLICULAR CENTER CELLS,
CAMERA LUCIDA
Normal follicular center cells show a range in size and configuration of cleaved and noncleaved cells, as well as the amount of cytoplasm of the noncleaved cells. (Fig. 1 from Lukes, R.J. and Collins, R.D. New approaches to the classification of the lymphomata. Br. J. Cancer 31[Suppl. 2]:1-28, 1975.)

lymphocytes. Furthermore, follicular center cell lymphomas may change dramatically in histopathologic and clinical behavior due to the development of a high growth fraction. (4) Follicular center cell lymphomas rarely show significant plasma cell differentiation, although plasma cell precursors are produced in vivo in follicular centers. Tumorous accumulations of dormant nondividing small lymphocytic populations is a feature of cleaved follicular center cell processes, presumably by slow entry from a dividing pool, and there may be few neoplastic plasma cells in these tumors. There may also be slight evidence of plasmacytic differentiation in the rapidly growing processes. Neither of these groups of patients has clinical manifestations of paraproteinemia. (5) In general, the clinical behavior and histologic features of the follicular center cell lymphomas reflect the biologic characteristics of their normal cytologic counterparts. The lymphomas of the non-cleaved cells have a high proliferative and turnover rate, a diffuse histologic pattern, and a rapidly progressive course. Clinically, they are manifested by rapidly enlarging masses and aggressive symptomatic disease with short median survival. The small cleaved lymphomas are usually manifested by some degree of attempted follicle formation and slow progression. The small cleaved cells exhibit little cellular cohesion, may be found in the peripheral blood, and account for the widespread seeding of the marrow, spleen, and liver, possibly as a result of the normal homing of B cells to these sites. The small cleaved cell lymphoma is a slowly progressive disease with median survival often in excess of 5 years. (6) Consistent karyotypic abnormalities have been described in some types of follicular center cell lymphomas.

In summary, the analysis of follicular center cell lymphomas has provided a framework for understanding malignant lymphomas in general. It is apparent from these studies that malignant lymphomas of a completely different histopathologic appearance and clinical behavior may arise from a single functioning subpopulation of lymphocytes. Similar variations in the expression of other hematopoietic neoplasms may be expected. Furthermore, there is a direct correlation between the appearance and behavior of many follicular center cell lymphomas. We may anticipate refinement in our prognostic indicators as we broaden our analysis of lymphomas to include lymphocyte functional characteristics in addition to our present structural descriptions. Although the histopathologic appearance of some follicular center cell lymphomas is distinctive and specific as to cytologic and immunologic type, some prognostic indicators may require functional analyses as well as histopathology. Specific chromosomal abnormalities may delineate subpopulations of patients with variations in pathogenesis or prognosis.

Cell Types. Small cleaved cells are approximately the size of red cells. There is irregularity of the nuclei, dense nuclear chromatin, and very little cytoplasm, and the nuclei are elongated, indented, and clefted. Nucleoli are small or not apparent (plate XXVII-C,D).

Large cleaved cells are definitely larger than red cells. Nuclei may be very irregular and dysplastic, with clefting, nuclear protrusions, or considerable elongation. Chromatin is more dispersed than in the small cleaved cell type. Small nucleoli are present, and small amounts of cytoplasm may be seen (plate XXXI-D,E).

Small noncleaved cells are about the size of histiocytic or endothelial nuclei. Nuclear chromatin is less condensed than in cleaved cells, and several nucleoli are apparent. Cytoplasm is detectable, particularly on MGP stains (plate XXXII-A–C).

Large noncleaved cells are larger than endothelial or histiocytic nuclei and have small prominent nucleoli, often at the nuclear membrane. Nuclear chromatin is fine, and cytoplasm is abundant, particularly on MGP stains (plates XXXV-B,C; XXXVI-B).

Growth Pattern. These lymphomas may show marked variation in growth patterns (figs. 41, 42).

Discrete follicular growth exhibits follicles that are distinct and clearly defined from adjacent tissue. Lymphoid mantles may be present, and minimal infiltration of the capsule or the interfollicular areas may be demonstrated.

Infiltrative follicular growth yields follicles that are generally distinct, but some may be blurred. The follicular mantle is often absent. Infiltration of follicular center cells, either focal or widespread, should be demonstrated in the interfollicular areas, capsule, fat, or vessels. Capsular infiltration is the rule with this growth pattern.

Vague follicular growth produces follicles that are vague, indistinct, and may be apparent only under low magnification or when accentuated by PAS stains. Areas of diffuse growth are present. Marked infiltration of interfollicular areas, vessels, capsule, or fat may be demonstrated.

Minimal follicular growth has only a few follicles present in portions of the node. Growth is mostly diffuse and often of noncleaved cells.

Diffuse growth does not exhibit follicular nodulation in any section.

Histopathologic Features. The production of neoplastic follicular nodules is a specific marker of follicular center cell lymphomas (plates XXVII-A; XXVIII-C; XXIX-C; XXXI-B; figs. 43-45). Follicular nodules may be accepted as neoplastic if cleaved cells are present in excess and produce a monomorphic appearance; abnormal crowding and dysplastic features are often demonstrated by these cells as well (plate XXVII-C). The diagnosis of lymphoma may often be substantiated by demonstrating homogeneous infiltrates of cleaved cells in the interfollicular area (plate XXVII-C), into vessels or through the subcapsular sinus into adjacent soft tissue (plate XXVIII-A). Mitoses and macrophages are usually rare, and transformed cells are infrequent (plates XXVII-D; XXX-A). Rarely, follicular nodules contain a homogeneous population of transformed cells (fig. 44).

Neoplastic follicular nodules are usually found back-to-back across the section in association with marked distortion of nodal architecture (plates XXVII-A; XXXI-B; fig. 45). Similar nodules often extend into the pericapsular fat. Extensive infiltration of the interfollicular area may be associated with indistinct follicular nodules, with only a few nodules remaining in some cases. Careful low magnification examination of PAS stained sections may be required to recognize vague or focal neoplastic follicles.

Diffuse processes may be recognized as follicular center cell in origin if there is a significant population of neoplastic-appearing cleaved cells. In some cases, only cleaved cells will be present, but most diffuse processes show frequent transformed cells (plate XXXV-D). Diffuse processes are much more difficult to recognize with assurance as follicular center cell lymphomas than those with follicular

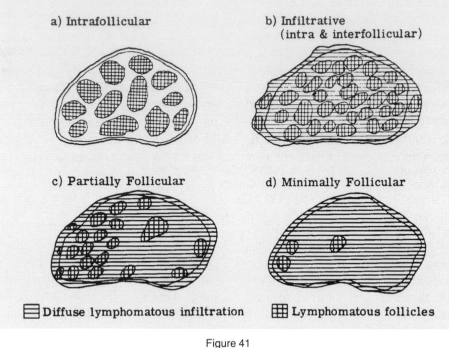

Figure 41
FOLLICULAR CENTER CELL LYMPHOMAS, GROWTH PATTERNS
Variations in follicular pattern in follicular center cell lymphomas are illustrated in this figure.

nodulation. The postulated relationship between growth patterns and cytological types of follicular center cell lymphomas is shown in figure 42.

Follicular center cell lymphomas often deviate in histopathology from the typical appearance. The many factors involved in this variation include: (1) change from a follicular to diffuse growth pattern; (2) sclerosing pattern or deposition of amorphous hyaline material; (3) change in predominant cell from cleaved to noncleaved type; (4) marked dysplasia and multinucleation of neoplastic cells; (5) cytoplasmic inclusions of immunoglobulin, plasmacytic differentiation; (6) massive necrosis; (7) partial involvement of node or spleen; and (8) development of composite neoplasms.

The loss of a follicular growth pattern occurs in approximately 80 percent of the follicular lymphomas by the time of autopsy. In fact, 22 of 30 sequential biopsies were reported by Wright to have lost the follicular pattern. Sclerosing lymphomas (other than Hodgkin's disease) are almost always follicular center cell in type, although they were initially viewed as a distinct neoplasm. Sclerosis may be so extensive that the neoplastic lymphoid component is obscured (plate XXXI-A–C). There are many different patterns of sclerosis with intrafollicular and perifollicular deposits noted (figs. 46, 47). PAS positivity may be intense. In addition to connective tissue deposition, other cases with amorphous hyaline material have been described.

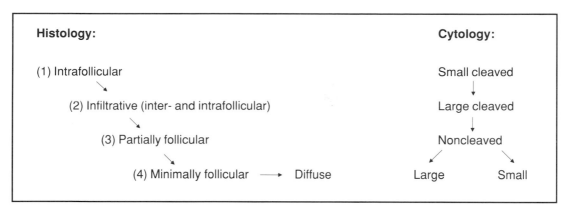

Figure 42
FOLLICULAR CENTER CELL LYMPHOMAS
The postulated relationship of the histologic pattern and cytologic types of follicular center cell lymphomas is schematized. (Fig. 4 from Lukes, R.J. and Collins, R.D. New approaches to the classification of the lymphomata. Br. J. Cancer 31[Suppl. 2]:1-28, 1975.)

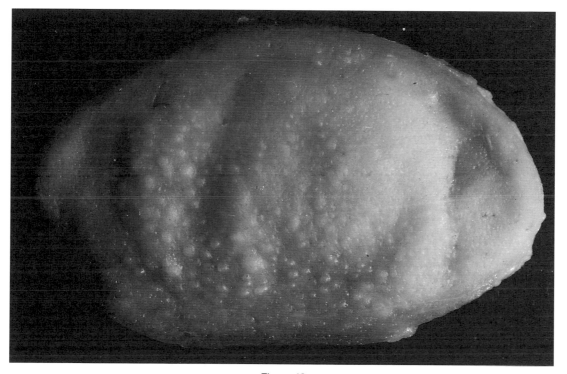

Figure 43
FOLLICULAR CENTER CELL LYMPHOMA, NODE
In this figure, a node measuring 4 cm in greatest dimension shows follicular nodulation of the cut surface. This node was fixed in formalin before photography.

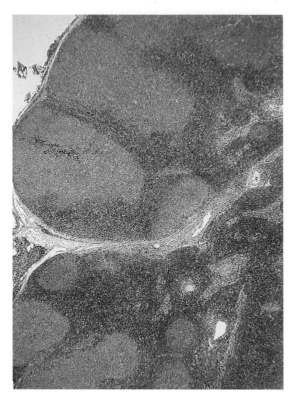

Figure 44
(Figure 44 and plate XXXVI-A,B are from the same patient)
FOLLICULAR CENTER CELL LYMPHOMA, LARGE
NONCLEAVED CELL, LYMPH NODE
This case shows partial node involvement with large, pale, neoplastic follicular nodules under the capsule and an uninvolved medullary area. Large noncleaved cell lymphomas occasionally present with follicular nodulation. X20.

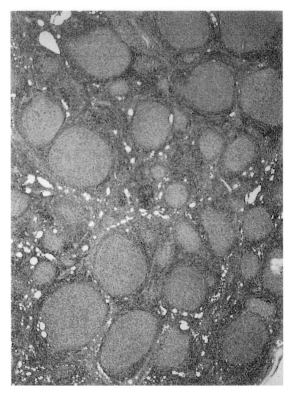

Figure 45
FOLLICULAR CENTER CELL LYMPHOMA, LARGE
CLEAVED CELL, LYMPH NODE
A lymph node at low magnification shows back-to-back pale follicular nodules with complete alteration of the nodal architecture. X25.

Rarely, follicular center cell lymphomas contain PAS positive extracellular material (often in follicular nodules) that may be mistaken for amyloid. Many follicular center cell lymphomas with sclerosis involve the retroperitoneum and inguinal nodes. Retroperitoneal masses in older adults frequently represent sclerosing follicular center cell lymphomas. Judicious biopsies with node sampling may be required in these cases to establish the diagnosis because superficial biopsies often show essentially acellular connective tissue.

A change in the predominant cell has been reported in approximately 34 percent of cases at autopsy and in 42 percent in sequential biopsies. Marked dysplasia of follicular center cell lymphomas with multinucleated cells resembling Reed-Sternberg cells has been repeatedly described. Large cells may be present singly in predominantly cleaved cell processes or in large numbers (plate XXVII-D).

Approximately 5 percent of the follicular lymphomas exhibit recognizable plasmacytic differentiation with plasma cells between, and often within, the follicles. Monoclonal paraproteins may be identified

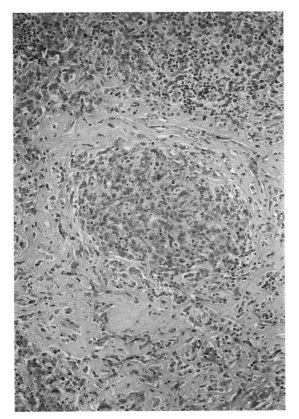

Figure 46
FOLLICULAR CENTER CELL LYMPHOMA, LARGE
CLEAVED CELL, LYMPH NODE
A lymphomatous nodule is surrounded by dense, eosinophilic connective tissue. This sclerosing feature is
often seen in follicular center cell lymphomas of the large
cleaved cell type. H&E. X140.

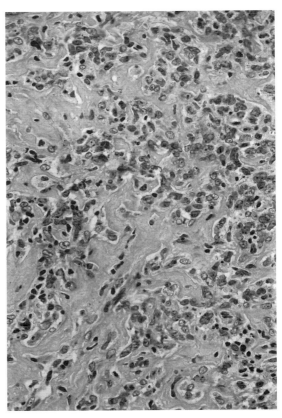

Figure 47
FOLLICULAR CENTER CELL LYMPHOMA, LARGE
CLEAVED CELL, LYMPH NODE
A higher magnification shows the large cleaved cells
interspersed in the sclerotic tissue with some areas virtu-
ally free of lymphocytes. H&E. X280.

in some of these patients. Because reactive plasma cells are also present in follicular lymphomas, immunophenotypic studies
are required to determine if the plasma
cells are part of the neoplastic process.
Another type of immunoglobulin accumulation present in approximately 10 percent of
the follicular lymphomas includes nuclear
and/or cytoplasmic inclusions in follicular
center cells. Associated plasmacytic differentiation may or may not be present. The
cytoplasmic inclusions may be small and
multiple or massive, with single globules

that give the cells a signet-ring appearance. Most reported cases of "signet-ring
cell" lymphomas have been follicular lymphomas. Cases with eosinophilic PAS
positive inclusions have been associated
with IgM, and those with clear vacuolated
cytoplasm have been associated with IgG.
The nuclear inclusions are usually single.
Massive necrosis, probably due to isch-
emia, occasionally occurs in follicular center cell lymphomas. Necrosis may involve
most of the node. The capsule is usually
intact and often contains a few neoplastic

lymphocytes. In distinction, necrosis in other lymphomas is often focal. Partial involvement of the nodes and spleen has been noted (rarely) in a variety of biopsy or staging procedures. Partial involvement is noteworthy because it may result in a mixture of benign and neoplastic follicular structures and is often unrecognized. Neoplastic follicles may be diagnosed by their homogeneity in comparison to the adjacent reactive structures.

Many patients presenting with cleaved follicular center cell lymphomas have evidence of marrow involvement (plate XXIX-A) or liver involvement (plate XXIX-B). Extranodal presentations of follicular center cell lymphomas are frequent (plates XXXII-A,B; XXXV-A).

Coincidental carcinomas have been noted at Vanderbilt University, but case numbers have been inadequate to determine significance. We have had three patients with follicular center cell lymphoma who developed a simultaneous lymphoma of transformed T lymphocytes and two patients who developed malignant histiocytosis.

Bone Marrow and Peripheral Blood Involvement. Follicular center cell lymphomas frequently involve the marrow and peripheral blood. Approximately 80 percent of the small cleaved cell type and small noncleaved cell type neoplasms show marrow lesions (plate XXIX-A). Peripheral blood involvement ("lymphosarcoma cell leukemia") has been recognized for years when the leukemic phase was massive, and most patients with small cleaved cell processes have circulating tumor cells. Marrow lesions are usually similar cytologically to the nodes, although proportionally more cleaved cells may be found in the marrow. Some patients with

large noncleaved cell type lymphomas in the nodes will have peritrabecular marrow lesions composed almost exclusively of small cleaved cell type. This process may be confused with prolymphocytic leukemia when there is extensive peripheral blood involvement by the lymphoma.

The surface immunoglobulin present on marrow and peripheral blood neoplastic cells is identical to that on the nodal material. The amount of surface immunoglobulin is typically greater than in small B cell neoplasms (including chronic lymphocytic leukemia).

Transformation of Small Cleaved Cell Changing to Noncleaved Lymphoma. The duration from diagnosis to transformation in various series has ranged from 8 to 120 months (with a mean of 52 months). The incidence of evolution is difficult to assess, but in our experience, cytologic transformation has occurred in 40 percent of the patients with follicular center cell lymphomas of small cleaved cell type.

Transformation was characterized by new or persistent adenopathy, visceral disease, or marrow involvement. A leukemic phase occurs rarely and may be confused with acute leukemia. Despite aggressive chemotherapy, median survival after transformation averages 7 months (with a range of <1 month to 23 months).

Transformation may be seen in the nodes, marrow, and extranodal tissue (plate XXIX-D). Histopathologically, most cases at transformation demonstrated a diffuse lymphoma composed of uniform large noncleaved follicular center cells (plate XXX-B–D) with scattered small cleaved cells, and rarely is there extreme lobation or marked nuclear irregularity. This uniform morphology is in contrast to other B cell neoplasms (small B cell neoplasms, plasmacytoid lymphocytic lymphoma, and multiple myeloma) undergoing transformation in which a pleomorphic pattern with bizarre large cells is common. In some cases, follicular small cleaved cell type lymphomas evolve into a diffuse small noncleaved cell lymphoma similar to Burkitt's lymphoma.

Several studies have demonstrated the monotypic B cell nature of these diffuse large cell lymphomas. In some cases, immunologic studies have been performed on the small cleaved cells before transformation and on the large cells after the morphologic change. The surface immunoglobulin class remained constant before and after transformation.

Mixed Types of Lymphoma in the Working Formulation

Our concepts of mixed cell lymphoma have changed since Rappaport and colleagues described it as mixed cell type (lymphocytic and reticulum cell) occurring in either nodular or diffuse histologic patterns. This lymphomatous proliferation was considered to be a combination of two separate neoplastic cell types, the lymphocyte and reticulum cell, without either cell type predominating, but with a common origin in an undifferentiated lymphoma cell. In the First Series Fascicle (Rappaport), this lymphoma was termed mixed cell, histiocytic-lymphocytic, and described as a mixture of atypical histiocytes and poorly differentiated lymphocytes, with the histiocytic component equivalent to reticulum cell sarcoma. The atypical histiocytes varied widely in size and shape presumably related to the degree of differentiation. The mixed cell type usually exhibited a nodular histologic pattern, but rarely retained the mixed composition in its diffuse form.

The mixed cell type reappeared in the Working Formulation as follicular mixed, small cleaved and large cell in the low grade clinical group, and as diffuse mixed, small and large cell in the intermediate grade. The follicular mixed, small cleaved and large cell designation was created for those cases with a follicular histologic pattern without a preponderance of either small or large cells. The large cells were described as having cleaved or noncleaved nuclei which are commonly two or three times the size of a lymphocyte nucleus. These nuclei have a vesicular appearance with two or three nucleoli often on the nuclear membrane. The large cells as described closely resemble noncleaved follicular center cells.

According to Mann and Berard, there has been discrepancy among pathologists in applying the follicular mixed type of the Working Formulation. This difficulty in classification has led to conflicting data on the response to therapy and survival reported from large treatment centers. It seems likely that even greater classification problems will be encountered with diffuse mixed cell type. Depending on their background and experience, pathologists might erroneously include a variety of cytologic types in the diffuse mixed cell type. The mixed type presents a special problem in classification because all lymphomas in our experience are comprised of a mixture of cells. There are varying numbers of T cells in most B cell lymphomas, and variations in cell size and configuration in most T cell lymphomas. The presence of numerous reactive histiocytes in T cell lymphomas is an additional complicating feature.

Mann and Berard believed that the follicular mixed classification problem resulted from an increase in the number of large cells in the follicles. In an attempt to bring precision and reproducibility to the classification of follicular mixed lymphoma, Mann and Berard proposed counting the large cells within the lymphomatous follicular centers. They suggested examining 20 fields using 10X ocular and 40X objective lenses, and if 5 to 15 large neoplastic cells (noncleaved cells) are found per magnification field, a lymphoma with a follicular pattern would qualify as follicular mixed lymphoma. If less than 5 large cells are identified, the case is classified as a follicular small cleaved; if more than 15 large cells are found, the case is classified as follicular large cell. No guidelines were provided for classifying the diffuse mixed type.

From our experience with follicular center cell lymphomas, it is likely that at least two of our follicular center cell types (the small cleaved follicular center cell with increased numbers of noncleaved follicular center cells and the large cleaved follicular center cell type) may be included in the follicular mixed category, thereby accounting for the problem with this classification. In the early 1970s, we appreciated the difficulty of classifying increased numbers of large cells in lymphomatous follicular centers. In cases with sequential biopsies, we noted that the number of noncleaved follicular center cells might remain fairly constant over long periods of time. Progression was usually noted clinically and pathologically only when solid "colony-like" aggregates of noncleaved follicular center cells were found. As a result, in our approach, cases are classified as follicular, small cleaved cell until the number of noncleaved follicular center cells exceeds 25 percent per high magnification field. A diagnosis of noncleaved follicular center cell is ideally based on a dominance of noncleaved cells or the presence of homogeneous aggregates of noncleaved cells. Data from the international study (The Non-Hodgkin's Lymphoma Classification Project) that provided the foundation for the Working Formulation has supported our approach. All of the cases with follicular or follicular and diffuse patterns of the small cleaved follicular center cell type were identified as "Lukes cases" and classified using our approach. The median survival for small cleaved follicular center cell, follicular and small cleaved follicular center cell, follicular and diffuse was 7.3 and 6.2 years, respectively. These results are not significantly different from the median survival of 7.2 years for the 259 cases that were used as the basis of the Working Formulation, in which 10 cases were apparently moved out and placed in the follicular mixed, small cleaved and large cell group. From these data it seems that the problem with the diagnosis of follicular mixed lymphoma is not the increased number of noncleaved follicular center cells, but the failure to consider another large cell group, the large cleaved cell type of follicular lymphoma.

The large cleaved cell type in the Lukes-Collins approach closely resembles a reactive follicle having both a lymphocytic mantle and a center of variable cellular composition. The latter exhibits a range in nuclear size and configuration and includes both small and large cleaved and noncleaved follicular center cells, most being larger than the tingible body macrophage nucleus. The large cleaved nucleus is commonly elongated, bent, curved, or cleaved (fig. 48). Mitoses are usually frequent and considerably more numerous than in the small cleaved follicular center

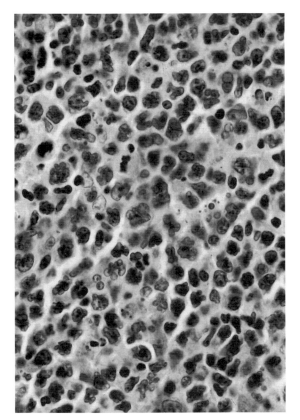

Figure 48
FOLLICULAR CENTER CELL LYMPHOMA, LARGE
CLEAVED CELL, LYMPH NODE
This high magnification photograph shows the very
irregular, polyploid, hyperlobated appearance of large
cleaved cells. A few small cells are also present, particularly at the bottom of the figure. H&E. X565.

cell type. The variable follicular center cell
population is commonly situated in an acidophilic intercellular matrix that results in
the follicular centers presenting a "pink,"
appearance in contrast to the blue of the
small cleaved follicular center cell follicles.
This pink intercellular material stains for
acid mucopolysaccharide, and it is also
found in cases without a follicular histologic pattern often in association with varying degrees of sclerosis. From our experience, evidence of these cytologic features
together with the "pink" appearance of the

follicles facilitates identification of large
cleaved follicular center cell type and
makes its recognition much simpler than
is the case with the controversial mixed
cell, follicular of the Working Formulation.

**Extranodal Follicular Center Cell
Lymphomas**. The cytologic subtypes of
nodal follicular center cell lymphomas
are found in similar lymphomas originating
in extranodal sites. Follicular center cell
lymphomas arising in lymphoid tissue
other than the nodes (e.g., gastrointestinal
tract, spleen) are also similar to nodal
processes. The same general criteria
for the diagnosis of follicular center cell
lymphomas apply to both nodal and
extranodal processes. Follicular nodulation per se in extranodal biopsies does
not force the diagnosis of a benign reactive process. Lymphomas with follicular
nodulation occur in virtually all non-nodal
tissues, and residual benign follicular
structures are often seen in association
with overt lymphoma. In fact, it is likely
that most extranodal lymphomas develop
in sites of prolonged immunologic stimulation. For example, in the thyroid, there is
evidence that most of the lymphomas are
follicular center cell in type and that they
arise in a setting of Hashimoto's thyroiditis.

**Immunologic and Karyotypic Fea-
tures.** Most follicular center cell lymphomas of all types may be readily shown to
represent clonal B cell proliferations by
use of anti-B cell antisera in flow studies,
by finding monotypic surface/cytoplasmic
immunoglobulin, or by showing that clonal
immunoglobulin gene rearrangements
have occurred. Occasionally, follicular
center cell lymphomas lack a demonstrable
population of light chain class-restricted
B cells in cell suspension studies due
to numerous polyclonal interfollicular B

cells or undetectable surface/cytoplasmic immunoglobulin.

With paraffin immunoperoxidase, follicular center cells usually show distinct marking with CDw75, whether in follicular nodules (plate XXVIII-D) or growing diffusely (plates XXXIV-D; XXXVI-C). CD74 may mark large noncleaved cells (plate XXXVI-D). The distribution of T cells is particularly apparent with the pan-T antibody CD45RO (plate XXVIII-E).

Cleaved cell lymphomas are usually CD10 positive (common acute lymphocytic leukemia antigen) and CD5 negative. Cleaved cell lymphomas usually express IgM ± IgD or IgG with a smaller number of IgA-positive cases. "Centrocytic" type cleaved cell lymphomas (Lennert, 1981) are CD10 negative and often CD5 positive. IgM ± IgD is almost always the type of immunoglobulin expressed. Follicles occasionally present in these lymphomas may be polyclonal in frozen section immunoperoxidase studies.

Small noncleaved cell malignant lymphomas usually express SIgM and are CD5 negative. Cytoplasmic immunoglobulin may be present, and CD10 positivity is reported in 50 to 100 percent of the cases. Large noncleaved malignant lymphomas, in contrast to cleaved follicular center cell lymphomas, are more likely to be SIg negative and less likely to be CD10 positive. The type of immunoglobulin expressed includes IgM, IgD, IgG, and IgA. CD5 positivity is generally not identified. CIg is present in 90 percent of the cases.

Reactive T cells are often numerous (20-30 percent) and sometimes predominate in cleaved cell lymphomas (plate XXVIII-E). The T cells have a normal T helper to T suppressor ratio. In follicular lymphomas, frozen section immunoperoxidase studies show that the majority of T cells are located in the interfollicular area. Neoplastic follicles from patients with HIV infection may contain more CD8 positive cells than most reactive follicles. Large noncleaved malignant lymphoma contains approximately 10 percent T cells. Small noncleaved malignant lymphoma has very few admixed T cells.

Cytogenetic studies show that up to 85 percent of all follicular lymphomas have a characteristic t(14;18) translocation; all follicular small cleaved cell types have this karyotypic abnormality. Diffuse lymphomas with this translocation are much less common, are reported to be of large cell type, and at least some have a prior history of follicular lymphoma. Numerous other recurrent chromosomal defects have been described in follicular lymphomas. Some are associated with an increased number of large noncleaved cells, a leukemic blood picture, and/or a poor prognosis. The t(8;14) (q24;q32) is characteristic of B cell lymphomas of small noncleaved cell types, but translocations with chromosome 14 may also occur with chromosomes 2 and 22.

Differential Diagnosis. The difficulties in diagnosing follicular center cell lymphomas may be grouped into three general categories: (1) differentiation of follicular center cell lymphoma from exuberant follicular hyperplasia; (2) categorization of follicular center cell lymphomas in terms of growth pattern and predominant cell; and (3) separation of follicular center cell lymphomas from other lymphomas.

Histopathologic features favoring follicular center cell lymphomas include architectural effacement with numerically increased, crowded follicles detected throughout the node; monomorphic follicular centers with excessively homogeneous populations of cleaved or transformed cells; and infiltration of cleaved follicular center cells into interfollicular areas or capsules. The presence of benign follicular centers does not exclude follicular center cell lymphoma, because nodes may show partial involvement in lymphoma (fig. 44). Follicle size and shape are not reliable diagnostic criteria for malignancy nor is the presence or absence of the mantle layer. In cases suspected to be follicular center cell lymphomas, individual follicles from several areas must be examined cytologically. If diagnostic changes are not revealed, the interfollicular area, capsule, and sinuses must be examined for invasion by follicular center cells. Plasma cells in large numbers in follicular processes usually indicate a benign state. However, approximately 5 percent of follicular lymphomas contain numerous plasma cells that may be differentiated components of the neoplastic proliferation.

Follicular center cell lymphomas should be called follicular (nodular) if an interfollicular infiltrate is not present, and follicular and diffuse if any neoplastic follicles are detected. Some follicular center cell lymphomas are essentially diffuse in growth, and neoplastic follicular nodulation may be focal or indistinct. Designation of cell type in follicular center cell lymphomas is somewhat arbitrary, controversial, and judgmental. MGP stains highlight noncleaved follicular center cells and aid in estimating their number. Lymphomas are diagnosed as the large noncleaved type if aggregates of large cells are detected or if their percentage is estimated at greater than 25 percent. Differentiation between small and large cleaved cells may be very difficult if formalin fixation causes artifactual changes, or quite

easy if the large cleaved cells are dysplastic. Such differentiation may not be clinically significant because there is evidence that large cleaved cell lymphomas are also indolent processes.

Follicular center cell lymphomas may be confused with Hodgkin's disease if there is extensive sclerosis, if the neoplastic follicles are not recognized, and if transformed follicular center cells are mistaken for Reed-Sternberg cells. Follicular center cell lymphomas may be misdiagnosed as peripheral T cell lymphomas because of the former's high content of reacting T cells, occasional intermixed macrophages, and small population of transformed B cells. Paraffin immunoperoxidase or gene rearrangement studies are helpful in these cases in recognizing the neoplastic follicular center cell component.

CENTROCYTIC LYMPHOMA

Lennert (1981) has used the term "centrocytic lymphoma" to refer to a type of follicular center cell lymphoma. His reasons for considering centrocytic lymphoma as a distinct entity are given essentially verbatim in the following sections from his 1981 book.

Definition. Centrocytic lymphoma is derived from the centrocytes of germinal centers. Thus, it is always a B cell lymphoma. The tumor consists exclusively of centrocytes and contains no centroblasts. In this definition, the Kiel classification differs from that of Lukes and Collins, who apply the term "cleaved follicular center cell lymphoma" to all lymphomas that consist chiefly of centrocytes, irrespective of whether there is an admixture of centroblasts. In centrocytic lymphomas, there are also virtually no lymphocytes among the tumor cells, and immunologic analysis reveals a correspondingly small number of T lymphocytes. In our opinion, these features are important in differential diagnosis and in determining the nature of the disease.

Histology. Even at a low magnification, it is possible to make a tentative diagnosis of centrocytic lymphoma on Giemsastained slides: there is a monotonous proliferation of small to, at most, medium sized cells whose nuclei show weaker (grayer) staining than do those of chronic lymphocytic leukemia or immunocytoma. The nuclei are also irregularly shaped and occasionally cleaved. The cytoplasm of the tumor cells shows practically no staining with Giemsa. There are no blasts (basophilic cells) of any type, including centroblasts. The number of mitotic figures varies from case to case. The tumor cells are interspersed with a small number of reticulum cells, mostly of the dendritic and histiocytic types. In occasional cases, there are some reactive plasma cells (PIP immunostaining reveals both κ-positive and λ-positive cells), especially near small blood vessels with hyalinized walls.

The reticulin fibers are usually thick and form a coarse alveolar network that surrounds large solid groups of tumor cells. Band-forming sclerosis or a diffuse increase in fibers is also found occasionally. The growth patterns are usually diffuse, as can be seen with silver impregnation. In occasional cases, however, there is a vaguely, or even a markedly, nodular pattern (we avoid using the term "follicular" to emphasize the fact that not all components of germinal centers are present in centrocytic lymphoma).

The neoplasia appears to begin within or around (pre-existent) germinal centers. In any event, newly infiltrated lymph nodes often show a wide mantle of centrocytes around residual germinal centers. The centrocytes in the germinal centers are isomorphic, with the tumor cells outside.

It might be helpful to distinguish a small cell and a large cell ("anaplastic") type of centrocytic lymphoma, although the borderline between the two types would not be distinct.

Prognosis. Centrocytic lymphoma shows a much poorer prognosis than chronic lymphocytic lymphoma B, LP immunocytoma, and centroblastic-centrocytic lymphoma. The median survival time of 45 patients studied by the Kiel Lymphoma Study Group was 48 months.

FOLLICULAR CENTER CELL LYMPHOMAS, SMALL CLEAVED CELL TYPE

Clinical Features. Small cleaved follicular center cell lymphoma is the most common lymphoid malignancy in the United States and constitutes 20 to 30 percent of all such tumors.

Patients are usually 50 to 60 years of age, with males affected slightly more frequently than females. The usual presentation is asymptomatic peripheral lymph node enlargement, but the vast majority of the patients on initial staging have advanced disease, with involvement of bone marrow in 60 to 80 percent, liver in approximately 20 percent, and lung or pleura in approximately 10 percent of the patients.

Although this disease is usually disseminated at diagnosis, the natural history is indolent in spite of the presence of active and disseminated disease. Asymptomatic individuals, if initially untreated, may be expected to remain asymptomatic for approximately 3 to 4 years before therapy is considered necessary. The average life expectancy is approximately 7 to 10 years, with survival in excess of 10 years in some patients in whom initial therapy was withheld. Progression of the disease to a noncleaved lymphoma occurs in 40 percent of the patients and is accompanied by a poor response to subsequent therapy.

Histopathologic Features (Table 33). The growth pattern is follicular in 75 to 80 percent of the cases, and there is clear infiltration of small cleaved cells into the interfollicular areas and capsule in most of these cases. Partial nodal involvement occasionally occurs, as evidenced by coexisting benign and malignant follicles. Massive necrosis is occasionally observed, presumably due to vascular involvement.

Follicular and interfollicular infiltrates are typically homogeneous, with only scattered macrophages, mitoses, and noncleaved cells. Some follicular small cleaved cell lymphomas contain 5 to 10 percent large noncleaved cells, a number that may remain stable for several years in subsequent biopsies (plate XXVII-D). Transformation to a higher-grade lymphoma is most easily recognized when discrete aggregates or masses of large noncleaved cells develop (plate XXX-B–D).

FOLLICULAR CENTER CELL LYMPHOMAS, LARGE CLEAVED CELL TYPE

Clinical Features. Large cleaved cell lymphomas account for approximately 5 percent of the lymphoid malignancies in the United States and 10 percent of the follicular center cell lymphomas. The mean age is approximately 50 years, with males comprising about 60 percent of the patient population.

Common modes of presentation include peripheral lymphadenopathy, but "B" symptoms occur in approximately 20 percent of these patients. Some patients present with retroperitoneal masses. Lymphadenopathy is expected on physical examination, but splenomegaly and/or hepatomegaly may also be apparent. Gastrointestinal or retroperitoneal involvement may be indicated by palpable abdominal masses.

A full staging evaluation reveals widely disseminated disease in many patients. Bone marrow involvement has been reported in 30 percent, and a similar percentage of patients have gastrointestinal tract disease.

Optimal therapy in the disease is not yet clearly defined. Stein and associates have recently presented evidence that this lymphoma may be more indolent in clinical behavior than indicated by the Working Formulation categorization as an intermediate grade lymphoma.

Histopathologic Features (Table 34). The growth patterns are follicular in 40 to 50 percent of the cases and are often mixed with areas of diffuse growth (figs. 45, 46). Sclerosis is a prominent part of the low magnification appearance and may be distributed in a follicular, perifollicular, or apparently random distribution (plate XXXI-A,B; figs. 46, 47). When follicular in distribution, sclerosis may facilitate the recognition of these lymphomas, whereas other patterns may obscure the underlying follicular center cell lymphoma.

Large cleaved cells show an impressive range in nuclear size and configuration (fig. 48). Dysplastic cells are often apparent in well-prepared material. MGP or Giemsa stains facilitate the differentiation of large cleaved from large noncleaved cells; the latter have distinct cytoplasm and nucleoli.

Table 33

FOLLICULAR CENTER CELL, SMALL CLEAVED CELL TYPE

PATTERN	

	• Follicular in 75-80 percent of the cases
	   Infiltrative
	   Partial
	   Minimal
	
	• Diffuse in 20-25 percent of the cases
	
	• Perinodal extension frequent
	
	• Sclerosis may be seen

CYTOLOGY — NEOPLASTIC	MARKERS — NEOPLASTIC

• Scant cytoplasm; nuclei range in size from small lymphocyte up to size of histiocyte nucleus; nuclei are irregular, angulated, indented, may have deep cleavage planes
 	
• Cleaved follicular center cell: MGP (–); Giemsa (–)
 	
• Noncleaved follicular center cell: MGP (+); Giemsa basophilic cytoplasm
 	
• Large noncleaved vary in number; >5, <15/hpf: mixed in WF
	• Flow, FSIP: SIg monoclonal in 90 percent of the cases; CD10 (+), CD5 (–), most cases
	
	• PIP:
	   CIg (±)
	   CD20 (+)
	   CDw75 (+)
	
	• Typically have 14;18 translocation

INVOLVED SITES	CLINICAL FEATURES

• Lymph nodes, generalized adenopathy
 	
• Spleen and portal areas of liver
 	
• Bone marrow frequently involved
 	
• Other uncommon sites of involvement include nasopharynx, gastrointestinal tract, lung, skin
	• Presenting sites: Lymph nodes in >90 percent of the cases
	
	• Many patients are essentially asymptomatic at presentation
	
	• Stage III or IV in >80 percent of the cases
	   Enlarged spleen
	   Bone marrow positive in 55-80 percent of the cases
	
	• Evolution to noncleaved in >40 percent of the cases

REACTIVE COMPONENTS	DIFFERENTIAL DIAGNOSIS
• Intrafollicular, T helper:suppressor ratio of 3:1; interfollicular, large numbers of T helper cells • Plasma cells are usually reactive and contain polyclonal immunoglobulin, but in approximately 5 percent of the cases, plasma cells are monotypic and presumably part of the neoplasm	• Small B/T cell neoplasms • Mantle zone lymphoma • Plasmacytoid lymphocytic lymphoma • Follicular center cell lymphoma, large cleaved cell • Follicular hyperplasia

Table 34

FOLLICULAR CENTER CELL, LARGE CLEAVED CELL TYPE

PATTERN	
	• Follicular in 40-50 percent of the cases, often partial • Diffuse in 50-60 percent of the cases • Sclerosis frequent

CYTOLOGY — NEOPLASTIC	MARKERS — NEOPLASTIC

• Indistinct cytoplasm and cell borders
• Nuclei range upward in size from diameter of histiocyte nucleus; nuclear configurations vary from oval to polypoid and at times are hyper-lobated
• Large cleaved follicular center cells may inter-mingle with sclerosing components
• Mitoses and large noncleaved cells may be frequent
	• Cell suspensions difficult to obtain when sclerosis present
	
	• FSIP: Monoclonal SIg or CIg
	
	• PIP:
	    CD20 (+)
	    CDw75 (+)

INVOLVED SITES	CLINICAL FEATURES
• Superficial lymph nodes • Mesenteric and retroperitoneal masses • Extranodal masses in wide variety of sites, usually with sclerosis	• Asymptomatic lymphadenopathy • Asymptomatic mesenteric or retroperitoneal masses frequent • Lower incidence of bone marrow involvement • Stages I and II frequent with sclerosis • Growth rate: Moderate/low

REACTIVE COMPONENTS	DIFFERENTIAL DIAGNOSIS
• T cells in interfollicular and intrafollicular sites • Plasma cells polyclonal, in variable frequency	• Follicular center cell lymphoma, small cleaved cell, follicular or diffuse • Follicular center cell lymphoma, large noncleaved cell, follicular or diffuse • Hodgkin's disease, nodular sclerosing • Metastatic carcinoma with sclerosis

PLATE XXVII
FOLLICULAR CENTER CELL LYMPHOMA, SMALL CLEAVED CELL, LYMPH NODE
(Plate XXVII is from the same patient)

A. This lymph node shows back-to-back follicular nodules with moderate variation in the size of the follicular nodules. Sinuses are not apparent, and there are several extremely large follicular nodules. H&E. X25.

B. A single follicular nodule and the edges of adjacent follicles are shown at higher magnification. The cellular homogeneity apparent at this magnification is characteristic of small cleaved follicular center cell lymphomas. There is no mantle zone, and only scattered macrophages are present. H&E. X160.

C. The homogeneous infiltrate of small cleaved cells is apparent on oil immersion examination. These cells show an irregular irregularity and nuclear cleavage planes. Note the density and the relative homogeneity of this infiltrate. H&E. X1000.

D. A Giemsa stain of a follicular nodule shows that, in some areas, there is a mixture of cleaved and noncleaved (transformed) follicular center cells. This lesion is still classified as small cleaved cell predominant. The number of noncleaved cells is much more apparent in Giemsa or MGP stains than in H&E stained sections. This number of noncleaved cells may persist in subsequent biopsies without significant change in clinical status. Giemsa. X1000.

PLATE XXVII

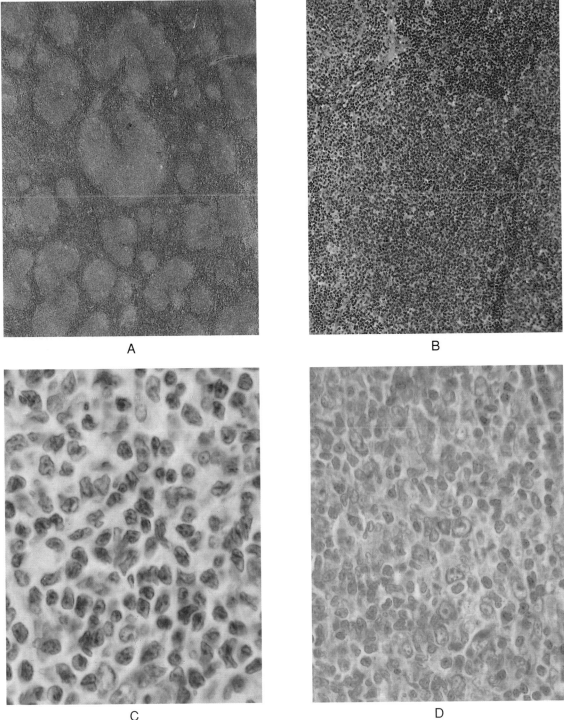

A

B

C

D

PLATE XXVIII
FOLLICULAR CENTER CELL LYMPHOMA, SMALL CLEAVED CELL, NODE
(Plate XXVIII-C and D are from the same patient)

A. This low magnification photomicrograph shows the extensive infiltration of the capsule and the extracapsular area by ill-defined nodular aggregates of cleaved cells. This type of capsular infiltration is characteristic of cleaved follicular center cell lymphomas. H&E. X25.

B. An inguinal node shows separated follicular nodules. This degree of separation is occasionally seen in follicular center cell lymphomas along with dilated sinuses in inguinal and retroperitoneal nodes. Focal areas of hyalinized connective tissue are also present. This patient presented with unilateral edema due to lymphatic obstruction. H&E. X32.

C. This photograph shows vague follicular nodules closely packed in the node and extending into adjacent fat. Neoplastic follicular nodules in these lymphomas vary widely in their distribution in individual patients and their ease of recognition from patient to patient. X32.

D. Immunoperoxidase may facilitate definition of follicular nodules. Note how clearly demarcated the follicular nodules are with this preparation. PIP with CDw75. X32.

E. A pan-T cell antibody shows the large number of T cells present in the interfollicular area with scattered T cells in the follicular centers. PIP with CD45RO. X64.

PLATE XXVIII

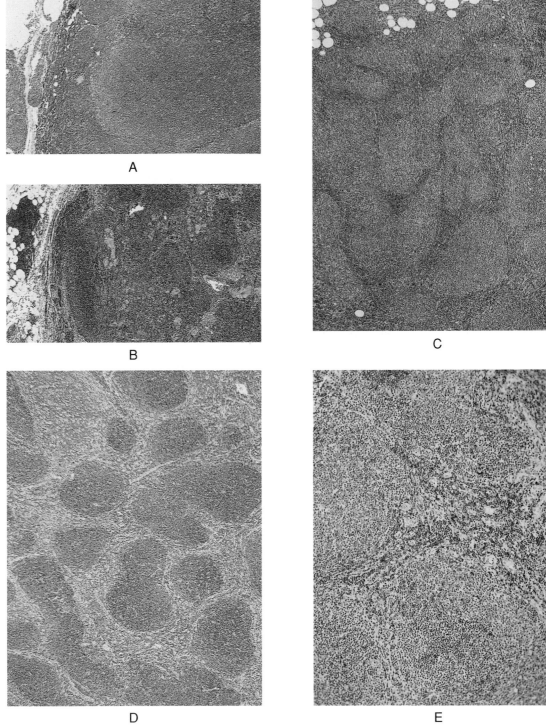

A

B

C

D

E

PLATE XXIX

A. FOLLICULAR CENTER CELL LYMPHOMA, SMALL CLEAVED CELL, BONE MARROW
This bone marrow biopsy shows many lymphoid nodules. These nodules often have a paratrabecular distribution. H&E. X25.

B. FOLLICULAR CENTER CELL LYMPHOMA, SMALL CLEAVED CELL, LIVER
This wedge biopsy shows numerous follicular nodules with some associated sclerosis. Hepatic involvement in follicular center cell lymphomas may be limited to portal areas without the more diffuse infiltrate shown in this photograph. H&E. X40.

C. FOLLICULAR CENTER CELL LYMPHOMA, SMALL CLEAVED CELL, INTESTINE
Typical involvement of the small intestine is illustrated in this photograph, with numerous follicular nodules extending from the mucosa to the serosa. H&E. X20.

D. FOLLICULAR CENTER CELL LYMPHOMA, SMALL CLEAVED CELL WITH TRANSFORMATION, SPLEEN
This enlarged spleen is involved with two types of follicular center cell lymphoma: a small cleaved component that is uniformly distributed throughout the Malpighian bodies and a large noncleaved component found in a large single mass. The two types of follicular center cell proliferation are evident at low magnification. The edge of the mass of large noncleaved cells is at the edge of the photomicrograph, and the small cleaved cells have replaced all of the Malpighian bodies. X20.

PLATE XXIX

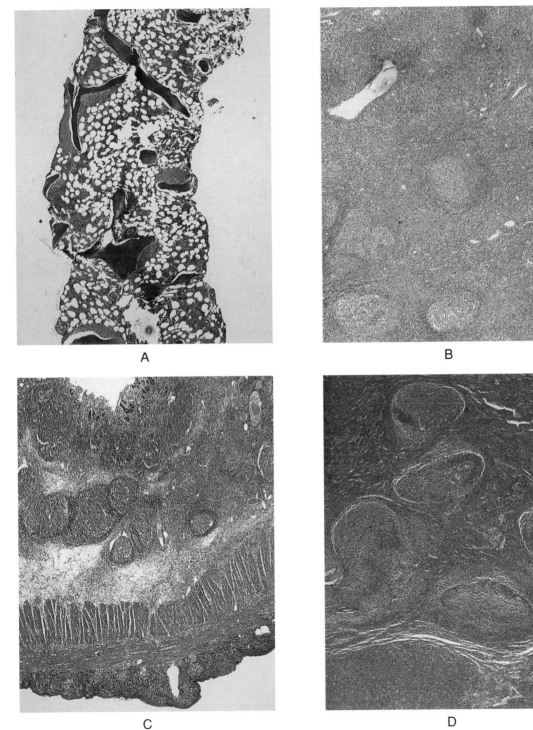

A

B

C

D

PLATE XXX

A. FOLLICULAR CENTER CELL LYMPHOMA, SMALL CLEAVED CELL, LYMPH NODE
An intrafollicular area shows a mixture of cleaved and noncleaved cells, with cleaved cells dominating. Meaningful transformation is evidenced by monomorphic aggregates (compare with plate XXX-B–D). The number of large noncleaved cells shown in this photograph may persist in sequential biopsies for several years. X600.

B. FOLLICULAR CENTER CELL LYMPHOMA WITH BOTH SMALL CLEAVED AND LARGE NONCLEAVED CELLS IN FOLLICULAR AGGREGATIONS, LYMPH NODE
(Plate XXX-B–D are from the same patient)
This low magnification photograph shows follicular nodules at the bottom composed predominately of small cleaved cells. At the top, lighter-staining follicular nodules are composed predominantly of transformed or noncleaved cells. H&E. X25.

C. FOLLICULAR CENTER CELL LYMPHOMA, SMALL CLEAVED CELL, LYMPH NODE
One of the follicular nodules at the bottom of Plate XXX-B is shown here at higher magnification. The homogeneous population of small cleaved cells is apparent. H&E. X250.

D. FOLLICULAR CENTER CELL LYMPHOMA, LARGE NONCLEAVED CELL, LYMPH NODE
This is one of the lighter-staining follicular nodules in Plate XXX-B shown at higher magnification. Many noncleaved or transformed cells are seen in this photograph. H&E. X250.

PLATE XXX

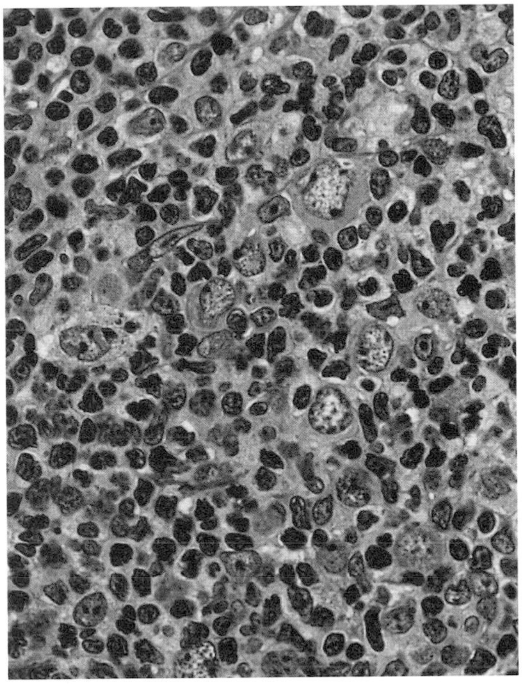

A

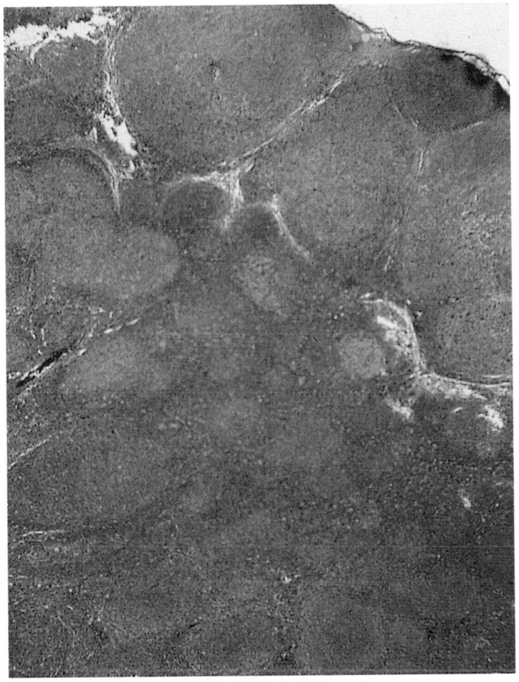

B

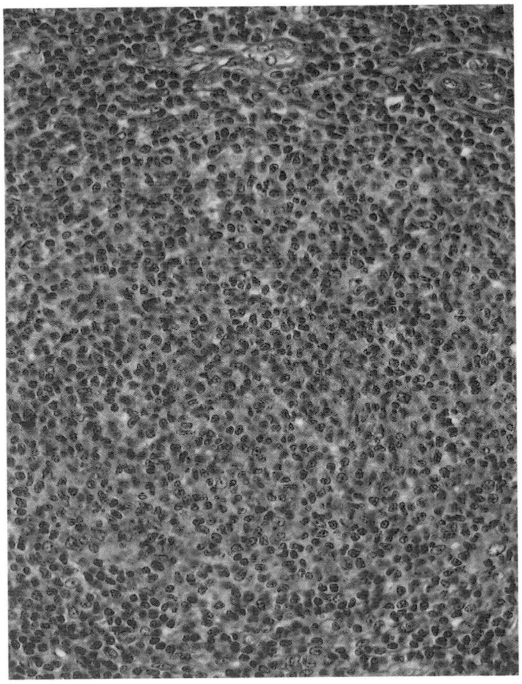

C

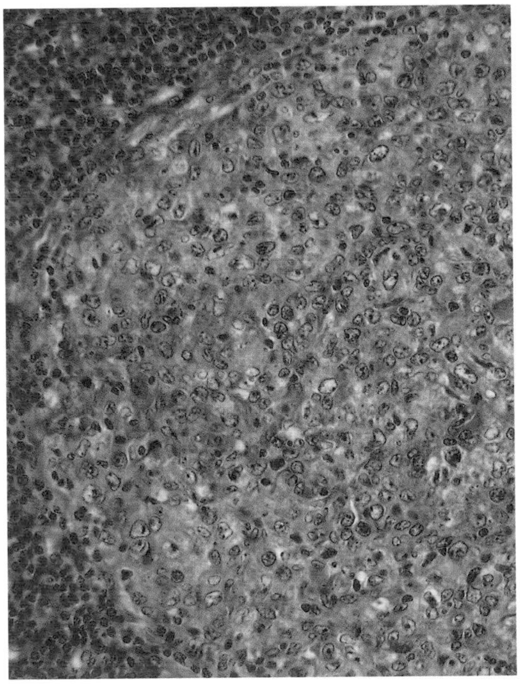

D

PLATE XXXI

A. FOLLICULAR CENTER CELL LYMPHOMA, LARGE CLEAVED CELL, ABDOMINAL MASS

Typical broad areas of acidophilic collagen subdivide this mass into varying size lymphomatous follicles. H&E. X20.

B. FOLLICULAR CENTER CELL LYMPHOMA, LARGE CLEAVED CELL, LYMPH NODE
(Plate XXXI-B and C are from the same patient)

The follicular nodules in large cleaved cell processes are often more eosinophilic than basophilic. Also note the eosinophilic sclerotic material around the follicular nodules. H&E. X25.

C. FOLLICULAR CENTER CELL LYMPHOMA, LARGE CLEAVED CELL, LYMPH NODE

This high magnification photomicrograph shows a follicular nodule surrounded by sclerosis. The larger cells with more irregular nuclei should be compared to small cleaved cells. H&E. X250.

D. FOLLICULAR CENTER CELL LYMPHOMA, LARGE CLEAVED CELL, LYMPH NODE, PLASTIC SECTION

The edge of a follicular area has small round mantle lymphocytes adjacent to medium to large cohesive cells with abundant cytoplasm. The large cleaved cells vary in size and configuration. Rare noncleaved cells are present with several mitoses. H&E. X400.

E. FOLLICULAR CENTER CELL LYMPHOMA, LARGE CLEAVED CELL, ABDOMINAL MASS

On high magnification, there is extraordinary variation in the nuclear configuration in this particular tumor. The cytoplasmic borders are not apparent. Nuclei are situated in loose, amorphous, almost mucinous material that sometimes stains with acid mucopolysaccharide. Flow studies of this case showed that 80 percent of the cells marked with IgA-λ. H&E. X800.

PLATE XXXI

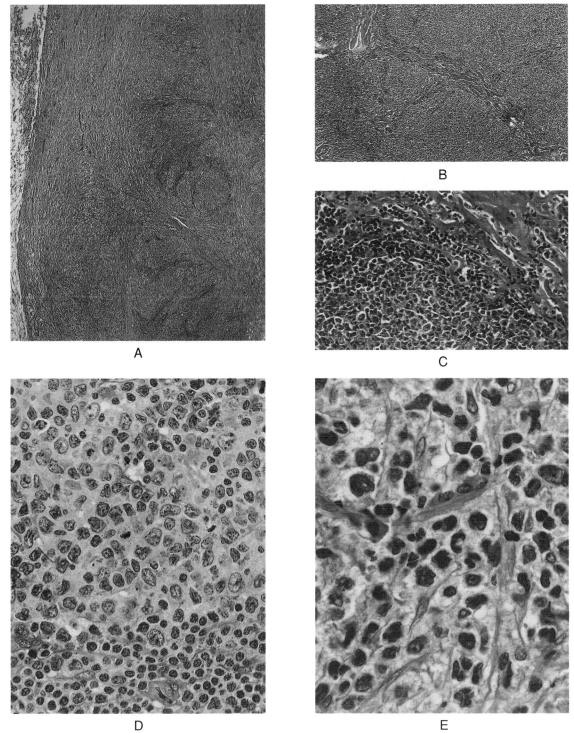

A

B

C

D

E

FOLLICULAR CENTER CELL LYMPHOMAS, SMALL NONCLEAVED CELL TYPE

Clinical Features. Small noncleaved lymphomas of Burkitt's type are endemic in equatorial Africa and are also found, but with much lower frequency, in the United States and Western Europe. In Africa, the disease is associated with the Epstein-Barr virus. High titers of antibody to the viral capsid antigen are found prospectively in patients who will develop Burkitt's lymphoma, and Epstein-Barr viral genomic material has been found, by DNA hybridization study, within the DNA of Burkitt's lymphoma cells. In Africa, the average age at onset is 7 years. Males are affected slightly more frequently than females. The most common site of initial involvement is the jaw, with 50 percent of the newly diagnosed cases occurring there. Involvement of the ovaries, kidneys, liver, and mesentery are also common. The central nervous system is often involved with lymphomatous meningitis, which occurs initially in 17 percent of the patients or, at the time of relapse, in 60 percent.

In the United States, Burkitt's lymphoma is rarely associated with the Epstein-Barr virus. The average age is 11 years. Males are affected twice as often as females. The most common site of presentation is the abdomen, with involvement of the ileocecal region in particular (plate XXXIII). The kidneys, ovaries, mesentery, and peripheral lymph nodes may also be involved. Bone marrow involvement occurs in approximately 15 to 30 percent of the cases. Central nervous system disease is expected less frequently than in the African variant.

The response to therapy and prognosis are dependent upon several factors. Most important, large tumor bulk is associated with a decreased survival rate. The level of serum lactic dehydrogenase correlates well with tumor bulk and with prognosis. Furthermore, patients over the age of 13 years have a poorer prognosis than younger individuals.

Small noncleaved lymphomas of non-Burkitt's type comprise 6 percent of the lymphoid malignancies in the United States. The median age at onset is in the fifth decade, with an age distribution ranging from pediatric to elderly individuals. Males are affected as frequently as females. Peripheral lymphadenopathy is the most common mode of initial presentation. Twenty-five percent of the patients first seek medical attention because of "B" symptoms.

Widespread disease is expected, with stage III or IV disease found in approximately 80 percent of the cases. Frequent sites of extranodal disease include the bone marrow, central nervous system, gastrointestinal tract, and liver. Bone marrow involvement has been reported in 40 to 60 percent of the patients. Frank leukemia has been noted occasionally. The therapeutic response to multiagent chemotherapy has been poor, with the median survival in the range of 1 year.

Histopathologic Features (Table 35). Tissue sections must be well-fixed (B5 or equivalent) for accurate diagnosis, and impression smears are useful. Growth patterns are usually diffuse and infiltrative (plate XXXIV); neoplastic cells rarely form or home to follicular structures (plate XXXIV-A) (Mann et al.). The neoplastic cells are small transformed lymphocytes, and 2 to 5 nucleoli are usually present. MGP stain shows a moderate amount of

Table 35

FOLLICULAR CENTER CELL, SMALL NONCLEAVED CELL TYPE — BURKITT'S AND NON-BURKITT'S

PATTERN	
	• Follicular in 10 percent of the cases; usually partial or minimal • Diffuse in 90 percent of the cases • Tumor masses usually have no discernible architecture or, at times, appear as a widely infiltrated structure such as in the wall of the intestine, in which only residual structures are discernible • Necrotic areas are sometimes extensive

CYTOLOGY — NEOPLASTIC	MARKERS — NEOPLASTIC

• Small noncleaved follicular center cells are small transformed cells that vary in nuclear size and amount of cytoplasm and are a high-grade neoplasm with numerous mitoses
 	
• Burkitt's variant: Uniform sized transformed follicular center cells with nuclei no larger than tingible body macrophage nuclei; cytoplasm MGP 2+ to 3+, lipid vacuoles
 	
• Non-Burkitt's variant: Variable sized transformed follicular center cells with some nuclei larger than tingible body macrophage nucleus; cytoplasm MGP 2+ to 3+; lipid vacuoles
	• Flow, FSIP: SIg monotypic in 85-90 percent of the cases May express CD10
	
	• PIP:
	    CD45 (+)
	    CD20 (+)
	    CDw75 (+)
	
	• TdT (−)
	
	• Typically show translocation involving chromosome 8

INVOLVED SITES	CLINICAL FEATURES
• Burkitt's variant: In the Northern Hemisphere, Burkitt's involves the abdominal tissues, terminal ileum, cecum, mesenteric lymph nodes, and rarely the facial bones, paranasal sinuses, or orbit—as in Burkitt's of Africa • Non-Burkitt's variant: Predominantly involves lymph nodes and bone marrow	• Dramatic presentation of rapidly enlarging lymph nodes or masses • Burkitt's variant occurs in children and young adults, whereas non-Burkitt's has a wide age range but generally involves older adults • Symptoms and signs of abdominal mass or obstruction with an intussusception at the ileocecal valve, usually with Burkitt's variant • Leukemic expression as "B cell acute lymphocytic leukemia" may occur • Stage variable in abdomen or extensive; may be localized (stage 1R)

REACTIVE COMPONENTS	DIFFERENTIAL DIAGNOSIS
• "Starry-sky" macrophages are common but not always present • T cells and plasma cells occur in small numbers • Mature granulocytes uncommon	• Follicular center cell lymphoma, large noncleaved cell • Immunoblastic lymphoma B • Convoluted (lymphoblastic) T lymphoma • Granulocytic sarcoma • Carcinomas with "starry-sky" phagocytes

positively staining cytoplasm. Mitoses and macrophages are abundant, with the macrophages producing the nonspecific "starry sky" appearance. Electron microscopy shows rounded nuclei and abundant polyribosomes.

Burkitt's type. Neoplastic cells are uniform in size and shape (plate XXXII-A,B).

Non-Burkitt's type. Neoplastic cells are distinctly variable in nuclear size and configuration (plate XXXII-C). Large noncleaved cells may be present in low numbers.

Comment. Burkitt's lymphoma is one of the first human malignancies in which chromosomal translocation and oncogene activation have been related. Two studies have recently shown that the human oncogene, c-*myc*, is located on the region of chromosome 8 (q24-qter) that is commonly translocated in Burkitt's lymphoma to the long arm of chromosome 14 (Dalla-Favera et al.; Taub et al.). In this translocation, the segment of chromosome 8 carrying the c-*myc* gene is brought into close proximity with the locus on chromosome 14, which encodes immunoglobulin heavy chains. Similar observations have been made in mouse plasmacytomas, where the most common translocation, t(12;15), involves a transfer of the region of chromosome 15 containing the c-*myc* gene to the immunoglobulin heavy chain gene locus on chromosome 12 (Crews et al.). Because transcription of the c-*myc* gene is amplified in a number of human malignancies, it is speculated that the translocation to the switch site of a gene active in B cells, the immunoglobulin heavy chain gene, may serve to promote c-*myc* gene expression above levels present in normal mature cells. A related promotion of oncogene expression with the development of B cell lymphomas has been demonstrated by inserting the c-*myc* gene into the mouse genome (Adams et al.). However, most investigators feel that activation of the c-*myc* gene represents only one event in a multistep pathway to oncogenesis in these cells. These observations founded in molecular genetics are certainly important clues to the basic mechanisms of neoplastic transformation in these and many other malignancies.

FOLLICULAR CENTER CELL LYMPHOMAS, LARGE NONCLEAVED CELL TYPE

Clinical Features. Large noncleaved cell lymphomas account for 6 percent of all lymphoid malignancies in the United States and for approximately 12 percent of all follicular center cell lymphomas. The median age of onset is 54 years (with a range of 18-90 years). Males are affected more frequently than females (3:2). The most common presenting complaints include lymphadenopathy (in 40 percent of the patients), pain (in 34 percent of the patients), and systemic "B" symptoms (in 40 percent of the patients). Approximately 75 percent of the patients present with stage III and IV disease, and stage I is seen in 10 percent. Common sites of involvement include the gastrointestinal tract, which is involved in approximately 30 percent of the patients. Common sites of disease within the alimentary tract include the small intestine, stomach, and large intestine. The naso- or oropharynx may also be involved. Central nervous system involvement is reported in approximately 10 percent of the patients, most commonly at the time of relapse. Disease in the nervous system may also be seen at the time of diagnosis, presenting as a mass lesion, lymphomatous meningitis, or an extradural mass. Bone marrow involvement is seen in approximately 10 percent of the patients at diagnosis.

Complete remission is achieved in approximately 60 to 70 percent of the patients with disseminated disease who are treated with multiagent combination chemotherapy (i.e., bleomycin, adriamycin, cyclophosphamide, vincristine, prednisone). Prolonged disease-free survival is reported in the majority of those achieving complete response, although late relapses may occur.

Pathologic Features (Table 36). The growth pattern is diffuse in 90 percent of the cases. Follicular nodulation may be atypical and difficult to detect (fig. 49) or obvious (plate XXXVI-A,B; fig 50). Previous or concurrent biopsies may show follicular lymphomas composed of small or, less frequently, large cleaved cells. Large noncleaved cells are usually mononuclear (plate XXXV-B–D), but binuclear and multinuclear variants may be confused with Reed-Sternberg cells. Nuclei usually show dispersed chromatin, and nucleoli are distinct. Giemsa and MGP stains highlight the abundant cytoplasm. Large noncleaved cells typically have prominent nucleoli and polyribosomes by electron microscopy.

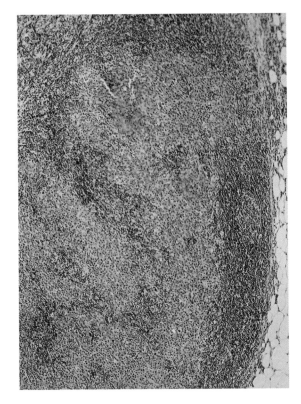

Figure 49
(Figure 49 and plate XXXV-B,C are from the same patient)
FOLLICULAR CENTER CELL LYMPHOMA,
LARGE NONCLEAVED CELL, LYMPH NODE
This perigastric lymph node shows a single uninvolved follicular center beneath the capsule and numerous adjacent ill-defined neoplastic follicular nodules. X60.

Table 36

FOLLICULAR CENTER CELL, LARGE NONCLEAVED CELL TYPE

PATTERN	
	• Follicular in 10 percent of the cases, usually partial or minimal • Diffuse in 90 percent of the cases • Occasionally occurs as an area of transformation with single or multiple nodules in follicular center cell lymphoma, small cleaved cell or as mass in subsequent lymph node biopsies on these patients
CYTOLOGY — NEOPLASTIC	**MARKERS — NEOPLASTIC**

• Large noncleaved follicular center cells are large transformed lymphocytes that have nuclei larger than 10-12 µm (macrophage nucleus diameter). Nucleoli are multiple, small, and usually located on the nuclear membrane but at times are large and central. Cytoplasm is pale but distinct; MGP positive and Giemsa basophilic	• Flow, FSIP: SIg monotypic in 85-90 percent of the cases
	
	• PIP: CIg usually monotypic, occasionally scant, absent, or polytypic
	    CD45 (+)
	    CD20 (+)
	    CDw75 (+)

INVOLVED SITES	**CLINICAL FEATURES**
• Lymph nodes • Tonsil • Gastrointestinal tract • Thyroid	• Commonly presents as rapidly enlarging lymph nodes or masses • B symptoms frequent • Tonsillar, abdominal, or thyroid mass frequent • Approximately 40 percent of the patients with follicular center cell lymphoma, small cleaved cell undergo transformation to large noncleaved cell
REACTIVE COMPONENTS	**DIFFERENTIAL DIAGNOSIS**
• "Starry-sky" macrophages found but are less frequent than in small noncleaved cell or convoluted (lymphoblastic) T lymphoma • T cells and plasma cells present in small numbers	• Follicular center cell lymphoma, small noncleaved cell • Follicular center cell lymphoma, large cleaved cell • Immunoblastic lymphoma B • Immunoblastic lymphoma T • Granulocytic sarcoma • Carcinoma

Figure 50
(Figure 50 and plate XXXV-D are from the same patient)
FOLLICULAR CENTER CELL LYMPHOMA,
LARGE NONCLEAVED CELL, LYMPH NODE
An unusual type of follicular nodulation is seen in this lymphoma. A large area shows a more diffuse pattern in which there are partial linear subdivisions by small lymphocytes, but no definite follicular nodules are seen. In the other portion of the node, the various sized aggregates more closely resemble follicular structures. X40.

PLATE XXXII

A. FOLLICULAR CENTER CELL LYMPHOMA, SMALL NONCLEAVED CELL, BOWEL
(Plate XXXII-A,B, plate XXXIII-A, and plate XXXIV-A–C are from the same patient)

This high magnification photomicrograph shows the pyroninophilia and regular nuclei characteristic of a small noncleaved cell lymphoma of the Burkitt's type. Small dice-like nucleoli are apparent. MGP. X630.

B. FOLLICULAR CENTER CELL LYMPHOMA, SMALL NONCLEAVED CELL, BOWEL

This high magnification photomicrograph shows a Giemsa stain with the dispersed nuclear chromatin, small nucleoli, and amphophilic cytoplasm typically seen in this neoplasm. Giemsa. X630.

C. FOLLICULAR CENTER CELL LYMPHOMA, SMALL NONCLEAVED CELL, NON-BURKITT'S TYPE
(Plate XXXII-C and plate XXXIV-D are from the same patient)

This high magnification photomicrograph shows irregular nuclei and prominent cytoplasm, to be contrasted with the regular uniform nuclei seen in photomicrographs of the Burkitt's variant. The tumor cells usually have a single central nucleolus. Several large noncleaved cells are situated in a predominantly small noncleaved cell population. The presence of such large cells may lead to a misclassification as a large noncleaved cell type. Giemsa. X400.

D. FOLLICULAR CENTER CELL LYMPHOMA, SMALL NONCLEAVED CELL, ASCITIC FLUID

This is a cytospin of ascitic fluid from a patient with an abdominal mass in which flow studies revealed monotypic B cells. The cells vary somewhat in size and nuclear configuration, and nuclear chromatin is slightly clumped. A single mitotic figure is present. The cytoplasm is azurophilic and contains several vacuoles. A single tingible body macrophage is seen in the upper left corner. Wright's stain. X1000.

E. FOLLICULAR CENTER CELL LYMPHOMA, SMALL NONCLEAVED CELL, CEREBROSPINAL FLUID

This cytospin shows a cluster of lymphoma cells with azurophilic cytoplasm containing clear vacuoles. This patient had a relapse in the cerebellum after therapy for a primary tumor in the abdomen. Wright's stain. X625.

PLATE XXXII

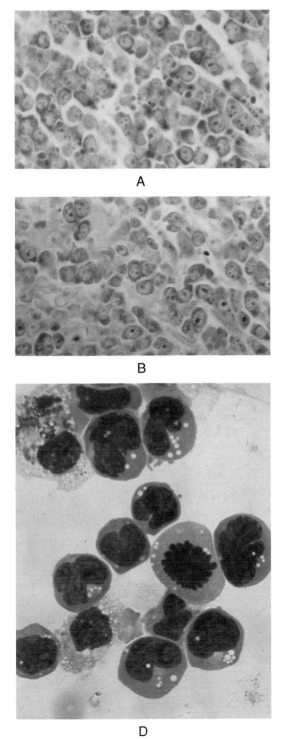

A

B

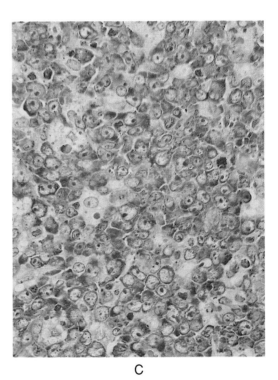

C

D

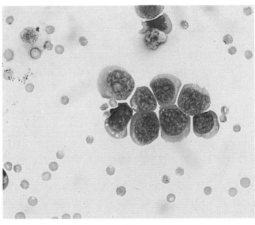

E

PLATE XXXIII
FOLLICULAR CENTER CELL LYMPHOMA, SMALL NONCLEAVED CELL, BOWEL
(Plate XXXIII-A, plate XXXII-A,B, and plate XXXIV-A–C are from the same patient,
and plate XXXIII-B and C are from the same patient)

A. This gross photograph shows a mass of the ileum intussuscepting into the lumen of the cecum in a 22 year old man. Burkitt's variants of small noncleaved cell lymphoma diagnosed in the United States commonly involve the ileocecal area.

B. In this gross photograph, the exterior of an ilial tumor mass with adjacent mesenteric involvement is shown.

C. After formalin fixation, this cut section shows the tumor extending from the bowel wall into an adjacent mesenteric mass. There was no apparent intraluminal extension.

PLATE XXXIII

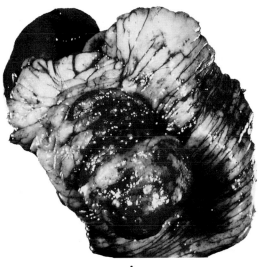

A

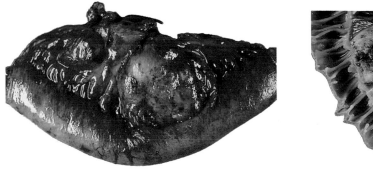

B

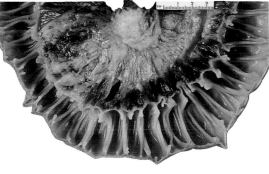

C

PLATE XXXIV

A. FOLLICULAR CENTER CELL LYMPHOMA, SMALL NONCLEAVED CELL, LYMPH NODE, HOMING OF A BURKITT'S TUMOR
(Plate XXXIV-A–C, plate XXXII-A,B, and plate XXXIII-A are from the same patient)

Two follicular lymphomatous nodules show extensive infiltration of the soft tissue adjacent to the lymph node capsule. In the node, a single benign-appearing follicular nodule is apparent at the top. Several neoplastic follicular structures are apparent at the bottom. X60.

B. FOLLICULAR CENTER CELL LYMPHOMA, SMALL NONCLEAVED CELL, BOWEL

A low magnification photomicrograph shows the extensive infiltration of the bowel wall often seen in this neoplasm. Giemsa. X15.

C. FOLLICULAR CENTER CELL LYMPHOMA, SMALL NONCLEAVED CELL, BOWEL

A high magnification photomicrograph of the submucosal area shows the extensive infiltration by neoplastic cells into the lamina propria. Giemsa. X160.

D. FOLLICULAR CENTER CELL LYMPHOMA, SMALL NONCLEAVED CELL, NON-BURKITT'S, PIP, WITH CDw75

In this illustration, a typical pattern of reactivity is shown. There is usually a single punctate paranuclear globule of positivity, presumably in the Golgi zone, as shown in this case.

PLATE XXXIV

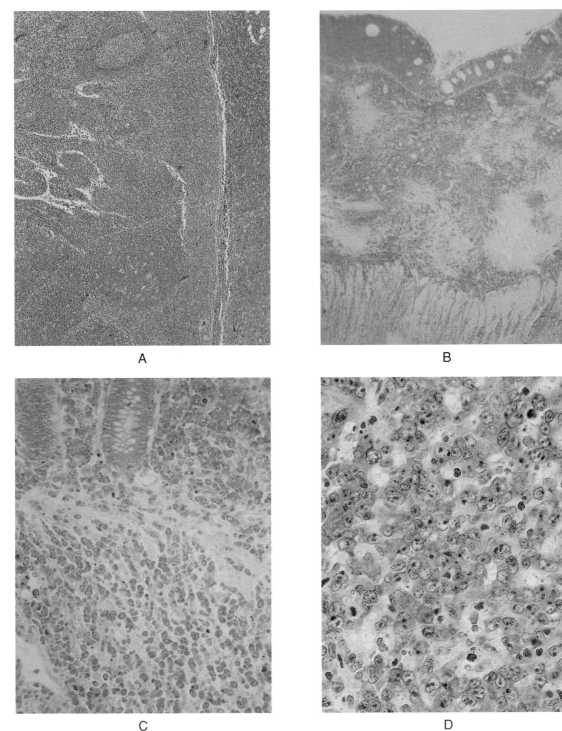

PLATE XXXV
FOLLICULAR CENTER CELL LYMPHOMA, LARGE NONCLEAVED CELL

A. STOMACH
This patient presented with an ulcerating gastric mass.

B. LYMPH NODE
(Plate XXXV-B,C and figure 49 are from the same patient)
At high magnification, typical large noncleaved cells with distinct nucleoli and dispersed nuclear chromatin are apparent. X1000.

C. LYMPH NODE
Pyroninophilia is apparent in this illustration. The nuclei are large, with dispersed chromatin and prominent nucleoli. MGP. X1000.

D. LYMPH NODE
(Plate XXXV-D and figure 50 are from the same patient)
A mixture of medium to large pale cytoplasmic cells and numerous small irregular lymphocytes is apparent. The cellular borders are not well demarcated, and mitoses are uncommon. The majority of the large cells marked with CD20 in flow cytometry studies but showed scant surface immuno-globulin, as is often noted with large noncleaved cell processes. X600.

PLATE XXXV

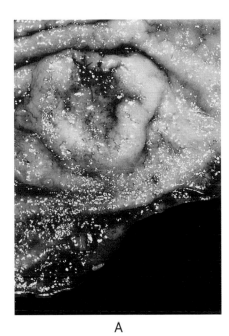

A

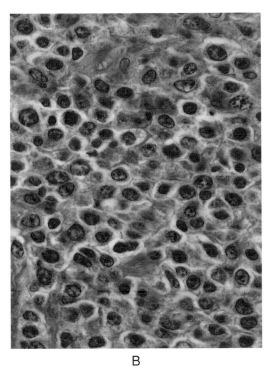

B

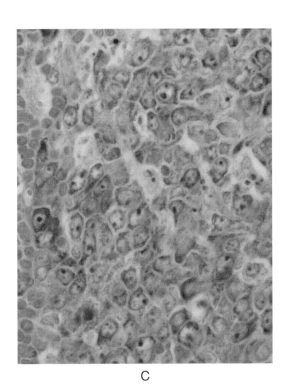

C

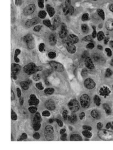

D

PLATE XXXVI

FOLLICULAR CENTER CELL LYMPHOMA, LARGE NONCLEAVED CELL, LYMPH NODE

(Plate XXXVI-A,B and figure 44 are from the same patient, and plate XXXVI-C and D are from the same patient)

A. The junction between a neoplastic follicle and residual lymphocytic mantle is shown. Note the homogeneous population of large noncleaved cells with only scattered mitoses. Tingible body macrophages are not present and are usually not seen in large noncleaved cell processes. X320.

B. This high magnification photomicrograph shows pale cytoplasmic cells that vary considerably in size. Many of the medium and large cells show nuclear features of transformed lymphocytes with finely dispersed chromatin, several dice-like nucleoli, and thin nuclear membranes. Mitoses in large noncleaved cell processes are infrequent, in contrast to their frequency in the small noncleaved cell lymphomas. H&E. X800.

C. Most of the large cells have diffuse cytoplasmic positivity in this immunoperoxidase preparation; only occasional membrane positivity and rare cytoplasmic globules are noted. The pattern of single globular positivity with CDw75 is noted in only a few cells, although it is the expected pattern of reactivity in these lymphomas. PIP with CDw75. X320.

D. All of the large cells have marked cytoplasmic labeling in this immunoperoxidase preparation. Small cells marked with a pan-T antibody (not shown). PIP with CD74. X320.

PLATE XXXVI

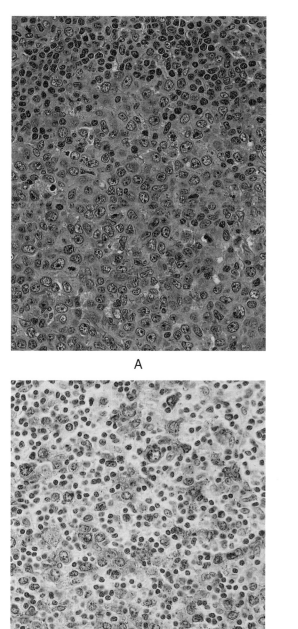

A

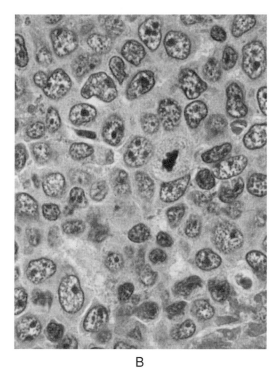

B

C

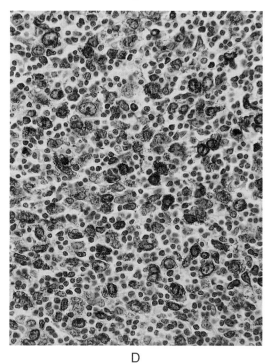

D

MEDIASTINAL LARGE CELL LYMPHOMA

Definition. Except for Hodgkin's disease, large cell lymphomas in the mediastinum are, with very rare exceptions, B cell neoplasms of follicular center cell origin. There is some evidence that these lymphomas arise in thymic B tissue (Addis and Isaacson).

Clinical Features. Mediastinal large cell lymphoma is associated with an anterior mediastinal mass that often produces shortness of breath, superior vena caval syndrome, cough, weight loss, fatigue, or pleural effusions. In rare instances, patients are asymptomatic. In the largest series (Perrone et al.), approximately 85 percent of the patients were 35 years of age or younger at the time of diagnosis, and many of the women were in their mid-twenties. Chest wall extension is frequent, and approximately 25 percent of the patients show extension of the tumor outside the thorax at presentation.

Pathologic Features. This tumor is often described as large or extensive with dimensions of up to 26.5 cm and weights up to 736 g. Thymic involvement is often noted at exploratory thoracotomy, and in one case the tumor was confined by the thymic capsule (Lamarre et al.). Growth patterns are entirely diffuse with no follicular nodulation and have frequently been associated with deposition of connective tissue ranging from thin hyaline bands to broad bands of connective tissue. In some cases the connective tissue deposition is fine and interstitial. Necrosis may be present. These have been uniformly large cell processes composed of cells ranging in appearance from large cleaved to non-cleaved to immunoblastic in type. Most cases have the usual features associated with large noncleaved follicular center cell lymphomas. Rare cells resembling Reed-Sternberg cells have been noted. Some cases have had clear cells of variable size (Möller et al.).

Immunologic Features. Most of the cases of mediastinal large cell lymphoma have had a B cell phenotype, either marking in paraffin immunoperoxidase with pan-B markers or showing a monotypic surface immunoglobulin. A few cases have had heavy or light chain immunoglobulin gene rearrangement.

Differential Diagnosis. Intermixed thymic epithelium may be found, leading to some confusion with malignant thymomas. Other neoplasms to be excluded include metastatic carcinoma or melanoma, seminomas, and nodular sclerosing Hodgkin's disease. An awareness of the occurrence of this lymphoma in young females and the availability of diagnostic immunophenotypic studies usually leads to the correct diagnosis.

References

Adams, J.M., Harris, A.W., Pinkert, C.A., et al. The c-*myc* oncogene driven by immunoglobulin enhancers induces lymphoid malignancy in transgenic mice. Nature 318:533-535, 1985.

Addis, B.J. and Isaacson, P.G. Large cell lymphoma of the mediastinum: a B-cell tumour of probable thymic origin. Histopathology 10:379-390, 1986.

Crews, S., Barth, R., Hood, L., Prehn, J., and Calame, K. Mouse c-*myc* oncogene is located on chromosome 15 and translocated to chromosome 12 in plasmacytomas. Science 218:1319-1321, 1982.

Dalla-Favera, R., Bregni, M., Erikson, J., et al. Human c-*myc onc* gene is located on the region of chromosome 8 that is translocated in Burkitt lymphoma cells. Proc. Natl. Acad. Sci. USA 79:7824-7827, 1982.

Lamarre, L., Jacobson, J.O., Aisenberg, A.C., and Harris, N.L. Primary large cell lymphoma of the mediastinum. A histologic and immunophenotypic study of 29 cases. Am. J. Surg. Pathol. 13:730-739, 1989.

Lennert, K. Germinal centers and germinal center neoplasms. Nippon Ketsueki Gakkai Zasshi 32:495-500, 1969.

_____ . Follicular lymphomas—a tumor of the germinal centers. Gann Monogr. Cancer Res. 15:217, 1973.

_____ . Histopathology of Non-Hodgkin's Lymphomas (Based on the Kiel Classification). New York: Springer-Verlag, 1981.

Lukes, R.J. and Collins, R.D. New approaches to the classification of the lymphomata. Br. J. Cancer 2(Suppl.):1-28, 1975.

Mann, R.B. and Berard, C.W. Criteria for the cytologic subclassification of follicular lymphomas: a proposed alternative method. Hematol. Oncol. 1:187-192, 1983.

_____ , Jaffe, E.S., Braylan, R.C., et al. Nonendemic Burkitt's lymphoma. A B-cell tumor related to germinal centers. N. Engl. J. Med. 295:685-691, 1976.

Möller, P., Moldenhauer, G., Momburg, F., et al. Mediastinal lymphoma of clear cell type is a tumor corresponding to terminal steps of B cell differentiation. Blood 69:1087-1095, 1987.

The Non-Hodgkin's Lymphoma Classification Project. National Cancer Institute sponsored study of classifications of non-Hodgkin's lymphomas: summary and description of a working formulation for clinical usage. Cancer 49:2112-2135, 1982.

Perrone, T., Frizzera, G., and Rosai, J. Mediastinal diffuse large-cell lymphoma with sclerosis. A clinicopathologic study of 60 cases. Am. J. Surg. Pathol. 10:176-191, 1986.

Rappaport, H. Tumors of the Hematopoietic System. Fascicle 8, First Series. Atlas of Tumor Pathology. Washington: Armed Forces Institute of Pathology, 1966.

_____ , Winter, W.J., and Hicks, E.B. Follicular lymphoma. A re-evaluation of its position in the scheme of malignant lymphoma, based on a survey of 253 cases. Cancer 9:792-821, 1956.

Stein, R.S., Magee, M.J., Lenox, R.K., et al. Malignant lymphomas of follicular center cell origin in man. VI. Large cleaved cell lymphoma. Cancer 60:2704-2711, 1987.

Taub, R., Kirsch, I., Morton, C., et al. Translocation of the c-myc gene into the immunoglobulin heavy chain locus in human Burkitt lymphoma and murine plasmacytoma cells. Proc. Natl. Acad. Sci. USA 79:7837, 1982.

Wright, C.J. Macrofollicular lymphoma. Am. J. Pathol. 32:201-233, 1956.

Additional References

Arseneau, J.C., Canellos, G.P., Banks, P.M., et al. American Burkitt's lymphoma. I. Clinical factors relating to prolonged survival. Am. J. Med. 58:314-321, 1975.

Bennett, M.H. and Millett, Y.L. Nodular sclerotic lymphosarcoma. Clin. Radiol. 20:339-343, 1969.

Berard, C.W., O'Conor, G.T., Thomas, L.B., and Torloni, H. Histopathological definition of Burkitt's tumour. Bull. WHO 40:601-607, 1969.

Bloomfield, C.D., Gajl-Peczalska, K.J., Frizzera, G., Kersey, J.H., and Goldman, A.I. Clinical utility of lymphocyte surface markers combined with the Lukes-Collins histologic classification in adult lymphoma. N. Engl. J. Med. 301:512-518, 1979.

Burke, J.S., Butler, J.J., and Fuller, L.M. Malignant lymphomas of the thyroid. Cancer 39:1587-1602, 1977.

Burkitt, D. A sarcoma involving the jaws in African children. Br. J. Surg. 46:218-223, 1958.

Cullen, M.H., Lister, T.A., Brearley, R.I., Shand, W.S., and Stansfeld, A.G. Histological transformation of non-Hodgkin's lymphoma. Cancer 44:645-651, 1979.

Gall, E.A., Morrison, H.R., and Scott, A.T. The follicular type of malignant lymphoma. Ann. Intern. Med. 14:2073, 1940.

Glick, A.D., Leech, J.H., Waldron, J.A., et al. Malignant lymphomas of follicular center cell origin in man. II. Ultrastructural and cytochemical studies. J. Natl. Cancer Inst. 54:23-36, 1975.

Horning, S.J. and Rosenberg, S.A. The natural history of initially untreated low-grade non-Hodgkin's lymphomas. N. Engl. J. Med. 311:1471-1475, 1984.

Jaffe, E.S., Shevach, E.M., Frank, M.M., Berard, C.W., and Green, I. Nodular lymphoma. N. Engl. J. Med. 290:813-819, 1974.

Kim, H., Dorfman, R.F., and Rappaport, H. Signet ring cell lymphoma. A rare morphological and functional expression of nodular (follicular) lymphoma. Am. J. Surg. Pathol. 2:119-132, 1978.

Kojima, M., Imai, Y., and Mori, N. A concept of follicular lymphoma—a proposal for the existence of a neoplasm originating from the germinal center. Gann Monogr. Cancer Res. 15:195, 1973.

Leech, J.H., Glick, A.D., Waldron, J.A., et al. Malignant lymphomas of follicular center cell origin in man. I. Immunologic studies. J. Natl. Cancer Inst. 54:11-22, 1975.

Levine, A.M., Pavlova, Z., Pockros, A.W., et al. Small noncleaved follicular center cell (FCC) lymphoma: Burkitt and non-Burkitt variants in the United States. I. Clinical features. Cancer 52:1073-1079, 1983.

_____ , Goldstein, M., Meyer, P.R., et al. Heterogeneity of response and survival in diffuse histiocytic lymphomas after BACOP therapy (bleomycin, doxorubicin, cyclophosphamide, vincristine, prednisone). Hematol. Oncol. 3:87-98, 1985.

Lukes, R.J. and Collins, R.D. New observations on follicular lymphoma. Gann Monogr. Cancer Res. 15:209, 1973.

_____ and Collins, R.D. Immunologic characterization of human malignant lymphomas. Cancer 34(Suppl. 4):1488-1503, 1974.

_____ , Parker, J.W., Taylor, C.R., et al. Immunologic approach to non-Hodgkin lymphomas and related leukemias. Semin. Hematol. 15:322-351, 1978.

Maurer, R., Taylor, C.R., Terry, R., and Lukes, R.J. Non-Hodgkin lymphomas of the thyroid. A clinico-pathological review of 29 cases applying the Lukes-Collins classification and an immunoperoxidase method. Virchows Arch. [Pathol. Anat.] 383:293-317, 1979.

Millett, Y.L., Bennett, M.H., Jelliffe, A.M., and Farrer-Brown, G. Nodular sclerotic lymphosarcoma. Br. J. Cancer 23:683-692, 1969.

Qazi, R., Aisenberg, A.C., and Long, J.C. The natural history of nodular lymphoma. Cancer 37:1923-1927, 1976.

Spiro, S., Galton, D.A., Wiltshaw, E., and Lohmann, R.C. Follicular lymphoma: a survey of 75 cases with special reference to the syndrome resembling chronic lymphocytic leukemia. Br. J. Cancer 2(Suppl.):60-70, 1975.

Stein, H., Siemssen, U., and Lennert, K. Complement receptor subtypes C3b and C3d in lymphatic tissue and follicular lymphoma. Br. J. Cancer 37:520-529, 1978.

_____, Bonk, A., Tolksdorf, G., et al. Immunohistologic analysis of the organization of normal lymphoid tissue and non-Hodgkin's lymphomas. J. Histochem. Cytochem. 28:746-760, 1980.

Stein, R.S., Cousar, J., Flexner, J.M., et al. Malignant lymphomas of follicular center cell origin in man. III. Prognostic features. Cancer 44:2236-2243, 1979.

Stewart, M.L., Felman, I.E., Nichols, P.W., Pagnini-Hill, A., Lukes, R.J., and Levine, A.M. Large noncleaved follicular center cell lymphoma. Clinical features in 53 patients. Cancer 57:288-297, 1986.

Sweet, D.L., Collins, R.D., Stein, R.S., and Ultmann, J.E. Prognostic significance of the Lukes and Collins classification in patients treated with COMLA. Cancer Treat. Rep. 66:1107-1111, 1982.

Taylor, C.R. Classification of lymphoma. Arch. Pathol. Lab. Med. 102:549-554, 1978.

_____. Immunocytochemical methods in the study of lymphoma and related conditions. J. Histochem. Cytochem. 26:496-512, 1978.

Tolksdorf, G., Stein, H., and Lennert, K. Morphological and immunological definition of a malignant lymphoma derived from germinal-centre cells with cleaved nuclei (centrocytes). Br. J. Cancer 41:168-182, 1980.

van den Tweel, J.G., Taylor, C.R., Parker, J.W., and Lukes, R.J. Immunoglobulin inclusions in non-Hodgkin's lymphomas. Am. J. Clin. Pathol. 69:306-313, 1978.

_____, Lukes, R.J., and Taylor, C.R. Pathophysiology of lymphocyte transformation. A study of so-called composite lymphomas. Am. J. Clin. Pathol. 71:509-520, 1979.

Warnke, R. and Levy, R. Immunopathology of follicular lymphomas. A model of B-lymphocyte homing. N. Engl. J. Med. 298:481-486, 1978.

Woda, B.A., and Knowles, D.M., Jr. Nodular lymphocytic lymphoma eventuating into diffuse histiocytic lymphoma. Cancer 43:303-307, 1979.

Ziegler, J.L. Burkitt's lymphoma. N. Engl. J. Med. 305:735-745, 1983.

IMMUNOBLASTIC LYMPHOMA, B TYPE

SYNONYMS AND RELATED TERMS: Working Formulation: large cell, immunoblastic; large cell, plasmacytoid. Kiel: malignant lymphoma, immunoblastic. Rappaport: diffuse histiocytic.

Definition. Immunoblastic lymphoma, B type is a neoplastic proliferation of immunoblasts that exhibit plasmacytic differentiation (Lukes and Collins, 1974, 1975). The presence of plasmacytic differentiation is one of the features distinguishing immunoblastic lymphoma, B type from follicular center cell lymphomas of large cell type. Immunoblastic lymphoma, B type often arises from small cell lymphoid neoplasms (with and without plasmacytic differentiation) or from previous chronic abnormal immune disorders. For pathologic details, see Plates XXXVII and XXXVIII.

Clinical Features. Immunoblastic lymphoma, B type comprises approximately 3 to 4 percent of all lymphoid malignancies in the United States. The usual age of onset is the fifth decade, although pediatric and elderly patients have been described. Males and females are affected equally. As many as one-third of the patients may have histories of prior immune disease, including congenital immune deficiency syndromes (Wiskott-Aldridge, X-linked lymphoproliferative disease, acquired auto-immune disease, Sjögren syndrome, rheumatoid arthritis, acquired immune deficiency syndromes, organ transplantation, and immunoblastic lymphadenopathy) (Levine et al.). Furthermore, approximately 10 percent of the newly diagnosed patients with immunoblastic lymphoma B may have had histories of prior lymphoproliferative reaction or malignancy, including B chronic lymphocytic leukemia (Richter's syndrome) or plasmacytoid lymphocytic lymphoma.

Approximately 50 percent of all patients initially seek medical attention because of peripheral lymphadenopathy; extranodal presentations, including the gastrointestinal tract (plate XXXVIII-A–C), lung, and brain, may be seen in the remainder. "B" symptoms, including fever, night sweats, and weight loss, are present in 60 percent of the patients.

Stage III or IV disease has been found in approximately 80 percent of the newly diagnosed cases, with the gastrointestinal tract, lung, and bone marrow as prominent sites of stage IV involvement. Mild anemia (with a mean hemoglobin of 11.8 g/dl) is expected at diagnosis, with 35 percent of the patients demonstrating absolute lymphocytopenia and approximately 25 percent presenting with bone marrow involvement. Some patients may have monoclonal paraproteins or hypogammaglobulinemia on serum protein electrophoresis.

Approximately 50 percent of all patients will achieve complete remission with multi-agent chemotherapy such as bleomycin, adriamycin, vincristine, cyclophosphamide, and prednisone. Long-term disease-free survival may be expected in the majority of complete responders, with a median survival of approximately 2 years in the group as a whole.

Pathologic Features (Table 37). Histopathologic sections show a relatively monomorphic growth of large transformed lymphocytes, plasmacytic intermediates, and plasma cells (plates XXXVII; XXXVIII-D). Giemsa and MGP stains are strongly positive (plate XXXVII-B). Plasmacytic differentiation may be subtle (plate XXXVII-A,B) or overt (plates XXXVII-C,D; XXXVIII-A). Numerous segments of rough endoplasmic reticulum shown by electron microscopy are further manifestations of plasmacytic

differentiation. Most of these neoplasms have a diffuse growth pattern. Immunoblastic lymphoma B arising from previous lymphoid neoplasms probably represents a transformational phenomenon in the kinetics of the neoplasm. Immunoblastic lymphoma B arising from abnormal immunologic reactions may represent a response to chronic abnormal immunologic stimulation. It is of interest that immunoblastic lymphoma B has rarely been described as a transformational process in cleaved follicular center cell lymphomas.

Immunologic Features. Neoplastic cells often have monotypic surface and cytoplasmic immunoglobulin, but some clearly neoplastic cases do not mark distinctly with immunoperoxidase procedures for CIg or have bitypic or polyclonal SIg (Lukes et al.).

Differential Diagnosis. Immunoblastic lymphoma B should be diagnosed when the predominant cell is a large transformed lymphocyte with amphophilic, strongly pyroninophilic cytoplasm. Nuclei should be large and generally mononuclear in configuration with prominent nucleoli. PIP should show a monotypic or bitypic CIg.

Malignant lymphoma, immunoblastic lymphoma, T type. Cytoplasm is usually water clear, and plasmacytic differentiation is not apparent in this neoplasm. PIP does not show CIg. Neoplastic cells mark as T cells.

Malignant lymphoma, follicular center cell, large cleaved cell type, small noncleaved cell type, and large noncleaved cell type. In these lymphomas, follicular nodulation may be quite focal but is nevertheless diagnostic of the follicular center nature of the process. Large cleaved cells show very irregular nuclear configurations, usually with inapparent cytoplasm and

213

Table 37

IMMUNOBLASTIC LYMPHOMA B

PATTERN

- Focal or multifocal nodules of immunoblasts in abnormal immune reactions of lymph nodes and other tissues or in small B cell neoplasms; plasmacytoid lymphocytic lymphoma; and multiple myeloma

- Diffusely involved lymph nodes and masses

CYTOLOGY — NEOPLASTIC	MARKERS — NEOPLASTIC

• Immunoblasts, including plasmacytoid forms, range in size and appearance from 10-12 μm to pleomorphic dysplastic Reed-Sternberg-like cells
• Nucleoli usually small, multiple, scattered; may be single, large, amphophilic
• Mitoses frequent and abnormal
• Cytoplasm amphophilic in plasmacytoid forms; pale in some cases
	• Flow, FSIP: SIg often monotypic, at times scant
	• PIP: CIg often monotypic but may be bitypic
	   CD45 (+)
	   CD20 (+)
	   CDw75 (−)

INVOLVED SITES	CLINICAL FEATURES
• Lymph nodes • Various sites, including lung, thyroid, gastro-intestinal tract, skin, and central nervous system	• Commonly reflects underlying abnormal immune process or prior small B cell lymphoma (i.e., plasmacytoid lymphocytic lymphoma) • Conditions complicated by the development of immunoblastic lymphoma B include Hashimoto's disease, asthma, malabsorption, and AIDS; in AIDS, central nervous system lymphomas develop

REACTIVE COMPONENTS	DIFFERENTIAL DIAGNOSIS
• Residual uninvolved lymph node in abnormal immune process • "Starry-sky" phagocytes are uncommon • Macrophages in small clusters or as giant cells	• Immunoblastic lymphoma T • Follicular center cell lymphoma, large noncleaved cell, diffuse • Follicular center cell lymphoma, small noncleaved cell, diffuse • Follicular center cell lymphoma, large cleaved cell, diffuse • Granulocytic sarcoma • Carcinoma • Abnormal immune processes with prominent immunoblastic component

indistinct nucleoli. Small noncleaved cells demonstrate an extremely infiltrative growth pattern with large numbers of mitoses and macrophages and a consistently smaller cell than in immunoblastic lymphoma, B type with very few (if any) plasma cells. Large noncleaved cells closely resemble the immunoblasts of immunoblastic lymphoma B but do not exhibit plasmacytic differentiation.

Granulocytic sarcoma. Neoplastic cells may be distinctly cytoplasmic, but nuclei are often medium sized, and nucleoli are small or inconspicuous. PIP fails to reveal monotypic CIg, and other markers show the myeloid differentiation of these cells.

Carcinomas. Neoplastic cells in carcinomas usually show more cohesion than the growth patterns in immunoblastic lymphoma B and often have a sinus component. PAS stains may be strongly positive and PIP shows clear marking with epithelial or keratin antibodies.

Abnormal immune reaction with prominent immunoblastic component. The diagnosis of immunoblastic lymphoma evolving from abnormal immune reaction should only be made when there are unequivocal aggregates of immunoblasts or when monotypism is demonstrated. Clusters of immunoblasts less than a high magnification field in diameter do not justify the diagnosis of immunoblastic lymphoma.

References

Levine, A.M., Taylor, C.R., Schneider, D.R., et al. Immunoblastic sarcoma of T-cell versus B-cell origin: I. Clinical features. Blood 58:52-61, 1981.

Lukes, R.J. and Collins, R.D. Immunologic characterization of human malignant lymphomas. Cancer 34(Suppl. 4):1488-1503, 1974.

Lukes, R.J. and Collins, R.D. New approaches to the classification of the lymphomata. Br. J. Cancer 2(Suppl.):1-28, 1975.

_____, Parker, J.W., Taylor, C.R., et al. Immunologic approach to non-Hodgkin lymphomas and related leukemias. Semin. Hematol. 15:322-351, 1978.

Additional References

Anderson, L.G. and Talal, N. The spectrum of benign to malignant lymphoproliferation in Sjögren's syndrome. Clin. Exp. Immunol. 10:199-221, 1972.

Kurtz, D.M. Immunoblastic sarcoma. Am. J. Clin. Pathol. 67:227-229, 1977.

Lichtenstein, A., Levine, A.M., Lukes, R.J., et al. Immunoblastic sarcoma. Cancer 43:343-352, 1979.

Schneider, D.R., Taylor, C.R., Parker, J.W., Cramer, A.C., Meyer, P.R., and Lukes, R.J. Immunoblastic sarcoma of T- and B-cell types: morphologic description and comparison. Hum. Pathol. 16:885-900, 1985.

Schwartz, R.S. and Beldotti, L. Malignant lymphomas following allogenic disease: transition from an immunological to a neoplastic disorder. Science 149:1511-1514, 1965.

PLATE XXXVII
IMMUNOBLASTIC LYMPHOMA B
(Plate XXXVII-A and B are from the same patient)

A. Some of the variations in cytology encountered in immunoblastic lymphoma B are shown. Here there is a pleomorphic appearance to the tumor, with some polypoid features and other dysplastic changes in the larger cells. Plasmacytic differentiation is limited, although some nuclei have eccentric locations. The cytoplasm is lightly acidophilic. H&E. X1000.

B. Although plasmacytic differentiation is not readily apparent in H&E stained sections, Giemsa stain dramatically brings out the amphophilia and plasmacytoid appearance. Only a few nuclei are large and clearly immunoblastic. Nuclear membranes are slightly thickened. Giemsa. X600.

C. Amphophilia is very apparent in this H&E stained section. The amount of deeply staining cytoplasm varies, and nuclei are often eccentric in position. Both medium and large cells are present. Nuclear membranes are slightly to moderately thickened. H&E. X600.

D. This high magnification photomicrograph shows eccentric nuclei, amphophilic cytoplasm, and distinct plasmacytic differentiation of the immunoblastic cells. Nuclei are clearly immunoblastic in appearance, with thick nuclear membranes. H&E. X1000.

PLATE XXXVII

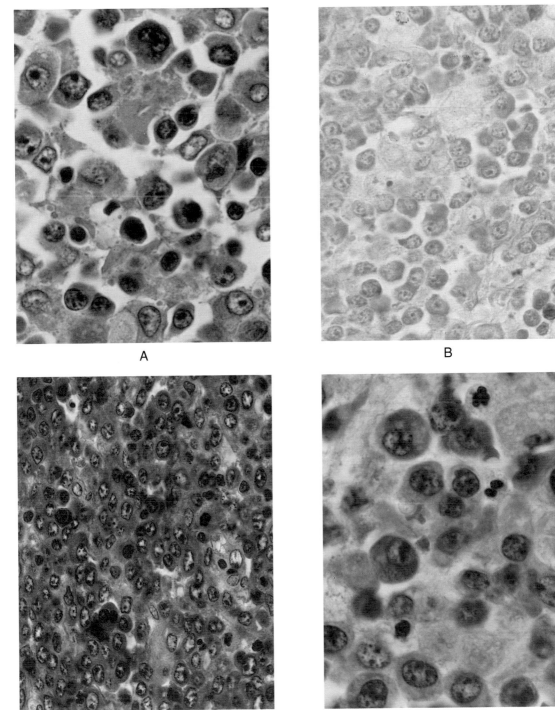

A

B

C

D

PLATE XXXVIII

A. IMMUNOBLASTIC LYMPHOMA B, STOMACH
In this case, plasmacytic differentiation is evidenced by the prominent Russell body formation. H&E. X100.

B. IMMUNOBLASTIC LYMPHOMA B, BOWEL
(Plate XXXVIII-B–D are from the same patient)
A diffuse mucosal and submucosal infiltrate is noted in this case of α-chain disease. H&E. X50.

C. IMMUNOBLASTIC LYMPHOMA B, BOWEL
A higher magnification photomicrograph shows numerous plasma cells in the submucosal area. These plasma cells are benign in appearance, pack the submucosa, and extend into the lamina propria. H&E. X400.

D. EVOLVING IMMUNOBLASTIC LYMPHOMA B, NODE
This high magnification photograph shows the large number of immunoblasts, numerous mitoses, and slight plasmacytic differentiation in the node. The number of immunoblasts varies widely. This process is not monomorphic in appearance, but a number of the immunoblasts exhibit atypical nuclear features and large central nucleoli, indicating an evolving immunoblastic lymphoma B. H&E. X400.

PLATE XXXVIII

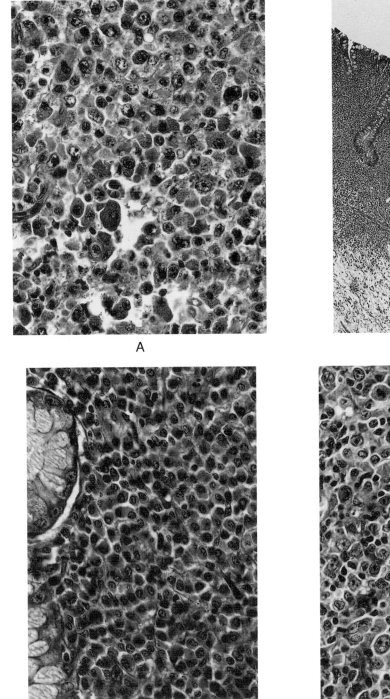

A

B

C

D

ANGIOTROPIC LARGE CELL LYMPHOMA

SYNONYMS AND RELATED TERMS: Angioendotheliomatosis proliferans systemisata; malignant angioendotheliomatosis; intravascular lymphomatosis.

Definition. This lymphoid neoplasm apparently arises outside of the marrow and is characterized by the presence of large lymphoid cells in small blood vessels throughout the body, often with occlusion. The lymphoma cells often have a B phenotype.

Clinical Features. Approximately 100 cases have been reported. Most patients are older adults of either sex, with an age range of 13-84 years (Domizio et al.). In the literature review by Domizio and colleagues, diagnosis was made at autopsy in 48 percent, skin biopsy in 38 percent, brain biopsy in 10 percent, and surgical resection in 4 percent of the cases. B symptoms alone are described in approximately 10 percent of the cases. Cutaneous and neurologic manifestations occur in 75 percent of the cases. Neurologic complaints include rapidly progressive dementia or nonlocalizing neurologic deficits (Wick et al.). Skin lesions may be disseminated, plaque-like, and hemorrhagic or hyperpigmented. Curiously, adrenal masses or adrenal involvement are frequently seen (Wick et al.). Some patients apparently have a coexistent or prior autoimmune disease.

Pathologic Features. Arterioles, venules, and capillaries contain numerous noncohesive tumor cells. Venules and capillaries may be distended, and tumor cells are usually enmeshed in thrombi. Individual tumor cells are large, with vesicular chromatin, prominent nucleoli, and frequent mitotic figures. Areas of diffuse lymphomatous growth are often seen in conjunction with the intravascular component (Ansell et al.; Bhawan et al.).

Immunologic Features. Most cases of angiotropic large cell lymphoma have shown a B phenotype when frozen or paraffin immunoperoxidase procedures are used (Carroll et al.; Domizio et al.; Sheibani et al.; Theaker et al.), although T cell lineage has been shown in two cases (Sepp et al.). Immunoglobulin or T receptor gene rearrangements have been found in a few cases (Domizio et al.; Sepp et al.).

Differential Diagnosis. Intravascular growths of carcinoma, melanoma, or endothelial cells should be considered and appropriate immunoperoxidase batteries used to establish a diagnosis.

References

Ansell, J., Bhawan, J., Cohen, S., Sullivan, J., and Sherman, D. Histiocytic lymphoma and malignant angioendotheliomatosis. One disease or two? Cancer 50:1506-1512, 1982.

Bhawan, J., Wolff, S.M., Ucci, A.A., and Bhan, A.K. Malignant lymphoma and malignant angioendotheliomatosis: one disease. Cancer 55:570-576, 1985.

Carroll, T.J., Schelper, R.L., Goeken, J.A., and Kemp, J.D. Neoplastic angioendotheliomatosis: immunopathologic and morphologic evidence for intravascular malignant lymphomatosis. Am. J. Clin. Pathol. 85:169-175, 1986.

Domizio, P., Hall, P.A., Cotter, F., et al. Angiotropic large cell lymphoma (ALCL): morphological, immunohistochemical and genotypic studies with analysis of previous reports. Hematol. Oncol. 7:195-206, 1989.

Sepp, N., Schyuler, G., Romani, N., et al. "Intravascular lymphomatosis" (angioendotheliomatosis): evidence for a T-cell origin in two cases. Hum. Pathol. 21:1051-1058, 1990.

Sheibani, K., Battifora, H., Winberg, C.D., et al. Further evidence that "malignant angioendotheliomatosis" is an angiotropic large-cell lymphoma. N. Engl. J. Med. 314:943-948, 1986.

Theaker, J.M., Gatter, K.C., Esiri, M.M., and Easterbrook, P. Neoplastic angioendotheliosis—further evidence supporting a lymphoid origin. Histopathology 10:1261-1270, 1986.

Wick, M.R., Mills, S.E., Scheithauer, B.W., Cooper, P.H., Davitz, M.A., and Parkinson, K. Reassessment of malignant "angioendotheliomatosis." Evidence in favor of its reclassification as "intravascular lymphomatosis." Am. J. Surg. Pathol. 10:112-123, 1986.

T CELL-RICH B CELL LYMPHOMA

Definition. T cell-rich B cell lymphomas are recently described, unusual lymphomas that have a diffuse morphology, a predominance of reactive T cells, and only a minority of neoplastic B cells. The B cells are usually large. These lymphomas may represent follicular center cell lymphomas with an unusual reactive component, or a large cell lymphoma evolving from lymphocyte predominant Hodgkin's disease.

Clinical Features. Very few cases of T cell-rich B cell lymphoma have been reported. In very small series, patients have ranged in age from 7.5 to 94 years, with a slight male preponderance. Most patients have extensive superficial adenopathy, but extranodal involvement in bone, brain, and skin has been described. "B" symptoms are frequent. Natural history and preferred treatment are unknown. We consider this process an intermediate grade lymphoma.

Pathologic Features. Growth patterns of T cell-rich B cell lymphoma are usually diffuse but may be interfollicular. Vessels (particularly high endothelial venules) are prominent. In some cases, previous or subsequent biopsies may show neoplastic follicular nodulation. These lymphomas may resemble peripheral T cell lymphomas in tissue sections (Mirchandani et al.).

Tumor cells are large, occasionally multinucleate and Reed-Sternberg-like (Ramsay et al.). Rare cases of a small lymphocyte type have been described.

Epithelioid macrophages are almost invariably present and may appear in clusters. Plasma cells may be noted, but eosinophils are rare. Most (>90 percent) cells in these lymphomas are small T lymphocytes.

Immunologic Features. By paraffin immunoperoxidase, the neoplastic B cell component is readily recognized by the prominent CD20 (L26) positivity (Osborne et al.). Tumor cells are strongly positive, often easily detected at 10X magnification, and evenly distributed throughout. CDw75 (LN-1) positivity may be noted. Monotypic cytoplasmic immunoglobulin (usually μ-heavy chain) is often detected. CD15 (Leu-M1) is usually negative, as is EMA.

By flow cytometry and frozen section immunoperoxidase, the neoplastic component may be obscured by the high number of T cells (Winberg et al.).

Immunoglobulin gene rearrangement has been noted in some of these lymphomas (Ng et al.).

Differential Diagnosis. These lymphomas are readily confused with peripheral T cell lymphomas if phenotyping is dependent on flow or frozen section immunoperoxidase. PIP shows large B cells that mark strongly and are usually evenly distributed throughout. Differentiation from Hodgkin's disease, especially lymphocyte predominant, may be particularly difficult, and in fact T cell-rich B cell lymphoma may represent an evolutionary phase of this type Hodgkin's disease. EMA and CD15 (Leu-M1) positivity are not expected in T cell-rich B cell lymphoma. Small cell lymphoid neoplasms have been incorrectly diagnosed when the large cell component is overlooked due to poor fixation or sectioning.

References

Mirchandani, I., Palutke, M., Tabaczka, P., Goldfarb, S., Eisenberg, L., and Pak, M.S.Y. B-cell lymphomas morphologically resembling T-cell lymphomas. Cancer 56:1578-1583, 1985.

Ng, C.S., Chan, J.K.C., Hui, P.K., and Lau, W.H. Large B-cell lymphomas with a high content of reactive T cells. Hum. Pathol. 20:1145-1154, 1989.

Osborne, B.M., Butler, J.J., and Pugh, W.C. The value of immunophenotyping on paraffin sections in the identification of T-cell rich B-cell large-cell lymphomas: lineage confirmed by J_H rearrangement. Am. J. Surg. Pathol. 14:933-938, 1990.

Ramsay, A.D., Smith, W.J., and Isaacson, P.G. T-cell–rich B-cell lymphoma. Am. J. Surg. Pathol. 12:433-443, 1988.

Winberg, C.D., Sheibani, K., Burke, J.S., Wu, A., and Rappaport, H. T-cell–rich lymphoproliferative disorders. Morphologic and immunologic differential diagnoses. Cancer 62:1539-1555, 1988.

MICROVILLOUS LYMPHOMA

SYNONYMS AND RELATED TERMS: Anemone or villiform lymphoma.

Definition. Microvillous lymphoma is a large cell lymphoma with a sinus growth pattern and cytoplasmic processes detectable only by electron microscopy.

Clinical Features. So few cases of microvillous lymphoma have been reported that clinical features have not been defined. All of our cases have been in adults, many of whom had superficial adenopathy.

Pathologic Features. Microvillous lymphomas have a diffuse growth pattern, with some involvement of sinuses (Kinney et al.; Osborne et al.). In some cases the sinus involvement may predominate (fig. 51A). Large areas of necrosis may be present.

Tumor cells are usually large (14-20 µm) and have round or slightly irregular nuclei with prominent nucleoli (fig. 51B). Cytoplasm may be abundant, and cell borders may stain with PAS. Polylobated nuclei have been seen, and a few tumor giant cells are present in all cases. Mitotic figures are frequent. By electron microscopy (fig. 52), tumor cells resemble transformed lymphocytes and have long thin surface microvilli (Azar et al.; Taxy and Almanaseer).

Immunologic Features. Virtually all cases show reactivity of tumor against CD45, CDw75 (LN-1), and CD20 (L26) (fig. 51C). By definition, CD30 is negative, as are T markers and EMA. CD15 (Leu-M1) rarely marks these cells. Monotypic cytoplasmic immunoglobulin may be detected by paraffin immunoperoxidase.

Differential Diagnosis. Sinus growth patterns are seen in anaplastic large cell Ki-1 lymphoma, melanomas, metastatic carcinoma, and malignant histiocytoses. Both Ki-1 malignant lymphoma and microvillous malignant lymphoma should be considered in patients with sinus growth patterns, clinical or pathologic suspicion of carcinoma, melanoma, and inapparent primary tumors. Ki-1 malignant lymphoma may be readily separated from microvillous malignant lymphoma in most cases by paraffin immunoperoxidase, the former being CD30 (Ber H2) positive, usually pan-T positive. Malignant histiocytoses are very rare and should not be diagnosed without ultrastructural confirmation.

References

Azar, H.A., Espinoza, C.G., Richman, A.V., Saba, S.R., and Wang, T. "Undifferentiated" large cell malignancies: an ultrastructural and immunocytochemical study. Hum. Pathol. 13:323-333, 1982.

Kinney, M.C., Glick, A.D., Stein, H., and Collins, R.D. Comparison of anaplastic large cell Ki-1 lymphomas and microvillous lymphomas in their immunologic and ultrastructural features. Am. J. Surg. Pathol. 14:1047-1060, 1990.

Osborne, B.M., Mackay, B., Butler, J.J., and Ordonez, N.G. Large cell lymphoma with microvillus-like projections: an ultrastructural study. Am. J. Clin. Pathol. 79:443-450, 1983.

Taxy, J.B. and Almanaseer, I.Y. "Anemone" cell (villiform) tumors: electron microscopy and immunohistochemistry of five cases. Ultrastruct. Pathol. 7:143-150, 1984.

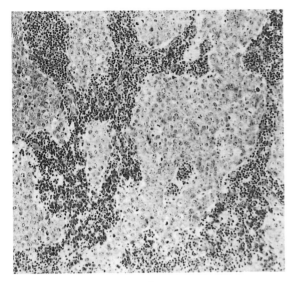

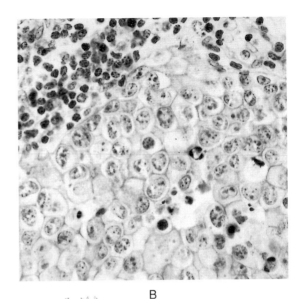

A   B

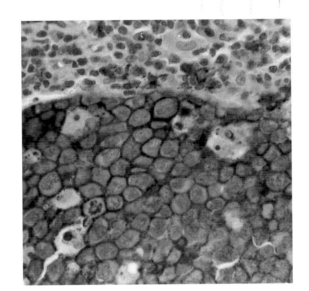

C

Figure 51
MICROVILLOUS LYMPHOMA, LYMPH NODE
A. Prominent involvement of sinuses by this lymphoma is demonstrated in this example. B. The tumor cells in this field have large round to slightly irregular nuclei and abundant cytoplasm. C. Immunoperoxidase stain for CD20 (L26) shows distinct membrane reactivity of tumor cells. This antibody is very useful in the recognition of B cell neoplasms. (Fig. 4 from Kinney, M.C., Glick, A.D., Stein, H., and Collins, R.D. Comparison of anaplastic large cell Ki-1 lymphomas and microvillous lymphomas in their immunologic and ultrastructural features. Am. J. Surg. Pathol. 14:1047-1060, 1990.)

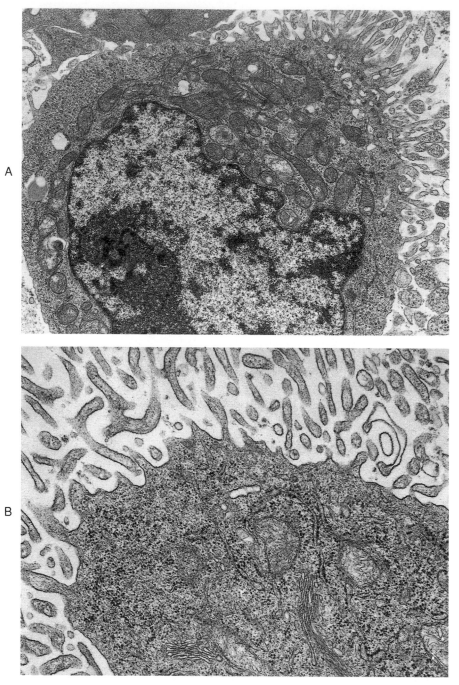

Figure 52
MICROVILLOUS MALIGNANT LYMPHOMA
A. This microvillous malignant lymphoma has a large nucleolus and surface microvilli. X12,300. B. Numerous long thin surface microvilli are demonstrated. X29,000. (Fig. 7 from Kinney, M.C., Glick, A.D., Stein, H., and Collins, R.D. Comparison of anaplastic large cell Ki-1 lymphomas and microvillous lymphomas in their immunologic and ultrastructural features. Am. J. Surg. Pathol. 14:1047-1060, 1990.)

HODGKIN'S DISEASE

Definition. The term Hodgkin's disease includes several lymphomas primarily affecting the lymph nodes, with later involvement of the liver, spleen, bone marrow, and lung. Proliferating cells seem to be mononuclear Reed-Sternberg cells, although the critical cells of recognition are binucleated or multinucleated types of Reed-Sternberg cells. Electron microscopy indicates that Reed-Sternberg cells are actually lobated or hyperlobated. For pathologic details, see Plates XXXIX-XLV and figures 53-88.

Hodgkin's disease has been controversial in the past because misdiagnoses and superinfections obscured the neoplastic nature of the process. It is controversial now because the nature of Reed-Sternberg cells has only been partially elucidated, despite extensive research. The failure to characterize Reed-Sternberg cells more completely is partly due to the heterogeneity of Hodgkin's disease, as well as to the difficulties in working with Reed-Sternberg cells in vitro. In addition, a laboratory model is not available.

In the past, Hodgkin's disease was considered an infectious rather than a neoplastic disease because of the unusual and extensive immunologic reactions associated with it and because of the frequent complicating infections. However, Hodgkin's disease is now recognized to be a malignant neoplasm for the following reasons: (1) the disease leads to death unless treated; (2) the disease apparently begins unifocally and spreads to distant sites (plate XXXIX); (3) tumorous masses are produced (plate XXXIX-B,C) that contain abnormal cells that display the usual cytologic features associated with neoplasia (cytologic atypia and dysplasia); (4) proliferating cells in a few cases have shown aneuploidy and chromosomal abnormalities, indicating clonal proliferation; and (5) no specific infectious agent has been uniformly demonstrated in patients with Hodgkin's disease; bacterial and fungal studies at diagnosis on affected nodes are almost always sterile. Viral agents have not been consistently isolated from affected nodes.

Nature of Reed-Sternberg Cells. Many of the reports in the literature concerning the structural, cytochemical, or immunologic features of Reed-Sternberg cells are difficult to evaluate. There is often inadequate proof that all of the case material studied was clearly Hodgkin's disease and that the individual cells studied were Reed-Sternberg cells. These difficulties might be avoided if cases selected for study included only those clearly meeting the standard histopathologic criteria for Hodgkin's disease and if the cells subjected to analysis have morphologic features diagnostic of Reed-Sternberg cells. In this regard, exceptionally large nucleoli are probably the most distinctive feature of Reed-Sternberg cells. Because of their size and multinucleation, activated histiocytes have often been confused with Reed-Sternberg cells, but they do not have exceptionally prominent nucleoli.

Mononuclear Reed-Sternberg and Reed-Sternberg cells are difficult to study in vitro because tissue from patients with Hodgkin's disease is not easily disrupted into single-cell suspensions. Furthermore, Reed-Sternberg cells tend to be

PLATE XXXIX

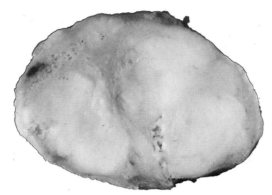

A. HODGKIN'S DISEASE, NODULAR SCLEROSIS
This is the gross appearance of a lymph node from a patient with Hodgkin's disease. The alteration of architecture and ill-defined nodules are shown.

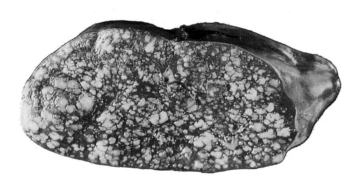

B. HODGKIN'S DISEASE, SPLEEN
Multiple nodules are present throughout the substance of this spleen. (Fig. 21 from Lukes, R.J. and Butler, J.J. The pathology and nomenclature of Hodgkin's disease. Cancer Res. 26:1063-1083, 1966.)

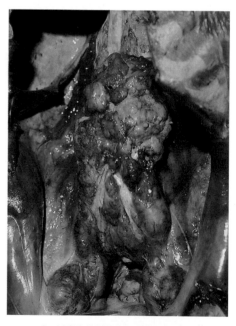

C. HODGKIN'S DISEASE
Massive retroperitoneal involvement is demonstrated in a patient with widely disseminated Hodgkin's disease at autopsy. (Fig. 20 from Lukes, R.J. and Butler, J.J. The pathology and nomenclature of Hodgkin's disease. Cancer Res. 26:1063-1083, 1966.)

preferentially lost in the various manipulations associated with immunologic testing. For these reasons, most of the studies of Reed-Sternberg cells have involved imprint cytochemistry, ultrastructure, or immunocytochemistry of tissue sections. These studies may be summarized as follows. (1) Reed-Sternberg cells do not mark cytochemically or by immunoperoxidase as histiocytes. (2) Reed-Sternberg cells do not contain the haloed granules by electron microscopy that are characteristic of mononuclear phagocyte system cells. In contrast, Reed-Sternberg cells have many of the ultrastructural characteristics of transformed lymphocytes (fig. 53) (Glick et al.). (3) Work with isolated or cultured cells has favored a macrophage lineage for the

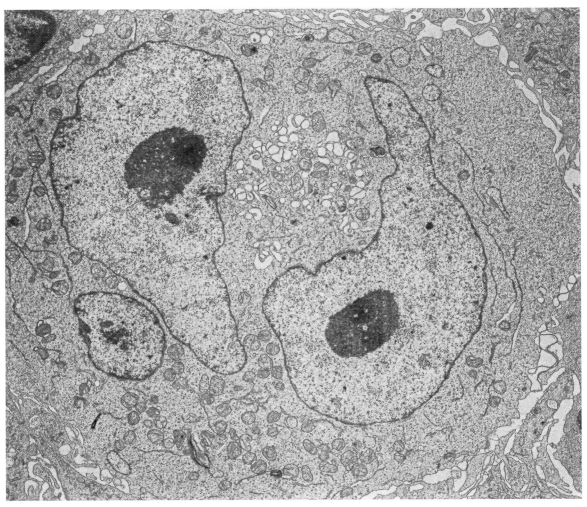

Figure 53
HODGKIN'S DISEASE, MIXED CELLULARITY, LYMPH NODE
This figure demonstrates the ultrastructure of a Reed-Sternberg cell. Note the huge nucleoli and cytoplasmic polysomes. Reed-Sternberg cells resemble transformed lymphocytes and do not contain the haloed granules typically seen in normal or activated macrophages. Uranyl acetate. X8400.

Reed-Sternberg cell. Kaplan and Gartner established long-term, but not permanent, cultures from 25 cases of Hodgkin's disease. Cells in these cultures were adherent, phagocytically active, heterotransplantable, and aneuploid. They had Fc and C3b receptors but no SIg or E-rosette receptors. These features were interpreted as indicating mononuclear phagocyte system origin, although there was no proof that Reed-Sternberg cells rather than a contaminating population were established in culture. (4) Immunocytochemical studies on tissue sections indicate that Reed-Sternberg cells are lymphocytic in nature rather than derived from the mononuclear phagocyte system. These results support the hypotheses based on the cytologic resemblance of Reed-Sternberg cells to transformed lymphocytes (Lukes and Collins; Tindle et al.). Furthermore, Reed-Sternberg cells in lymphocyte-predominant Hodgkin's disease have B features (Timens et al.), whereas Reed-Sternberg cells in nodular sclerosing Hodgkin's disease have shown T cell marking (Casey et al.; Kadin et al.; Stein et al.). (5) No absolutely specific immunocytochemical markers are available for the identification of Reed-Sternberg cells, but paraffin immunoperoxidase procedures often show that Reed-Sternberg cells mark with CD15 (Leu-M1) and CD30 (Ber H2). (6) Finally, gene rearrangement studies have not shown consistent rearrangements of either immunoglobulin or T-receptor genes in Hodgkin's disease.

In evaluating these observations, it is important to remember that Hodgkin's disease is diagnosed by the histopathologic features of a distinctive immunologic tissue reaction and the demonstration of Reed-Sternberg cells. It seems likely that different pathogenetic factors, different immune responses, or different target cells might be involved in producing what we now call Hodgkin's disease. It certainly seems possible that the distinctive immunologic reaction of Hodgkin's disease could be directed against altered T cells, B cells, or mononuclear phagocyte cells. These various activated dysplastic cells might be expected to have the light morphologic features of Reed-Sternberg cells. As our investigations become more sophisticated, therefore, we should anticipate discordant identification of Reed-Sternberg cells. The explanation for such discrepancies may not be in differing interpretations of the analyses of homogeneous case populations but instead may be attributable to a basic heterogeneity in cases diagnosed as Hodgkin's disease.

The identification of some cases of Hodgkin's disease as T cell or B cell type further confuses the distinction between Hodgkin's disease and non-Hodgkin's lymphoma. This distinction was primarily based on the extraordinary reactive component seen in Hodgkin's disease. Separation of Hodgkin's disease from non-Hodgkin's lymphoma may become even less distinct if studies clearly show the lymphocytic nature of Reed-Sternberg cells. Until markers with specificity for Hodgkin's disease become available, Hodgkin's disease should be diagnosed by following the more traditional steps of recognizing the reactive component specific for each type of Hodgkin's disease and detecting Reed-Sternberg cells in association with the appropriate reaction (Table 38). In borderline cases, immunocytochemistry with PIP that shows appropriate CD45, CD15, and CD30 reactions in Reed-Sternberg cells supports the diagnosis (Table 39).

Table 38

COMPARISON OF CLASSIFICATIONS OF HODGKIN'S DISEASE*

LUKES-BUTLER	RYE

Lymphocytic and/or histiocytic

    Nodular

                              Lymphocyte predominance

    Diffuse

Nodular sclerosis ———————————————— Nodular sclerosis

Mixed ———————————————— Mixed

Diffuse fibrosis

                              Lymphocyte depletion

Reticular

* Lukes, R.J., Craver, L.F., Hall, T.C., Rappaport, H., and Rubin, P. Report of the Nomenclature Committee. Cancer Res. 26(part 1):1311, 1966

Table 39

PARAFFIN IMMUNOPEROXIDASE* REACTIVITY EXPECTED IN HODGKIN'S DISEASE

Histologic Types	CD45 (Leuko-cyte Common Antigen)	CD15 (Leu-M1)	CDw75 (LN-1)	CD20 (L26)	CD30 (Ber H2)
L&H types					
Nodular	+	−	+	+	−
Diffuse	+	−	+	+	−
Mixed	−	+	−	−	+
Nodular sclerosing	−	+	−	−	+
Diffuse fibrosis	−	+	−	−	+
Reticular	−	+	−	−	+

* See Tables 7 and 8 for antibody descriptions

229

Thus, the heterogeneity of Hodgkin's disease is indicated by both immunologic and histopathologic features. Whether this apparent heterogeneity is a reflection of variation in host or oncogenic event is uncertain. Nevertheless, a distinctive feature of Hodgkin's disease is the immunologic reaction to the induction of neoplasia.

Clinical Features. The most common presenting symptom in Hodgkin's disease is painless peripheral lymphadenopathy. Cervical and supraclavicular nodes are involved most frequently, followed by axillary and inguinal involvement. "B" symptoms are prominent, particularly in older patients, and their presence implies a worse prognosis for any stage or pathologic subtype of the disease. Other systemic symptoms that do not imply unfavorable prognosis include pruritus and alcohol-related pain. Extranodal presentation of Hodgkin's disease is much less common than in the non-Hodgkin's lymphomas.

On physical examination, the most common abnormality is peripheral lymphadenopathy. Splenomegaly is found in approximately 16 percent of the cases.

Hodgkin's disease spreads in a fairly predictable manner from involved nodal sites either antegrade or retrograde to contiguous lymphoid tissue. Hodgkin's disease ultimately disseminates into the parenchymal organs, and the liver and lung are most commonly involved. Bone marrow involvement is observed in approximately 5 percent of the cases.

A full staging evaluation includes a physical examination, routine laboratory analysis, chest X ray, lymphangiogram, abdominal computerized axial tomography, and liver-spleen scan. Although a full-staging celiotomy has been routine in the past, the procedure has been ques-

tioned because of a small risk of surgical morbidity, mortality, or postsplenectomy sepsis. Currently, celiotomy is advised if subsequent therapy is dependent upon the surgical findings. After a staging evaluation, the patient is designated as having stage I, II, III, or IV disease by the criteria outlined in the Ann Arbor classification system. The specific treatment is dependent upon the stage of disease.

Long-term complications of combination radiation and chemotherapy do occur in the form of second malignancies, including acute granulocytic leukemia and non-Hodgkin's lymphoma. Other side effects of this therapy include infertility, hypothyroidism, and pulmonary or cardiac changes secondary to radiation and chemotherapeutic treatment.

Histopathologic Features. Nodular sclerosing Hodgkin's disease is the most common type and is often easily recognized. Some cases of nodular sclerosing Hodgkin's disease, lymphocyte-predominant Hodgkin's disease, and lymphocyte-depleted Hodgkin's disease are very difficult to diagnose.

The histopathologic features vary with the different types of Hodgkin's disease and indicate a marked immunologic reaction to neoplasm induction. The quality and quantity of these two elements, the immunologic reaction on the one hand and the Reed-Sternberg cells on the other, determine the histopathologic appearance and the classification.

The L&H, mixed cellularity, and lymphocyte-depleted forms of Hodgkin's disease are related. Progression from L&H Hodgkin's disease to the depleted forms has been clearly documented (fig. 54). Most of these progressions have apparently involved the diffuse form of

RELATIONSHIP OF HISTOLOGIC TYPES

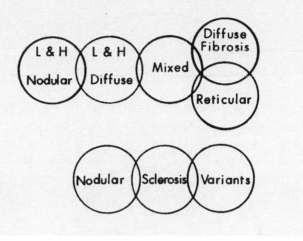

Figure 54
RELATIONSHIP OF HISTOLOGIC TYPES OF HODGKIN'S DISEASE
The parallel relationship of the nodular sclerosis variants and the remaining histologic types are illustrated by two parallel, overlapping series of circles. Diagnostic problems involve separating between the two series, as well as the overlapping circles. (Chart 1 from Lukes, R.J. Criteria for involvement of lymph node, bone marrow, spleen, and liver in Hodgkin's disease. Cancer Res. 31:1755-1767, 1971.)

lymphocyte-predominant Hodgkin's disease in that there is some evidence that the nodular form persists unchanged for long periods. Some patients present with mixed cellularity Hodgkin's disease or with one of the lymphocyte-depleted Hodgkin's disease types, without a demonstrable progression through this sequence. Nodular sclerosing Hodgkin's disease apparently remains purer in histopathologic expression (fig. 54), although the number of Reed-Sternberg cells in proportion to the reacting component may vary widely.

Patterns of nodal involvement are characteristic for each type of Hodgkin's disease, and they are illustrated schematically (figs. 55, 56) and in figures throughout this and the following sections (figs. 57, 58).

The cellular immunologic reaction is distinctive for each type of Hodgkin's disease and is more specific in appearance than individual Reed-Sternberg cells. The diagnosis and classification of Hodgkin's disease are made primarily by analyzing this reaction and secondarily by the cytologic features of Reed-Sternberg cells (figs. 59-64). The histologic character of the reactive features and Reed-Sternberg cells of each type of Hodgkin's disease are described in the following section.

Mononuclear Reed-Sternberg and Reed-Sternberg cells vary in appearance in the different types of Hodgkin's disease (plates XL-A–C; XLI-A–C; figs. 59-64) and show considerable variation within a single node. They vary in number from case to case, from area to area in a single node, and on sequential biopsies in the same patient. Mononuclear Reed-Sternberg and Reed-Sternberg cells, with the exception of some cases of lymphocyte-depleted Hodgkin's disease, are always associated with a characteristic immunologic reaction. They are not found as isolated cells in an otherwise normal node and are rarely found in sinuses or vascular spaces. The size of Reed-Sternberg cells varies from

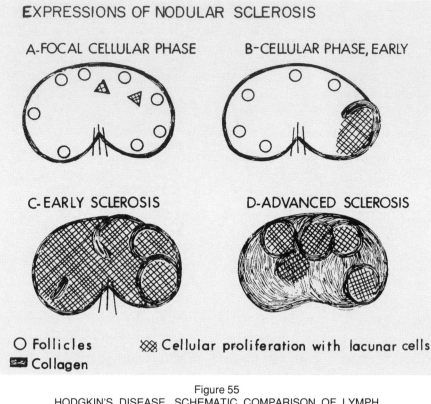

EXPRESSIONS OF NODULAR SCLEROSIS

A-FOCAL CELLULAR PHASE   B-CELLULAR PHASE, EARLY

C-EARLY SCLEROSIS   D-ADVANCED SCLEROSIS

○ Follicles   ⊗ Cellular proliferation with lacunar cells
▦ Collagen

Figure 55
HODGKIN'S DISEASE, SCHEMATIC COMPARISON OF LYMPH
NODE INVOLVEMENT IN NODULAR SCLEROSIS

A. Focal involvement, including lacunar cells on rare occasions, may be observed before any sclerosis. B. In the early cellular phase, there is a collagenous thickening of the capsule and extension of one band into the node. There is partial involvement by a cellular proliferation that includes lacunar-type Reed-Sternberg cells. C. Early sclerosis. The degree of sclerosis varies widely and may be limited to a small portion of the node that is totally involved by the typical cellular proliferation containing lacunar cells. D. Advanced sclerosis. The majority of the node or mass is replaced by dense collagen with residual nodular cellular portions containing typical lacunar-type Reed-Sternberg cells. (Chart 3 from Lukes, R.J. Criteria for involvement of lymph node, bone marrow, spleen, and liver in Hodgkin's disease. Cancer Res. 31:1755-1767, 1971.)

15 to 20 μm to giant forms of 200 to 300 μm. Mononuclear Reed-Sternberg cells as small as 10 μm may be found (fig. 60).

The appearance of mononuclear Reed-Sternberg and Reed-Sternberg cells is greatly affected by the type of fixative used. Formalin fixation produces poor nuclear detail and leads to a water-clear appearance of their cytoplasm (plates XL-C; XLI-A). In most cases of Hodgkin's dis-

ease, scattered Reed-Sternberg cells show degenerative or necrotizing changes. Mitotic figures, presumably in Reed-Sternberg cells, are often seen in Hodgkin's disease.

The Reed-Sternberg variants as we defined them (Lukes; Lukes and Butler) have proven to be extremely helpful in the diagnosis and classification of the histologic types of Hodgkin's disease. We described four variants of Reed-Sternberg

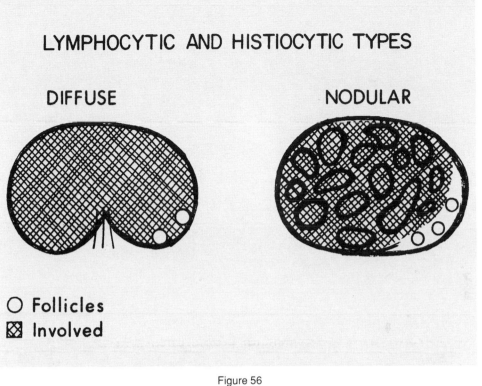

Figure 56
SCHEMATIC COMPARISON OF LYMPH NODE INVOLVEMENT
IN L&H TYPE, DIFFUSE AND NODULAR
Large irregular nodules extend throughout the node in the nodular form, whereas there is uniform involvement in the diffuse form. In each type, an occasional reactive follicle may remain at the periphery. (Chart 2 from Lukes, R.J. Criteria for involvement of lymph node, bone marrow, spleen, and liver in Hodgkin's disease. Cancer Res. 31:1755-1767, 1971.)

cells: (1) the diagnostic or marker Reed-Sternberg cell; (2) the L&H variant of the L&H types; (3) the lacunar cell of the nodular sclerosing type; and (4) the pleomorphic cell found in the bizarre sarcomatous form included in the reticular types. The diagnostic cell with bilobation or multilobation and huge nucleoli is found in all forms of Hodgkin's disease and is essential for the diagnosis of Hodgkin's disease when found in association with the histologic and cellular components of one of the histologic types. The diagnostic cell is the only type found in the mixed, diffuse fibrosis and nonsarcomatous reticular forms of Hodgkin's disease.

The L&H variant is essential for the recognition and diagnosis of both the nodular and diffuse L&H types of Hodgkin's disease (plate XL-C). The lacunar variant is an integral component of the nodular sclerosis type (plates XL-C; XLI-A) along with collagen band formation of varying degrees, whereas pleomorphic or bizarre Reed-Sternberg cells are found in the pleomorphic or sarcomatous variation of the reticular type (plate XLI-B). The lacunar cell of nodular sclerosing Hodgkin's

233

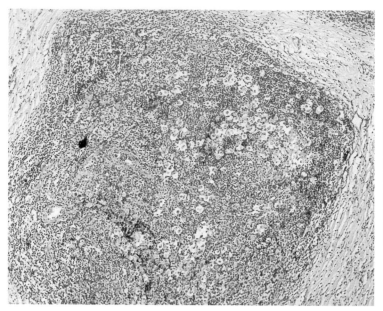

Figure 57
(Figures 57 and 72
are from the same patient)
HODGKIN'S DISEASE, NODULAR
SCLEROSIS, LYMPH NODE
The value of a histologic pattern in recognizing types of Hodgkin's disease is illustrated here and in figure 58. Large Reed-Sternberg cells are situated in lacunae. This cellular nodule is partially circumscribed by collagenous bands, an appearance that is virtually diagnostic of nodular sclerosing Hodgkin's disease. (Fig. 11 from Lukes, R.J. and Butler, J.J. The pathology and nomenclature of Hodgkin's disease. Cancer Res. 26:1063-1083, 1966.)

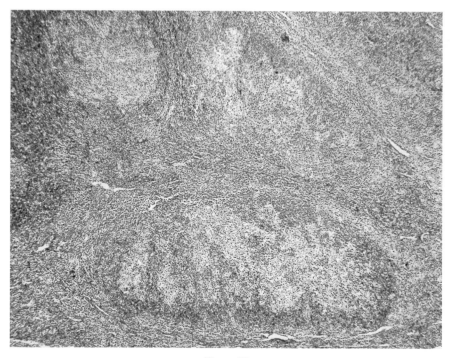

Figure 58
(Figure 58 and plate XLIII-A are from the same patient)
HODGKIN'S DISEASE, L&H NODULAR
Portions of three large lymphocytic nodules contain irregular large cell aggregates and resemble abnormal infiltrated follicular nodules. This low magnification appearance is virtually diagnostic of L&H nodular Hodgkin's disease. X30.

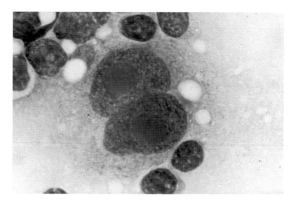

Figure 59
HODGKIN'S DISEASE, MIXED CELLULARITY,
TOUCH IMPRINT OF NODE
A diagnostic Reed-Sternberg cell is shown with its typical binucleate form and very large nucleoli. May-Gruenwald Giemsa. X1200.

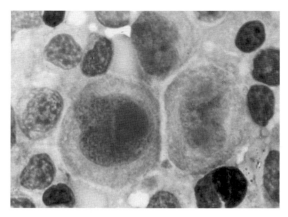

Figure 60
HODGKIN'S DISEASE, MIXED CELLULARITY,
TOUCH IMPRINT OF NODE
Several Reed-Sternberg variants show slight nuclear lobation. The largest cell in the center shows a large nucleolus. May-Gruenwald Giemsa. X1200.

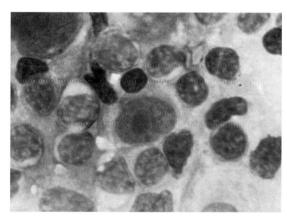

Figure 61
HODGKIN'S DISEASE, MIXED CELLULARITY,
TOUCH IMPRINT OF NODE
A small mononuclear variant is shown in the center of the field. The prominent nucleolus was taken as evidence that this was a mononuclear Reed-Sternberg cell. Note that this cell is only approximately twice as large in diameter as the adjacent small lymphocytes. May-Gruenwald Giemsa. X1200.

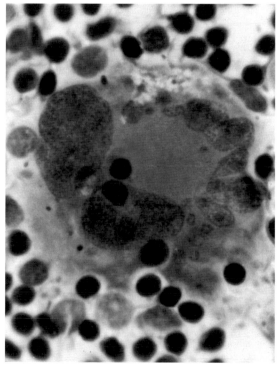

Figure 62
HODGKIN'S DISEASE, NODULAR SCLEROSING,
TOUCH IMPRINT OF NODE
An extremely polypoid Reed-Sternberg cell is seen with multiple nuclear indentations and lobations. May-Gruenwald Giemsa. X1200.

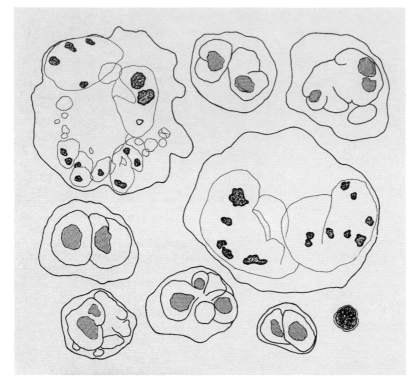

Figure 63
VARIATIONS IN REED-
STERNBERG CELLS
Variations in Reed-Sternberg cells
are shown in this composite prepared
from camera lucida drawings of touch
imprints. The two largest cells are
lacunar variants; the remainder are
from cases of mixed cellularity
Hodgkin's disease. Nucleoli are indicated by shading or scroll drawing. A
small lymphocyte at the lower right is
provided for size comparison.

Figure 64
MONONUCLEAR REED-
STERNBERG CELLS
Mononuclear Reed-Sternberg cells
are shown in this composite prepared
from camera lucida drawings of touch
imprints. All of these cells are from
cases of mixed cellularity Hodgkin's disease, with the exception of the large cell
in the upper row, center, which is from
nodular sclerosing Hodgkin's disease.
Nucleoli are shaded. A small lymphocyte at the lower left is provided for size
comparison.

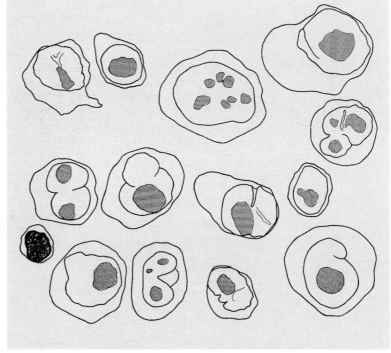

PLATE XL

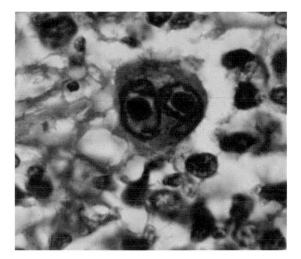

A. HODGKIN'S DISEASE, MIXED CELLULARITY
A diagnostic Reed-Sternberg cell is shown at high magnification. The huge inclusion-like nucleoli and binucleation are typical. X1210.

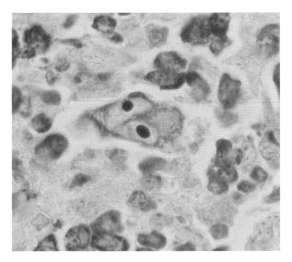

B. HODGKIN'S DISEASE, MIXED CELLULARITY
A binucleate Reed-Sternberg cell is shown in a sea of plasma cells. Giemsa. X1000.

C. HODGKIN'S DISEASE, REED-STERNBERG CELL VARIANTS
The L&H variants of Reed-Sternberg cells are compared with the lacunar variants in this composite. L&H variants are shown to the upper right and the bottom of this illustration. These cells have folded irregular nuclei with small nucleoli and scant cytoplasm. Numerous reactive histiocytes are also found. In contrast, the lacunar variant has nuclear forms that show extreme variation, from a mononuclear appearance to marked polypoidism, and has abundant pale cytoplasm. Upper left X300. Upper right X400. Bottom X300.

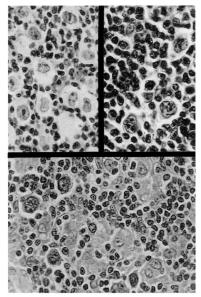

PLATE XLI

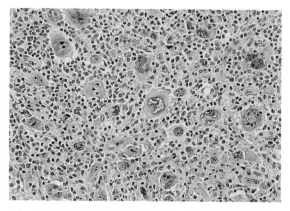

B. HODGKIN'S DISEASE, LYMPHOCYTE
DEPLETED, RETICULAR TYPE
An extremely dysplastic, bizarre, and sarcomatous variant of Reed-Sternberg cell is
shown. X600.

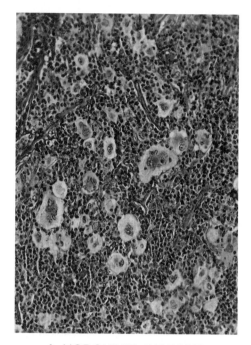

A. HODGKIN'S DISEASE,
NODULAR SCLEROSIS
(Plate XLI-A and figure 73
are from the same patient)
Lacunar variants of Reed-Sternberg
cells are seen in Zenker's fixed tissue.
The distinctive large variants of Reed-
Sternberg cells have abundant pale
cytoplasm, prominent lobation, and
sharp cellular borders. X300.

C. HODGKIN'S DISEASE, LYMPHOCYTE
DEPLETED, RETICULAR TYPE
Low magnification shows the hypocellular
appearance with numerous Reed-Sternberg
cells. X32.

disease and the L&H variants in L&H Hodgkin's disease are typically numerous and easily found, but diagnostic Reed-Sternberg cells in these two histologic types are uncommon or exceedingly rare. Because of this disparity in frequency of the critical Reed-Sternberg variants, the L&H and lacunar cells become especially important in considering the likelihood of Hodgkin's disease and its histologic types. Tissue must be ideally fixed and processed in order to recognize the subtle cytologic features of Reed-Sternberg variants. Poor handling may obscure the distinctive features of L&H, lacunar, and diagnostic Reed-Sternberg variants or produce artifactual changes that may simulate them. Therefore, when studying the pathologic features of the various histologic types of Hodgkin's disease, it is important to become familiar with the general components of each histologic type, as well as the cytologic characteristics of each Reed-Sternberg variant, including its manner of distribution, aggregation, and variation in frequency.

Differential Diagnosis. Hodgkin's disease has been confused with a variety of reactive and neoplastic conditions. Most of these mistakes are due to a lack of appreciation of the typical reactive changes seen in Hodgkin's disease and an inappropriate acceptance of binucleation or atypia of large cells as a diagnostic criterion per se of Hodgkin's disease. Hodgkin's disease should be diagnosed only when the characteristic reactive changes are detected and when Reed-Sternberg cells typical for the subclassification of Hodgkin's disease are demonstrated. Specific immunologic features may be added to our diagnostic criteria in the future.

Reactive states confused with Hodgkin's disease. Infectious mononucleosis produces architectural distortion and cytologic atypia, but the mixture of small and transformed lymphocytes, the presence of transformed lymphocytes in sinuses, the sparsity of Reed-Sternberg-like cells, and the lack of consolidation of the node should be taken as evidence against Hodgkin's disease. Immunoblastic lymphadenopathy produces architectural distortion and moderate cytologic atypia and may evolve into a malignant lymphoma. The pattern of nodal involvement, hypervascularization, and scarcity of Reed-Sternberg-like cells indicate immunoblastic lymphadenopathy rather than Hodgkin's disease. Rare patients with tuberculosis have fever, retroperitoneal adenopathy, and lymphangiographic changes confused with the clinical and radiographic findings in Hodgkin's disease (figs. 65, 66).

Non-Hodgkin's lymphomas confused with Hodgkin's disease. Peripheral T cell lymphomas, particularly those with a prominent epithelioid component (Lennert's lymphoma), are easily mistaken for Hodgkin's disease. Histopathologic differentiation between peripheral T cell lymphoma and Hodgkin's disease may be difficult. Immunologic studies showing a high percentage of T cells may be useful, particularly when the large cell component marks as T cell. CD15 (Leu-M1) reactivity is not expected in T cell lymphomas. Furthermore, Reed-Sternberg-like cells are rare in peripheral T cell lymphoma, as are plasma cells and eosinophils.

Follicular center cell lymphomas. Confusion with Hodgkin's disease may occur when dysplastic large noncleaved cells are mistaken for Reed-Sternberg cells. Lymphomas with neoplastic follicular nodulation are follicular center cell in type. Low magnification examination for follicular

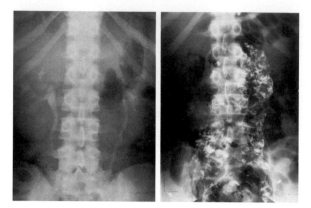

Figure 65
(Figures 65 and 66 are from the same patient)
HODGKIN'S DISEASE, DIFFERENTIAL DIAGNOSIS
This figure illustrates an intravenous pyelogram and lymphangiogram from a 20 year old black female nursing student with fever and lymphopenia. She had high fevers and other B symptoms. The lymphangiogram was thought to be typical of nodal involvement in Hodgkin's disease.

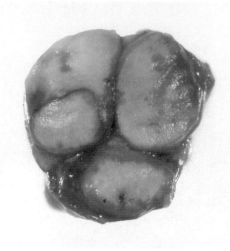

Figure 66
HODGKIN'S DISEASE,
DIFFERENTIAL DIAGNOSIS
This photograph demonstrates caseating necrosis in nodes obtained in an iliac dissection performed for diagnosis. The necrosis was shown to be due to tuberculosis.

nodulation in these cases is essential for an accurate diagnosis. Follicular center cell lymphomas also do not have the reaction mixture usually seen in Hodgkin's disease but may have high percentages of T cells on flow studies.

Epithelial neoplasms confused with Hodgkin's disease. The carcinoma most easily confused with Hodgkin's disease is a nasopharyngeal carcinoma that excites a prominent immunologic reaction (including plasma cells and eosinophils) and scarring. Some nasopharyngeal carcinomas have very large nuclei and small nucleoli but do not become multinucleated. Differentiation from Hodgkin's disease is based on the cytologic features of the neoplastic cells because the reaction patterns in both neoplasms are similar. Aggressive thymomas with dysplastic epithelial cells may be mistaken for Hodgkin's disease.

NODULAR SCLEROSING HODGKIN'S DISEASE

Clinical Features. Approximately 60 percent of the cases of Hodgkin's disease at referral centers are of the nodular sclerosing type, but the incidence is lower in impoverished populations. Nodular sclerosing Hodgkin's disease is most common in young adults and shows a predominance in females. Patients usually present with cervical or supraclavicular adenopathy and a mediastinal mass (figs. 67-69). Sixty percent of the patients are stage I or II at presentation.

Histopathologic Features (Table 40). The histopathologic criteria for nodular sclerosing Hodgkin's disease are prominent nodularity and architectural distortion due to birefringent broad collagen bands and the presence of lacunar variants of

Table 40

HODGKIN'S DISEASE, NODULAR SCLEROSIS

PATTERN
• Degree and pattern of involvement vary widely
• Focal involvement of reactive lymph nodes at times in paracortical area with thickened capsule and a single collagen band
• Collagen band formation or sclerosis varies greatly from a single band to advanced sclerosis
• Lacunar variants are scattered or in cohesive clusters
• Necrosis of lacunar clusters is frequent and occasionally extensive

CYTOLOGY — NEOPLASTIC	MARKERS — NEOPLASTIC
• Lacunar variant of Reed-Sternberg cell · High cytoplasmic to nuclear ratio · Water-clear granular cytoplasm · Prominent retraction of cytoplasmic membrane in formalin-fixed tissue; little retraction in B-5 fixed tissue · Nuclear hyperlobation typical, may be minor · Peripheral membrane acidophilic · Nucleoli usually small • Lacunar cells frequently numerous and cohesive around areas of necrosis • Large nucleated forms may be uncommon • Diagnostic Reed-Sternberg cells containing large nucleoli may be present	• PIP: Reed-Sternberg cells and variants mark as follows: 　CD45 (LCA) (−) 　CD15 (Leu-M1) (+) 　CDw75 (LN-1) (−) 　CD20 (L26) (−) 　CD30 (Ber H2) (+)

INVOLVED SITES	CLINICAL FEATURES
• Lymph nodes, supraclavicular, low cervical, axillary, lung hilar • Mediastinal (often thymic) mass • Bone marrow is uncommonly involved	• Asymptomatic state common • Anterior superior mediastinal mass often detected by X ray, at times with lung extension • All stages of disease at presentation but often stages I and II

REACTIVE COMPONENTS	DIFFERENTIAL DIAGNOSIS
• Numerous variations in the predominating cell population · Lymphocytic predominance · Lymphocytic predominance with eosinophils, plasma cells, and histiocytes · Mixed cellularity · Mixed cellularity with prominent lacunar cells · Lymphocytic depletion with pleomorphic lacunar cells • Numerous T cells usually present • Helper:suppressor ratio variable • Plasma cells show polyclonal cytoplasmic immunoglobulin	• Nodular sclerosing Hodgkin's disease may be confused with either L&H nodular, mixed cellularity, or lymphocyte-depleted Hodgkin's disease • Metastatic carcinoma

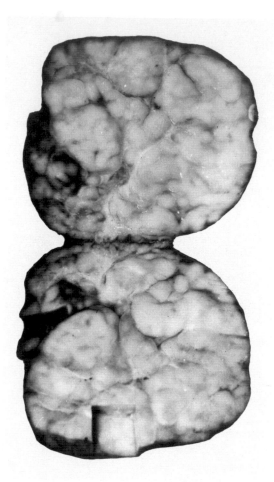

Figure 67
(Figures 67-69 are from the same patient)
HODGKIN'S DISEASE, NODULAR SCLEROSIS
A mediastinal mass was excised from the patient whose X rays are shown in figure 68. The cut surface of the mass had a bulging nodular character. (Fig. 19 from Lukes, R.J. and Butler, J.J. The pathology and nomenclature of Hodgkin's disease. Cancer Res. 26:1063-1083, 1966.)

Reed-Sternberg cells. The nodes are subdivided by single or multiple bands of polarizable connective tissue into nodules of varying size and configuration (figs. 70-72). These nodules do not conform to an anatomic structure and may be quite variable in size. Residual nodal tissue may be found in nodules, although the entire nodule usually shows changes of Hodgkin's disease. Residual normal node may be found adjacent to neoplastic nodules. On extension to adjacent nodes, nodular sclerosing Hodgkin's disease may involve only interfollicular areas. Capsular thickening is usually present and may be marked. In early lesions, fibrosis may involve only the capsule, but broad bands of sclerosis ultimately alter nodal architecture. Small and large areas of necrosis may be seen (plate XLII-C,D).

The cellular nodules isolated by connective tissue bands contain varying numbers of Reed-Sternberg cells (sheets of Reed-Sternberg cells are present in some cases) with intermixed small lymphocytes, plasma cells, macrophages (including foam cells), eosinophils, and neutrophils. Aggregates of eosinophils and neutrophils may be seen, but granulomas are unusual in nodular sclerosing Hodgkin's disease.

Reed-Sternberg variants in nodular sclerosing Hodgkin's disease are often called lacunar cells because their nuclei appear to sit in open spaces (plates XL-C; XLI-A). This artifact is usually due to formalin fixation (figs. 73, 74). Nodular sclerosing Hodgkin's disease variants often are multinucleated, show considerable range in nuclear size and shape, and have small nucleoli (plate XLII-A).

In summary, nodular sclerosing Hodgkin's disease is easily recognized when there are distinct fibrous bands, clearly defined nodules, and numerous lacunar variants. Diagnosis is much more difficult when only peripheral portions of mediastinal masses are available for sectioning. Some cases of nodular sclerosing Hodgkin's disease also appear atypical because of sheets of lacunar variants, the so-called

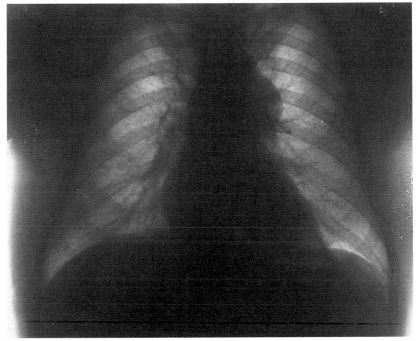

Figure 68
HODGKIN'S DISEASE,
NODULAR SCLEROSIS
This chest X ray shows a nodular superior mediastinal mass. (Courtesy of Andrews Air Force Base.)

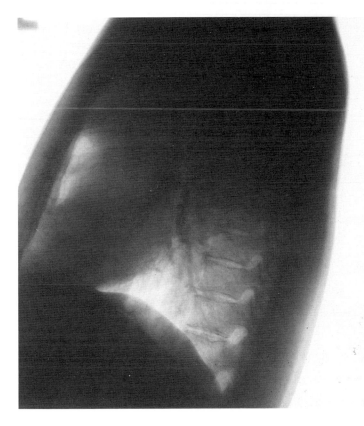

Figure 69
HODGKIN'S DISEASE, NODULAR SCLEROSIS
A lateral chest X ray shows an anterior-superior mediastinal mass. (Courtesy of Andrews Air Force Base.)

243

syncytial form (figs. 75, 76) (Strickler et al.), extensive necrosis (plate XLII-C), or exuberant acute inflammatory reactions. Nodular sclerosing Hodgkin's disease was initially not considered to show a progression to a mixed or lymphocyte-depleted phase, but another view has been proposed. On the basis of the extent of the reactive process, nodular sclerosing Hodgkin's disease has been subclassified into lymphocyte-predominant (lymphocytes predominate with few lacunar cells), mixed (numerous lacunar cells are intermixed with lymphocytes, plasma cells, eosinophils, and histiocytes), and lymphocyte-depleted nodular sclerosing Hodgkin's disease (lacunar cells predominate, and there is little reactive component) (Bennett et al.). The lymphocyte-depleted forms of nodular sclerosing Hodgkin's disease have a poorer prognosis.

Immunologic Features. Reed-Sternberg cells of nodular sclerosing Hodgkin's disease are usually positive on PIP for CD15 (Leu-M1) (plate XLII-B) and negative for CD45 (leukocyte common antigens). Monomorphic variants of nodular sclerosing Hodgkin's disease are usually CD15 positive and CD45 negative, thereby distinguishing them from non-Hodgkin's lymphomas, which are often CD15 negative and CD45 positive. The precise phenotype of the lacunar Reed-Sternberg cell is unclear, although there is evidence in a few cases that lacunar variants are activated T cells.

The reactive lymphocytes of nodular sclerosing Hodgkin's disease are primarily T cells, in contrast to lymphocyte predominant Hodgkin's disease, in which B cells predominate.

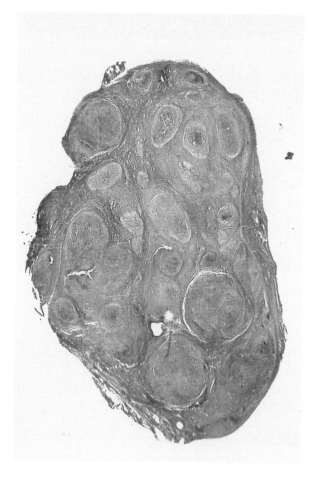

Figure 70
HODGKIN'S DISEASE, NODULAR SCLEROSIS
This mediastinal mass shows complete alteration of architecture with numerous ill-defined nodules outlined by bands of connective tissue. The sclerosing and nodular character of this disease is emphasized. H&E. X8. (Fig. 9 from Lukes, R.J. and Butler, J.J. The pathology and nomenclature of Hodgkin's disease. Cancer Res. 26:1063-1083, 1966.)

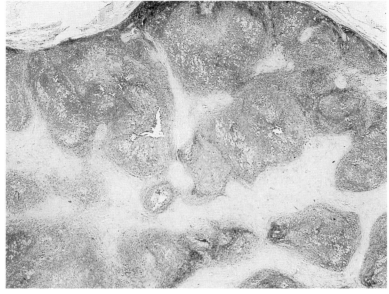

Figure 71
HODGKIN'S DISEASE, NODULAR
SCLEROSIS, LYMPH NODE
In this figure, there is partial sclerosis of the node by connecting collagen
bands. Nodular aggregates of lymphoid
tissue not clearly associated with collagen bands are apparent in the right-
hand portion of the field. H&E. X35.

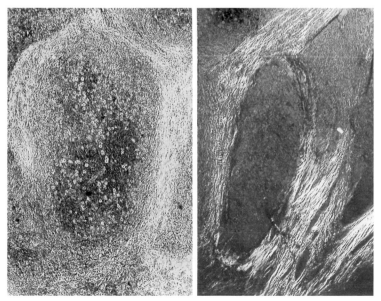

Figure 72
(Figures 72 and 57
are from the same patient)
HODGKIN'S DISEASE, NODULAR
SCLEROSIS, LYMPH NODE
These typical nodular cellular islands
are partially circumscribed by connective
tissue. Large pale cells situated in lacunae
are apparent at this magnification. At the
right, the birefringent character of the collagen is brought out by polarized light. H&E.
X35. (Fig. 10 from Lukes, R.J. and Butler,
J.J. The pathology and nomenclature of
Hodgkin's disease. Cancer Res. 26:1063-
1083, 1966.)

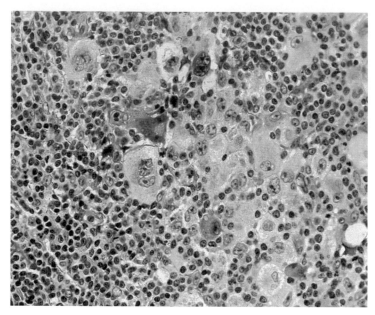

Figure 73
(Figure 73 and plate XLI-A
are from the same patient)
HODGKIN'S DISEASE, NODULAR
SCLEROSIS, LYMPH NODE
In Zenker's fixed tissue, artifactual retraction of the cytoplasm is minimized. The distinctive lacunar variants of Reed-Sternberg cells characteristically found in this type of Hodgkin's disease have abundant pale cytoplasm, prominent lobation, and sharp cellular borders. X350. (Fig. 13 from Lukes, R.J. and Butler, J.J. The pathology and nomenclature of Hodgkin's disease. Cancer Res. 26:1063-1083, 1966.)

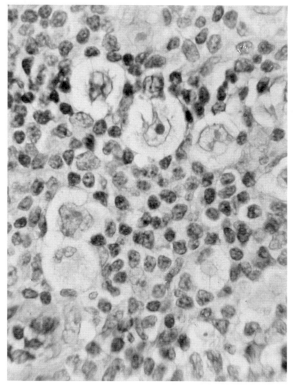

Figure 74
HODGKIN'S DISEASE, NODULAR SCLEROSIS,
LYMPH NODE
These lacunar cells exhibit the pale cytoplasm with artifactual vacuolization and peripheral cytoplasmic retraction that is typically found in tissue fixed in formalin. X700. (Fig. 2 from Lukes, R.J. Criteria for involvement of lymph node, bone marrow, spleen, and liver in Hodgkin's disease. Cancer Res. 31:1755-1767, 1971.)

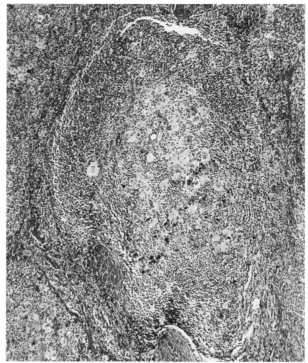

Figure 75
HODGKIN'S DISEASE, NODULAR SCLEROSIS,
CELLULAR PHASE WITH
FEW COLLAGENOUS BANDS
Collagen band formation was found elsewhere in this lymph node and is required for the diagnosis of nodular sclerosing Hodgkin's disease. No bands are shown in this illustration. X55. (Fig. 12 from Lukes, R.J. and Butler, J.J. The pathology and nomenclature of Hodgkin's disease. Cancer Res. 26:1063-1083, 1966.)

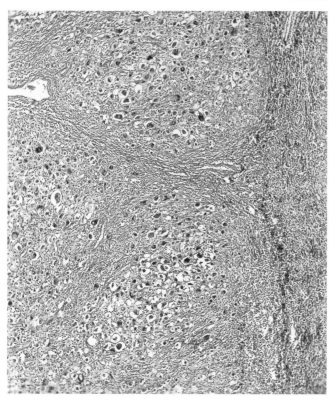

Figure 76
HODGKIN'S DISEASE, NODULAR SCLEROSIS,
LYMPH NODE
These ill-defined nodules contain large numbers of Reed-Sternberg cells of the lacunar type. There is only a narrow zone of connective tissue around the nodules, and the nodules are almost depleted of lymphocytes. H&E. X40.

PLATE XLII

A. NODULAR SCLEROSING HODGKIN'S DISEASE, LYMPH NODE
(Plate XLII-A and B are from the same patient)

This illustration shows the multiple appearances of lacunar cells in B5 fixed tissue. The cytoplasm is generally pale, acidophilic, and granular, with a high cytoplasmic/nuclear ratio. The nuclei are lobated and multilobated, at times in a horseshoe arrangement. Chromatin is generally finely dispersed, and the nuclear membranes are thin; nucleoli are generally small or inapparent. Small lymphocytes and eosinophils are interspersed. X400.

B. NODULAR SCLEROSING HODGKIN'S DISEASE, LYMPH NODE, PIP, WITH CD15 (LEU-M1)

Lacunar variants of Reed-Sternberg cells have various staining patterns. In many cells, there is a dark irregular mass of positivity, often in the perinuclear (Golgi) area. Many cells have intensely staining cytoplasmic membranes. X400.

C. NODULAR SCLEROSING HODGKIN'S DISEASE, LYMPH NODE

Massive necrosis was prominent in this node. In portions of the node (top), necrosis was so extensive as to suggest caseation. Elsewhere, sclerosis was noted with residual lymphoid tissue in which pale cytoplasmic lacunar variants were evident (lower portion). It is noteworthy that, in multiple sections of the node, only a few such cellular areas were found. X32.

D. NODULAR SCLEROSING HODGKIN'S DISEASE, LYMPH NODE
(Plate XLII-D and E are from the same patient)

In contrast to the process illustrated in Plate XLII-C, these sections have the more commonly observed small area of necrosis associated with nodular sclerosing Hodgkin's disease. The area of necrosis has ill-defined borders surrounded by a mass of lacunar cells of varying size and degree of nuclear lobation. X100.

E. NODULAR SCLEROSING HODGKIN'S DISEASE, LYMPH NODE

This lesion without obvious collagen bands may be confused with metastatic carcinoma. Collagen was apparent elsewhere in this section in both transsected and elongated bands. X435.

PLATE XLII

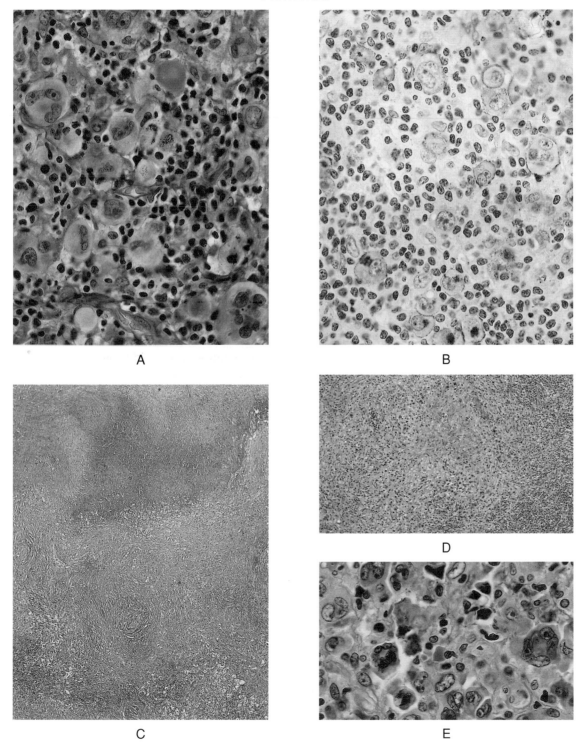

A

B

C

D

E

LYMPHOCYTE-PREDOMINANT HODGKIN'S DISEASE

Clinical Features. The lymphocyte-predominant form is rare, comprising approximately 5 percent of all Hodgkin's disease cases. The peak incidence occurs in young males. Cervical or axillary adenopathy is more frequent as a presenting manifestation than inguinal adenopathy. Intra-abdominal involvement is rare. Approximately 80 percent of the patients are stage I or II at presentation and are essentially asymptomatic, except for localized adenopathy. The prognosis of lymphocyte-predominant Hodgkin's disease is very favorable.

Histopathologic Features (Tables 41, 42). Lymphocyte-predominant Hodgkin's disease is divided into the two histopathologic subtypes L&H nodular and L&H diffuse. Small lymphocytes predominate in both types and are mixed with varying numbers of histiocytes. Eosinophils and polymorphonuclear neutrophils are rare. Diagnostic Reed-Sternberg cells are rare.

In lymphocyte-predominant Hodgkin's disease, L&H variants of Reed-Sternberg cells are numerous. These mononuclear cells resemble large transformed lymphocytes, with hyperlobated nuclei and finely granular chromatin ("popcorn nuclei"). These cells do not appear multinucleated, have a small amount of pale cytoplasm, and characteristically small nucleoli (plate XLIII-B,C).

In the L&H nodular subtype of lymphocyte-predominant Hodgkin's disease, there is almost total obliteration of the nodal architecture by a characteristic, yet vague, nodular process (plate XLIII-A,D). An attenuated rim of residual node is often compressed against the nodal capsule.

Necrosis is absent, and some cases may show a few delicate areas of hyalinization, but connective tissue deposition is insignificant. The nodules are chiefly composed of small round lymphocytes with varying numbers of epithelioid histiocytes. The histiocytes often form small aggregates and, in some cases, resemble small sarcoid granulomas. L&H variants of Reed-Sternberg cells are mainly seen in the nodules. Diagnostic Reed-Sternberg cells are rare, and step sections may be required for their identification.

In diffuse L&H Hodgkin's disease, a few residual germinal centers may remain, but a thin rim of compressed nodal tissue, as seen in nodular L&H Hodgkin's disease, is not seen (figs. 77, 78). Some cases of diffuse L&H Hodgkin's disease may contain a few ill-defined nodules that are difficult to identify without the aid of a reticulin or PAS stain. The reactive component is usually similar to that seen in nodular L&H Hodgkin's disease, although the histiocytic component may be more apparent (fig. 79). L&H variants are present, as in nodular L&H Hodgkin's disease. Cases with easily identified Reed-Sternberg cells are best classified as mixed cellularity Hodgkin's disease.

In summary, lymphocyte-predominant Hodgkin's disease is difficult to recognize unless slide preparations are thin and tissue is properly fixed. The macronodules present in the L&H nodular type and the compressed adjacent normal node are helpful low magnification clues. Diagnostic Reed-Sternberg cells may be extremely rare.

Nodes from patients with lymphocyte-predominant Hodgkin's disease may show the distinctive germinal center abnormality called progressive transformation of

Table 41

HODGKIN'S DISEASE, LYMPHOCYTIC AND HISTIOCYTIC NODULAR (LYMPHOCYTE PREDOMINANT)

PATTERN
• Large ill-defined nodules • Compressed atrophic node or atrophic follicular centers usually present in periphery • Progressively transformed follicles occasionally seen

CYTOLOGY — NEOPLASTIC	MARKERS — NEOPLASTIC

• Frequent L&H variants of Reed-Sternberg cells (large cells with polypoid nuclei, dot nucleoli, and scant cytoplasm)
 	
• Diagnostic Reed-Sternberg cells rare
	• PIP: Reed-Sternberg cells and variants mark as follows:
	  CD45 (LCA) (+)
	  CD15 (Leu-M1) (−)
	  CDw75 (LN-1) (+)
	  CD20 (L26) (+)
	  CD30 (Ber H2) (−)
	  EMA (+)
	  Monotypic B (±)
	
	• Nodules mark as B cells

INVOLVED SITES	CLINICAL FEATURES
• Superficial adenopathy (usually cervical)	• Usually stage I or II • Spleen, marrow involvement rare • May progress to mixed cellularity

REACTIVE COMPONENTS	DIFFERENTIAL DIAGNOSIS

• Plasma cells, eosinophils may be present in small numbers
 	
• Small lymphocytes in nodules and between nodules thought to be reactive
 	
• Macrophages in small clusters or as giant cells; sarcoid clusters of histiocytes
	• Hodgkin's disease, L&H diffuse
	
	• Follicular center cell lymphoma, small cleaved cell, follicular
	
	• Reactive states
	  Toxoplasmosis
	  Progressive follicular transformation
	
	• Chronic lymph node hyperplasia with small widely separated follicles

Table 42

HODGKIN'S DISEASE, LYMPHOCYTIC AND HISTIOCYTIC DIFFUSE (LYMPHOCYTE PREDOMINANT)

PATTERN	
• Diffuse alteration of architecture • Compressed adjacent atrophic node not seen • Follicles typically absent	
CYTOLOGY — NEOPLASTIC	**MARKERS — NEOPLASTIC**

• Frequent L&H variants of Reed-Sternberg cells (large cells with polypoid nuclei, dot nucleoli, and scant cytoplasm)
 	
• Diagnostic Reed-Sternberg cells rare; if easily found, classify as mixed
	• PIP: Reed-Sternberg cells and variants mark as follows:
	    CD45 (LCA) (+)
	    CD15 (Leu-M1) (−)
	    CDw75 (LN-1) (+)
	    CD20 (L26) (+)
	    CD30 (Ber H2) (−)
	    EMA (+), some cases

INVOLVED SITES	**CLINICAL FEATURES**
• Superficial lymphadenopathy	• Usually stage I or II • Spleen, marrow involvement rare • May progress to mixed cellularity
REACTIVE COMPONENTS	**DIFFERENTIAL DIAGNOSIS**
• Plasma cells, eosinophils may be present in small numbers • Small lymphocytes thought to be reactive • Macrophages in small clusters or giant cells • Sarcoid clusters of histiocytes at times	• Hodgkin's disease, L&H nodular • Small B/T cell neoplasms • Plasmacytoid lymphocytic lymphoma • Follicular center cell lymphoma, small cleaved cell, diffuse

252

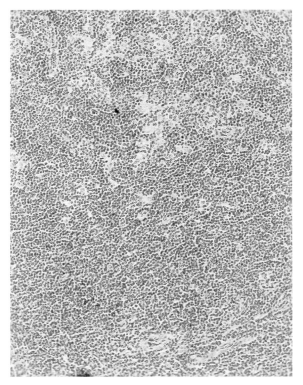

Figure 77
HODGKIN'S DISEASE, L&H DIFFUSE,
LYMPH NODE
Large histiocytes are scattered throughout this predominantly small lymphocytic proliferation. X130. (Fig. 5 from Lukes, R.J. and Butler, J.J. The pathology and nomenclature of Hodgkin's disease. Cancer Res. 26:1063-1083, 1966.)

Figure 78
HODGKIN'S DISEASE, L&H DIFFUSE,
LYMPH NODE
There is diffuse involvement by a lymphocytic population with numerous histiocytes occurring singly or in small clusters. Some of these clusters resemble epithelioid clusters, as in lymphoepithelioid lymphoma. Careful inspection reveals L&H and diagnostic Reed-Sternberg cells, whereas in lymphoepithelioid lymphoma, diagnostic Reed-Sternberg cells are not found. X70.

germinal centers (Poppema et al.). This abnormality may occur in patients with antecedent or concurrent lymphocyte-predominant Hodgkin's disease, as well as in patients who will develop lymphocyte-predominant Hodgkin's disease. There is also a subset of patients with progressive transformation who never have lymphocyte-predominant Hodgkin's disease. Transformed germinal centers are unusually large. The breakdown of the interface between the mantle zones and germinal centers produces a scalloped or serpentine border (plate XLIV-A,B,D; fig. 80). As the lesion progresses, there is extensive infiltration of the germinal center by small lymphocytes until small groups of large transformed cells or single large transformed cells are completely surrounded by small lymphocytes. The resultant progressively transformed germinal center

PLATE XLIII

A. HODGKIN'S DISEASE, L&H NODULAR, LYMPH NODE
(Plate XLIII-A and figure 58 are from the same patient)

The ill-defined nodules containing pale-staining histiocytes are characteristic of L&H nodular Hodgkin's disease as shown in this low magnification photomicrograph. X25.

B and C. HODGKIN'S DISEASE, L&H NODULAR, LYMPH NODE
(Plate XLIII-B,C, plate XLIV-A,B, and figure 80 are from the same patient)

In these illustrations, several L&H variants of Reed-Sternberg cells are found in a predominantly lymphocytic population. L&H variants vary in size and configuration. Nuclei are often indented, folded, or lobated and have finely dispersed chromatin, a delicate nuclear membrane, and small inapparent nucleoli. The cytoplasm is pale, acidophilic, and limited in amount. X600.

D. HODGKIN'S DISEASE, L&H NODULAR, LYMPH NODE
(Plate XLIII-D,E and plate XLIV-C,D are from the same patient)

In this illustration, a single ill-defined nodule contains numerous pink cytoplasmic histiocytes, lymphocytes, and scattered L&H variants. X132.

E. HODGKIN'S DISEASE, L&H NODULAR, LYMPH NODE, PIP, WITH CD45RO (UCHL-1)

A parallel section from the same nodule stained with a pan-T marker reveals many of the lymphocytes within the nodule are T cells, whereas histiocytes and L&H variants are unstained. X132.

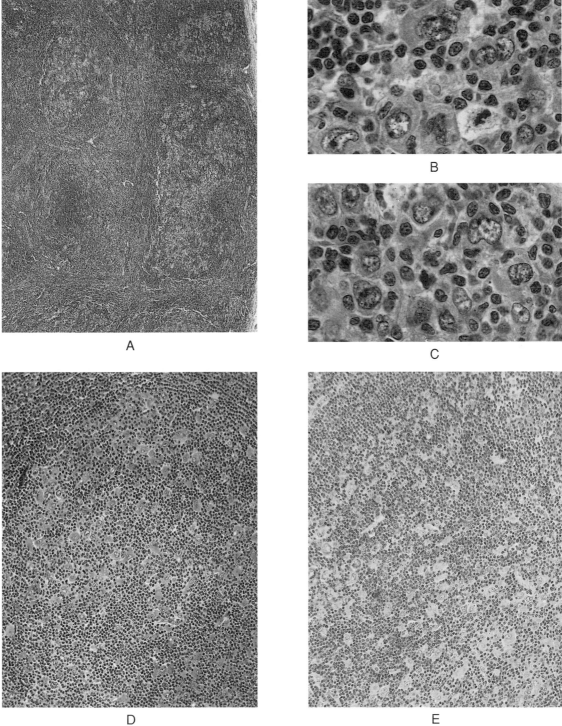

PLATE XLIII

A

B

C

D

E

255

Hodgkin's Disease

PLATE XLIV

A. PROGRESSIVE FOLLICULAR TRANSFORMATION, LYMPH NODE, PIP, WITH CDw75 (LN-1)
(Plate XLIV-A,B, plate XLIII-B,C, and figure 80 are from the same patient)

The follicular center cell antibody CDw75 marks a normal residual follicle on the bottom and an elongated, fragmented follicular center on the top. This type of fragmentation is typical of progressive follicular transformation. X80.

B. PROGRESSIVE FOLLICULAR TRANSFORMATION, LYMPH NODE, PIP, WITH CDw75

The edge of an infiltrated disrupted follicular center is stained, marking abnormal cells that extend into adjacent lymphoid tissue. Some of these abnormal large cells resemble L&H variants, which are often found in this location. X400.

C. HODGKIN'S DISEASE, L&H NODULAR, LYMPH, PIP, WITH CDw75
(Plate XLIV-C,D and plate XLIII-D,E are from the same patient)

The follicular center cell marking antibody CDw75 labels most of the L&H variants of Reed-Sternberg cells. Many have a single, large, deeply stained perinuclear globule and light-staining cytoplasm with distinctly positive membranes. Small lymphocytes are essentially unstained. X400.

D. HODGKIN'S DISEASE, L&H NODULAR, PIP, WITH CD74 (LN-2)

L&H variants principally stain with a single, intensely positive perinuclear globule, and the histiocytic cytoplasm is strongly and diffusely positive. The cytoplasm in a few cells stain slightly. The nuclei of a few lymphocytes are also positive. X400.

PLATE XLIV

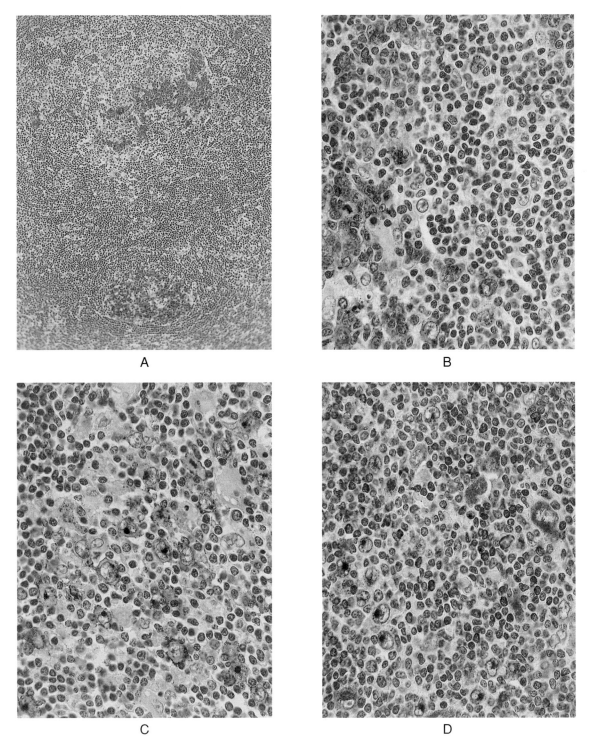

A

B

C

D

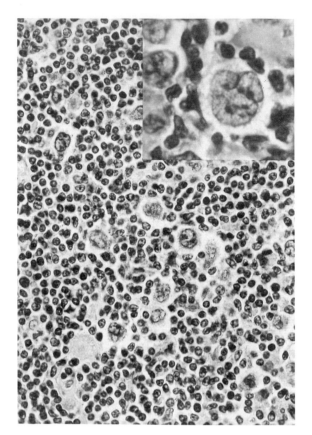

Figure 79
HODGKIN'S DISEASE, L&H DIFFUSE, LYMPH NODE
High magnification shows a mixture of small lymphocytes, histiocytes, and scattered L&H variants. The inset at the upper right is an L&H variant of a Reed-Sternberg cell. These fragile polypoid cells have large, convoluted, twisted, overlapping nuclear folds with finely distributed chromatin, small nucleoli, and a small amount of pale indistinct cytoplasm. X800. (Fig. 4 from Lukes, R.J. Criteria for involvement of lymph node, bone marrow, spleen, and liver in Hodgkin's disease. Cancer Res. 31:1755-1767, 1971.)

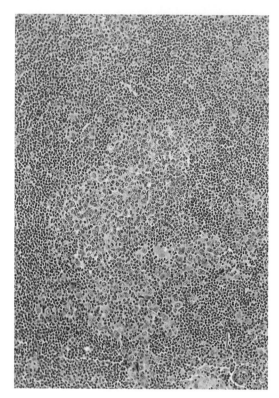

Figure 80
(Figure 80, plate XLIII-B,C, and plate XLIV-A,B are from the same patient)
PROGRESSIVE FOLLICULAR TRANSFORMATION, LYMPH NODE
These follicular centers have been infiltrated and fragmented by lymphocytes. The pattern of disruption of follicles varies considerably from case to case. X132.

is reminiscent of nodular lymphocyte-predominant Hodgkin's disease. However, lymphocyte-predominant Hodgkin's disease should not be diagnosed unless L&H variants and Reed-Sternberg cells are identified.

Immunologic Features. The association of lymphocyte-predominant Hodgkin's disease with progressive transformation of germinal centers suggests that lymphocyte-predominant Hodgkin's disease may be related to a germinal center proliferation and is therefore a B lymphocyte process. The reactive component of lymphocyte-predominant Hodgkin's disease is often B lymphocytic by immunological studies, and L&H variants in lymphocyte-predominant Hodgkin's disease mark with CD20, CDw75 (LN-1), and CD74 (LN-2) (plate LIV-C,D). Reed-Sternberg cells in most of the other subtypes of Hodgkin's disease are CDw75 negative. L&H variants differ immunohistochemically from other Reed-Sternberg cells in expressing common leukocyte antigens and epithelial membrane antigens, and failing to react with CD15 and CD30. These immunohistochemical differences indicate that lymphocyte-predominant Hodgkin's disease is a distinct entity, probably of B cell origin, and is different from the other subtypes of Hodgkin's disease.

MIXED CELLULARITY HODGKIN'S DISEASE

Clinical Features. Approximately 30 percent of the cases of Hodgkin's disease are mixed cellularity in type. A slight majority of these cases present with stage III or IV disease, and abdominal involvement is common. Prognosis is less favorable than in nodular sclerosing Hodgkin's disease.

Histopathologic Features (Table 43). The growth pattern is generally diffuse, with little residual node or capsular thickening. Partial or interfollicular involvement may be seen (plate XLV-A; fig. 81), and necrosis is unusual. Thin strands of connective tissue may be present. Macrophages, small lymphocytes, eosinophils, and plasma cells are evenly interspersed with mononuclear Reed-Sternberg and Reed-Sternberg cells (plate XLV-B,C).

The term "diagnostic" is applied to those Reed-Sternberg cells that are bilobated with huge inclusion-like nucleoli and amphophilic or clear cytoplasm. Such cells are rarely seen in lymphocyte-predominant Hodgkin's disease, are often present in nodular sclerosing Hodgkin's disease and some cases of lymphocyte-depleted Hodgkin's disease, and are required for

the diagnosis of mixed cellularity Hodgkin's disease (plate XLV-C). Cells that appear similar but occur in a completely different immunologic background may be seen in infectious mononucleosis, other benign reactive states, and a variety of non-Hodgkin's lymphomas. Thus, binucleate cells with large nucleoli are only "diagnostic" in the appropriate setting.

In summary, nodes are evenly involved in typical cases of mixed cellularity Hodgkin's disease and show similar changes in all sections. A consistent mixture of reacting and neoplastic components is present, with many of the latter having the typical appearance of diagnostic Reed-Sternberg cells.

Mixed cellularity Hodgkin's disease includes cases that are intermediate between lymphocyte-predominant Hodgkin's disease and lymphocyte-depleted Hodgkin's disease, as well as cases that do not fulfill all of the diagnostic criteria of the other subtypes. As a result, a wide spectrum of histopathologic features is seen in mixed cellularity Hodgkin's disease.

Cases that display a prominent lymphocytic-histiocytic reaction, as in lymphocyte-predominant Hodgkin's disease, but contain numerous diagnostic Reed-Sternberg cells are best categorized as mixed cellularity Hodgkin's disease (plate XLV-D). Nodes with a small amount of birefringent sclerosis should be diagnosed as mixed cellularity Hodgkin's disease rather than nodular sclerosing Hodgkin's disease if they do not contain lacunar Reed-Sternberg variants (Lukes). Partially involved nodes often do not display all features of lymphocyte-predominant, lymphocyte-depleted, or nodular sclerosing Hodgkin's disease. Such cases are categorized as mixed cellularity Hodgkin's disease if they are from the primary diagnostic biopsy.

Table 43

HODGKIN'S DISEASE, MIXED CELLULARITY

PATTERN
• Diffusely altered architecture, with residual follicles or adjacent compressed node • Focal involvement in interfollicular area • Foci of necrosis unusual • Collagen bands absent

CYTOLOGY — NEOPLASTIC	MARKERS — NEOPLASTIC

• Diagnostic Reed-Sternberg cells (binucleate in appearance; mirror-image nuclei, prominent large nucleoli) are frequent
 	
• Mononuclear Reed-Sternberg cells range upward in size from 10 μm
 	
• Mitoses unusual
 	
• Degeneration of Reed-Sternberg cells with condensation of cytoplasm and nuclear material often seen; "mummification"
	• PIP: Reed-Sternberg cells and variants mark as follows:
	    CD45 (LCA) (–)
	    CD15 (Leu-M1) (+)
	    CDw75 (LN-1) (–)
	    CD20 (L26) (–)
	    CD30 (Ber H2) (+)
	    CIg polytypic

INVOLVED SITES	CLINICAL FEATURES
• Superficial nodes • Marrow, liver, spleen • Mediastinum usually negative	• Superficial adenopathy • B symptoms • Hepatosplenomegaly ±

REACTIVE COMPONENTS	DIFFERENTIAL DIAGNOSIS
• Small lymphocytes, mostly T • B cells and plasma cells • Eosinophils • Macrophages, giant cells may be present	• Hodgkin's disease, nodular sclerosing • Hodgkin's disease, lymphocyte depleted • Hodgkin's disease, lymphocyte predominant • Peripheral T cell lymphoma • Reactive adenopathy • Immunoblastic lymphadenopathy

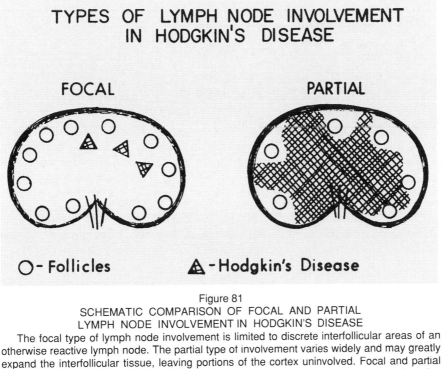

Figure 81
SCHEMATIC COMPARISON OF FOCAL AND PARTIAL
LYMPH NODE INVOLVEMENT IN HODGKIN'S DISEASE
The focal type of lymph node involvement is limited to discrete interfollicular areas of an otherwise reactive lymph node. The partial type of involvement varies widely and may greatly expand the interfollicular tissue, leaving portions of the cortex uninvolved. Focal and partial involvement are seen principally in mixed cellularity Hodgkin's disease and nodular sclerosing Hodgkin's disease. (Chart 4 from Lukes, R.J. Criteria for involvement of lymph node, bone marrow, spleen, and liver in Hodgkin's disease. Cancer Res. 31:1755-1767, 1971.)

Mixed cellularity Hodgkin's disease may also be associated with a prominent granulomatous reaction. These cases may be difficult to recognize because the reactive component may predominate. Focal consolidation of the node due to interfollicular infiltration of eosinophils, plasma cells, macrophages, and lymphocytes should suggest the diagnosis. Mononuclear and diagnostic Reed-Sternberg cells may be difficult to find. Appropriate immunoperoxidase studies often help in confirming the diagnosis.

Cases of mixed cellularity Hodgkin's disease may show foci of cellular depletion and diffuse fibrosis. Some cases may also show monomorphic growth of classic Reed-Sternberg cells. These changes, in the setting of mixed cellularity Hodgkin's disease, may be a harbinger of evolution to lymphocyte-depleted Hodgkin's disease.

Immunologic Features. As in nodular sclerosing Hodgkin's disease, the reactive component of mixed cellularity Hodgkin's disease contains numerous T lymphocytes. The Reed-Sternberg cells of mixed cellularity Hodgkin's disease are usually CD15 (Leu-M1) positive and CD45 (leukocyte common antigen) negative. CD15 negativity is encountered more often in mixed cellularity Hodgkin's disease than in nodular sclerosing Hodgkin's disease.

PLATE XLV

A. HODGKIN'S DISEASE, MIXED CELLULARITY WITH INTERFOLLICULAR INVOLVEMENT, LYMPH NODE

Areas of uninvolved lymphoid tissue containing reactive follicles with lymphocytic mantles are separated by the mixed cellular population of Hodgkin's disease. This type of lesion may be focal, multifocal, or partial and is best appreciated by careful low magnification examination of well-prepared material. X50.

B. HODGKIN'S DISEASE, MIXED CELLULARITY, LYMPH NODE

A variety of cellular components have a disorderly distribution. Note the fine, fibrillar connective tissue found in the mixed type, along with diagnostic Reed-Sternberg cells. H&E. X180.

C. HODGKIN'S DISEASE, MIXED CELLULARITY, LYMPH NODE

This high magnification photograph shows the characteristic mixture of eosinophils, plasma cells, and mononuclear and binucleate Reed-Sternberg cells. X400.

D. HODGKIN'S DISEASE, MIXED CELLULARITY, WITH PROMINENCE OF LYMPHOCYTES

This process is classified as the mixed type, even if lymphocytes predominate, when large nucleolated mononuclear and polypoid Reed-Sternberg cells are numerous, and no lacunar cells or L&H cells are identified. H&E. X600.

PLATE XLV

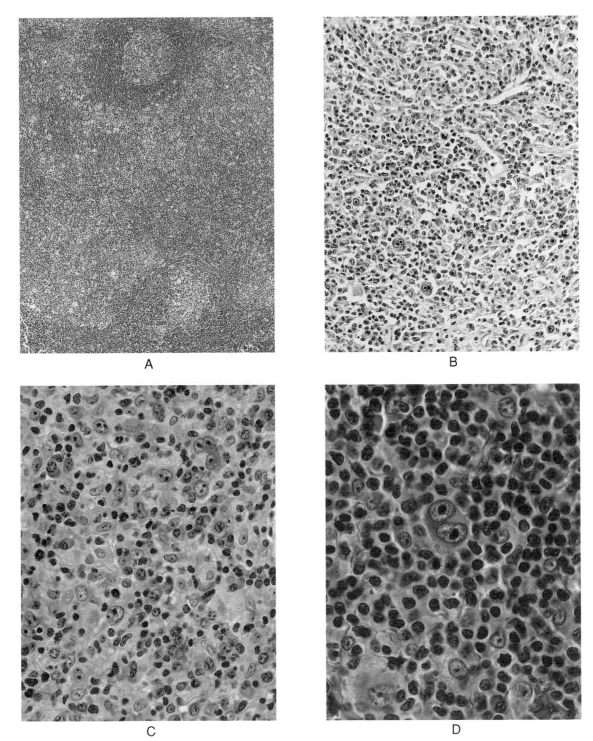

A

B

C

D

LYMPHOCYTE-DEPLETED HODGKIN'S DISEASE
(Including Diffuse Fibrosis and Reticular Histologic Types)

Clinical Features. Lymphocyte-depleted Hodgkin's disease comprises approximately 5 percent of all cases of Hodgkin's disease in the United States. The median age of onset is 55 years, and males are affected more commonly than females.

Most patients first seek medical attention because of "B" symptoms. Anorexia and weight loss occur in 67 percent of the patients, fever in 60 percent, and night sweats in 30 percent. Patients are often symptomatic 1 to 12 months prior to diagnosis.

The initial diagnosis of lymphocyte-depleted Hodgkin's disease may be made by biopsy of peripheral lymphadenopathy but may also require a prolonged evaluation for fever of unknown etiology in a patient whose Hodgkin's disease is located solely within the abdomen (liver, spleen) or bone marrow.

On physical examination, peripheral lymphadenopathy varies and occurs in as many as 70 percent of the patients. However, some series report a low incidence. Hepatomegaly alone is found in 25 percent of the cases, splenomegaly alone in 7 percent of the cases, and hepatosplenomegaly in 20 percent of the cases.

Laboratory analysis reveals anemia, thrombocytopenia, lymphopenia in over 50 percent of the cases, and abnormal liver function tests.

Disseminated disease is expected in the vast majority of the cases, with splenic involvement in 71 percent, liver involvement in 47 percent, and bone marrow involvement in 44 percent. In all, approximately 80 percent of the patients will be found to have stage III-B or IV disease at initial diagnosis.

In spite of the favorable therapeutic response for Hodgkin's disease of other pathologic types, lymphocyte-depleted Hodgkin's disease has an unfavorable prognosis, with a median survival of 2 years despite combination chemotherapy.

Histopathologic Features (Tables 44, 45). In the diffuse fibrosis type (figs. 82-84), hypocellularity is striking, with few lymphocytes, eosinophils, or plasma cells remaining. Diagnostic Reed-Sternberg cells are infrequent and may be difficult to identify. There is increased disorderly connective tissue, and fibrinoid changes may be seen. Lymph nodes are typically small.

The reticular type of lymphocyte-depleted Hodgkin's disease is characterized by a reduced immunologic reaction and numerous Reed-Sternberg cells, some of which are bizarre in size and appearance (plate XLI-B; figs. 85, 86). Small lymphocytes may be interspersed. Eosinophils and plasma cells are rare. Lymph nodes are characteristically large and may be massive in size.

Another type of lymphocyte-depleted Hodgkin's disease does not meet the criteria of diffuse fibrosis and reticular variants and is difficult to diagnose (Neiman et al.). This type often initially involves the liver, spleen, and marrow. In these organs, there may be a slight immunologic reaction associated with Reed-Sternberg cells, or small lymphocytes and plasma cells may be present. Eosinophils are unusual. This form of Hodgkin's disease typically involves the portal areas in the liver and the white pulp of the spleen (figs. 87, 88), and is apparently randomly distributed in the marrow. The suggestive granulomatous

Table 44

HODGKIN'S DISEASE, DIFFUSE FIBROSIS TYPE

PATTERN
• Diagnostic cells usually rare • Hypocellular, depleted small nodes • Amorphous, acidophilic fibrillar material throughout node • Disorderly reticulin fiber distribution • Areas of diagnostic or pleomorphic Reed-Sternberg cells on occasion

CYTOLOGY — NEOPLASTIC	MARKERS — NEOPLASTIC
• Diagnostic cells binucleate and have large or huge nucleoli	• PIP: Reed-Sternberg cells and variants mark as follows: CD45 (LCA) (+), some cases CD15 (Leu-M1) (+), most cases CDw75 (LN-1) (−) CD20 (L26) (+), some cases CD30 (Ber H2) (+), some cases CIg polytypic

INVOLVED SITES	CLINICAL FEATURES
• Abdominal lymph nodes • Spleen, liver • Bone marrow • Uncommon above the diaphragm	• B symptoms with wasting • Lymphopenia • Pancytopenia • Usually abdominal disease • Small lymph nodes • Stage III and IV usual

REACTIVE COMPONENTS	DIFFERENTIAL DIAGNOSIS
• Lymphocytes sparse • Plasma cells, eosinophils in small numbers • Follicular centers usually absent	• Postchemotherapy states • Immune deficient states, including lymphocyte depletion of AIDS

Table 45

HODGKIN'S DISEASE, RETICULAR TYPE

PATTERN
• Diagnostic cells are numerous or dominate the process • Node may be replaced by pleomorphic or sarcomatous aggregates • Areas of diffuse fibrosis and lymphocytic depletion often present

CYTOLOGY — NEOPLASTIC	MARKERS — NEOPLASTIC

• Lobated variation of Reed-Sternberg cell is common, and huge nucleoli are prominent, with deeply pyroninophilic cytoplasm
 	
• Sarcomatous or pleomorphic Reed-Sternberg cells are found at times
	• PIP: Reed-Sternberg cells and variants mark as follows:
	    CD45 (LCA) (+), some cases
	    CD15 (Leu-M1) (+), most cases
	    CDw75 (LN-1) (−)
	    CD20 (L26) (+), some cases
	    CD30 (Ber H2) (+), some cases
	    SIg, CIg polytypic

INVOLVED SITES	CLINICAL FEATURES
• Peripheral lymph nodes • Abdominal nodes	• Mass presentations in various sites • B symptoms and wasting with large tumor bulk • Lymphopenia and pancytopenia

REACTIVE COMPONENTS	DIFFERENTIAL DIAGNOSIS
• T cells and plasma cells sparse or in residual uninvolved node • Reactive follicles may remain in uninvolved portion of nodes	• Hodgkin's disease, mixed cellularity • Hodgkin's disease, nodular sclerosing with prominent lacunar cell component • Immunoblastic lymphoma B with pleomorphic B immunoblasts • Immunoblastic lymphoma T with pleomorphic T immunoblasts • Pleomorphic tumors including carcinomas

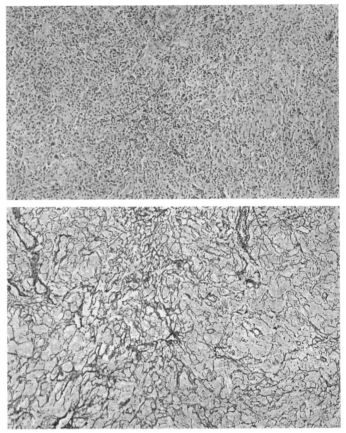

Figure 82
HODGKIN'S DISEASE, LYMPHOCYTE
DEPLETED (DIFFUSE FIBROSIS TYPE),
LYMPH NODE
This low magnification photomicrograph
shows the sparsity of cellular elements and diffuse effacement of architecture seen in this type
of Hodgkin's disease (top). X150. At the bottom,
a reticulin stain demonstrates the disorderly arrangement of connective tissue. Reticulin. X150.

features, coupled with small areas of necrosis, may lead to a mistaken diagnosis of
infection. These patients are often seriously and mysteriously ill, and the first diagnostic material may be from a marrow or
liver biopsy. The rarity of this disease, the
unusual reaction pattern, and the scarcity
of Reed-Sternberg cells often result in a
misdiagnosis, with correct diagnosis not
apparent until autopsy.

In summary, some cases of lymphocyte-
depleted Hodgkin's disease evolve from
a mixed cellularity presentation. In many
cases, it is difficult to separate treatment
effects with resultant hypocellularity from
the natural progression of the disease.

Reticular or sarcomatous variants are
extremely rare.

Immunologic Features. Comprehensive
phenotypic studies of the reactive component of lymphocyte-depleted Hodgkin's
disease have not been reported. In paraffin sections, Reed-Sternberg cells of
lymphocyte-depleted Hodgkin's disease
are usually CD15 (Leu-M1) positive and
CD45 (leukocyte common antigen) negative.
In some cases, the Reed-Sternberg cells
show an opposite phenotype, similar to the
Reed-Sternberg variants of lymphocyte-
predominant Hodgkin's disease, and
may also have CD20 and CDw75 (LN-1)
positivity.

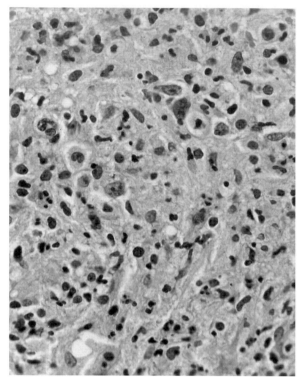

Figure 83
HODGKIN'S DISEASE, LYMPHOCYTE DEPLETED,
(DIFFUSE FIBROSIS), MARROW
A focus of diffuse fibrosis demonstrates the distinctive abnormal "precollagenous" character of the fibrosis typical of this type of Hodgkin's disease is seen in association with Reed-Sternberg variants. H&E. X435. (Fig. 7 from Lukes, R.J. Criteria for involvement of lymph node, bone marrow, spleen, and liver in Hodgkin's disease. Cancer Res. 31:1755-1767, 1971.)

Figure 84
HODGKIN'S DISEASE, LYMPHOCYTE DEPLETED,
(DIFFUSE FIBROSIS), MARROW
The marrow is diffusely altered in architecture due to the deposition of a prominent acidophilic interstitial material associated with diffuse fibrosis. This lesion may be focal or diffuse and is associated with decreased hematopoiesis, almost to the point of extreme hypocellularity. Reed-Sternberg cells may be difficult to find. The paradox in this lesion is that, with decreased cellularity, there is no increase in fat. H&E. X80.

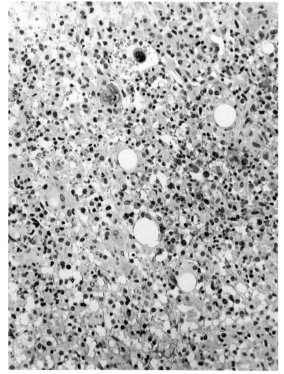

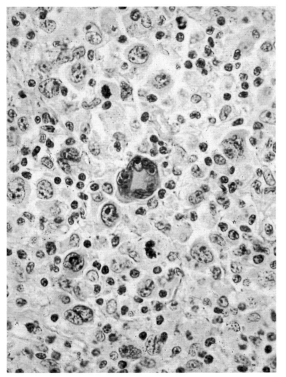

Figure 85
HODGKIN'S DISEASE, LYMPHOCYTE DEPLETED
(RETICULAR TYPE), LYMPH NODE
Various Reed-Sternberg cells are the prominent component
of this lesion. X530.

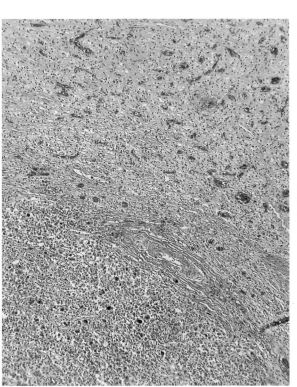

Figure 86
HODGKIN'S DISEASE, LYMPHOCYTE DEPLETED
(RETICULAR TYPE), LYMPH NODE
This illustration shows a nodule at the bottom containing
a large number of Reed-Sternberg cells and an area at the
top where there is a depletion of cellular elements and
diffuse fibrosis. This microscopic appearance is occasionally
seen in lymphocyte-depleted Hodgkin's disease. X135.

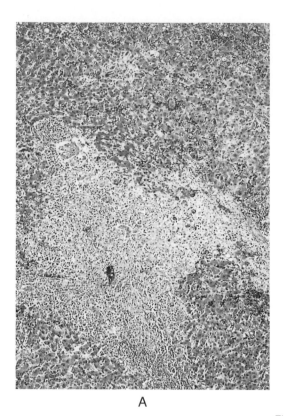

A

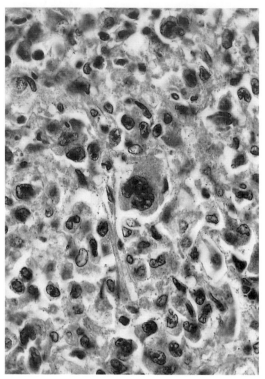

B

Figure 87
HODGKIN'S DISEASE, LYMPHOCYTE DEPLETED, LIVER
A. This biopsy shows an expanded portal area with a mixed infiltrate that often has a slightly depleted or granulomatous appearance. H&E. X60. B. Higher magnification shows the relative sparsity of cellular elements. In the center of the field, there is a single bizarre Reed-Sternberg cell. H&E. X620.

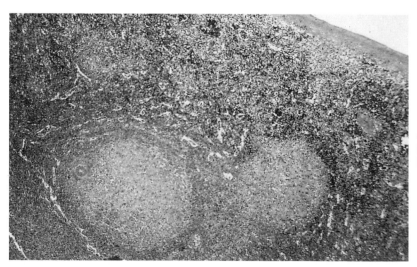

Figure 88
HODGKIN'S DISEASE, LYMPHO-
CYTE DEPLETED, SPLEEN
The Malpighian bodies of this spleen are almost depleted of lymphocytes and are replaced by acidophilic material of diffuse fibrosis. H&E. X90.

Histopathology of Hodgkin's Disease of Unclassified Type.

Some cases of Hodgkin's disease do not conform to any of the subclassifications stated above. This failure to conform to diagnostic criteria is particularly common in cases in which there are lacunar cells but no definite polarizable bands of connective tissue. Lukes classifies these cases as mixed cellularity Hodgkin's disease. Other cases of Hodgkin's disease may show striking granulomatous features but have too many mononuclear Reed-Sternberg and Reed-Sternberg cells to be classified as lymphocyte-predominant Hodgkin's disease. Such cases should be diagnosed as mixed cellularity Hodgkin's disease.

References

Bennett, M.H., Tu, A., and Hudson, G.V. Analysis of grade I Hodgkin's disease (Report no. 6). Clin. Radiol. 32:491-498, 1981.

Casey, T.T., Olson, S.J., Cousar, J.B., and Collins, R.D. Immunophenotypes of Reed-Sternberg cells: a study of 19 cases of Hodgkin's disease in plastic-embedded sections. Blood 74:2624-2628, 1989.

Glick, A.D., Leech, J.H., Flexner, J.M, and Collins, R.D. Ultrastructural study of Reed-Sternberg cells. Comparison with transformed lymphocytes and histiocytes. Am. J. Pathol. 85:195-208, 1976.

Kadin, M.E., Muramoto, M.S., and Said, J. Expression of T-cell antigens on Reed-Sternberg cells in a subset of patients with nodular sclerosing and mixed cellularity Hodgkin's disease. Am. J. Pathol. 130:345-353, 1988.

Kaplan, H.S. and Gartner, S. "Sternberg-Reed" giant cells of Hodgkin's disease: cultivation in vitro, heterotransplantation, and characterization as neoplastic macrophages. Int. J. Cancer 19:511-525, 1977.

Lukes, R.J. Criteria for involvement of lymph node, bone marrow, spleen, and liver in Hodgkin's disease. Cancer Res. 31:1755-1767, 1971.

_____ and Butler, J.J. The pathology and nomenclature of Hodgkin's disease. Cancer Res. 26:1063-1083, 1966.

_____ and Collins, R.D. The immunologic characterization of human malignant lymphomas. Cancer 31:1488-1503, 1974.

Neiman, R.S., Rosen, P.J., and Lukes, R.J. Lymphocyte-depletion Hodgkin's disease. N. Engl. J. Med. 288:751-755, 1973.

Poppema, S., Kaiserling, E., and Lennert, K. Hodgkin's disease with lymphocytic predominance, nodular type (nodular paragranuloma) and progressively transformed germinal centres—a cytohistological study. Histopathology 3:295-308, 1979.

Stein, H., Mason, D.Y., Gerdes, J., et al. The expression of the Hodgkin's disease associated antigen Ki-1 in reactive and neoplastic lymphoid tissue: evidence that Reed-Sternberg cells and histiocytic malignancies are derived from activated lymphoid cells. Blood 66:848-858, 1985.

Strickler, J.G., Michie, S.A., Warnke, R.A., and Dorfman, R.F. The "syncytial variant" of nodular sclerosing Hodgkin's disease. Am. J. Surg. Pathol. 10:470-477, 1986.

Timens, W., Visser, L., and Poppema, S. Nodular lymphocyte predominance type of Hodgkin's disease is a germinal center lymphoma. Lab. Invest. 54: 457-461, 1986.

Tindle, B.H., Parker, J.W., and Lukes, R.J. "Reed-Sternberg cells" in infectious mononucleosis? Am. J. Clin. Pathol. 58:607-617, 1972.

Additional References

Anagnostou, D., Parker, J.W., Taylor, C.R., Tindle, B.H., and Lukes, R.J. Lacunar cells of nodular sclerosing Hodgkin's disease. Cancer 39:1032-1043, 1977.

Bearman, R.M., Pangalis, G.A., and Rappaport, H. Hodgkin's disease, lymphocyte depletion type. Cancer 41:293-302, 1978.

Bernau, D., Feldmann, G., and Vorhauer, W. Hodgkin's disease: ultrastructural localization of intra-cytoplasmic immunoglobulins within malignant cells. Br. J. Haematol. 40:51-57, 1978.

Burns, B.F., Colby, T.V., and Dorfman, R.F. Differential diagnostic features of nodular L&H Hodgkin's disease, including progressive transformation of germinal centers. Am. J. Surg. Pathol. 8:253-261, 1984.

Carbone, P.P., Kaplan, H.S., Musshoff, K., Smithers, D.W., and Tubiana, M. Report of the Committee on Hodgkin's Disease Staging Classification. Cancer Res. 31:1860-1861, 1971.

Forni, M., Hofman, F.M., Parker, J.W., Lukes, R.J., and Taylor, C.R. B- and T-lymphocytes in Hodgkin's disease: an immunohistochemical study utilizing heterologous and monoclonal antibodies. Cancer 55:728-737, 1985.

Greer, J.P., Kinney, M.C., Cousar, J.B., et al. Lymphocyte-depleted Hodgkin's disease. Am. J. Med. 81:208-214, 1986.

Hsu, S.M., Yang, K., and Jaffe, E.S. Phenotypic expression of Hodgkin's and Reed-Sternberg cells in Hodgkin's disease. Am. J. Pathol. 118:209-217, 1985.

Kadin, M.E., Donaldson, S.S., and Dorfman, R.F. Isolated granulomas in Hodgkin's disease. N. Engl. J. Med. 283:859-861, 1970.

_____, Glatstein, E., and Dorfman, R.F. Clinicopathologic studies of 117 untreated patients subjected to laparotomy for the staging of Hodgkin's disease. Cancer 27:1277-1294, 1971.

Kant, J.A., Hubbard, S.M., Longo, D.L., et al. The pathologic and clinical heterogeneity of lymphocyte-depleted Hodgkin's disease. J. Clin. Oncol. 4:284-294, 1986.

Kaplan, H.S. Hodgkin's Disease. Cambridge: Harvard University Press, 1972.

_____. Hodgkin's disease. Cancer 45:2439-2474, 1980.

Keller, A.R., Kaplan, H.S., Lukes, R.J., and Rappaport, H. Correlation of histopathology with other prognostic indicators in Hodgkin's disease. Cancer 22:487-499, 1968.

Kinney, M.C., Greer, J.P., Stein, R.S., Collins, R.D., and Cousar, J.B. Lymphocyte-depletion Hodgkin's disease: histopathologic diagnosis of marrow involvement. Am. J. Surg. Pathol. 10:219-226, 1986.

Lennert, K., Kaiserling, E., and Müller-Hermelink, H.K. Malignant Lymphomas: Models of Differentiation and Cooperation of Lymphoreticular Cells, p. 897. In: Differentiation of Normal and Neoplastic Hematopoietic Cells. Cold Spring Harbor: Cold Spring Harbor Laboratory, 1978.

Lukes, R.J., Craver, L.F., Hall, T.C., Rappaport, H., and Rubin, P. Report of the Nomenclature Committee. Cancer Res. 26 (Part 1):1311, 1966.

Order, S.E. and Hellman, S. Pathogenesis of Hodgkin's disease. Lancet 1:571- 573, 1972.

Papadimitriou, C.S., Stein, H., and Lennert, K. The complexity of immunohistochemical staining pattern of Hodgkin and Sternberg-Reed cells—demonstration of immunoglobulin, albumin, alpha-1-antichymotrypsin and lysozyme. Int. J. Cancer 21:531-541, 1978.

Pinkus, G.S. and Said, J.W. Hodgkin's disease, lymphocyte predominance type, nodular—a distinct entity? Am. J. Pathol. 118:1-6, 1985.

_____, Thomas, P., and Said, J. Leu-M1—a marker for Reed-Sternberg cells in Hodgkin's disease. Am. J. Pathol. 119:244-252, 1985.

Poppema, S., Elema, J.D., and Halie, M.R. The localization of Hodgkin's disease in lymph nodes. A study with immunohistological, enzyme histochemical and rosetting techniques on frozen sections. Int. J. Cancer 24:532-540, 1979.

_____, Elema, J.D., and Halie, M.R. The significance of intracytoplasmic proteins in Reed-Sternberg cells. Cancer 42:1170-1176, 1981.

_____, Bhan, A.K., Reinherz, E.L., Posner, M.R., and Schlossman, S.F. In situ immunologic characterization of cellular constituents in lymph nodes and spleens involved by Hodgkin's disease. Blood 59:226-232, 1982.

Rappaport, H. Tumors of the Hematopoietic System. Fascicle 8, First Series. Atlas of Tumor Pathology. Washington: Armed Forces Institute of Pathology, 1966.

Sherrod, A.E., Felder, B., Levy, N., et al. Immunohistologic identification of phenotypic antigens associated with Hodgkin and Reed-Sternberg cells. A paraffin section study. Cancer 57:2135-2140, 1986.

Smithers, D.W. Spread of Hodgkin's disease. Lancet 1:1262-1267, 1970.

_____ and Fairly, G.H. Hodgkin's Disease. Edinburgh: Churchill Livingstone, 1973.

Stein, R.S. Clinical Features and Clinical Evaluation of Hodgkin's Disease and the Non-Hodgkin's Lymphomas, pp. 129-175. In: Lymphomas. Bennett, J.M. (Ed.). Netherlands: Martinus Nijhoff, 1981.

Swerdlow, S.H. and Wright, S.A. The spectrum of Leu-M1 staining in lymphoid and hematopoietic proliferations. Am. J. Clin. Pathol. 85:283-288, 1986.

Taylor, C.R. Upon the nature of Hodgkin's disease and the Reed-Sternberg cell. Recent Results Cancer Res. 64:214-231, 1978.

MONONUCLEAR PHAGOCYTE SYSTEM NEOPLASMS

Malignant mononuclear phagocyte system neoplasms include marrow-based acute and chronic monocytic leukemias, as well as various malignant histiocytoses arising from peripheral tissues (Chu et al.; Collins et al.). Considerable confusion has been associated with the classification of these neoplasms, in the past with separation of malignant histiocytoses from histiocytoses of varying aggressiveness such as Langerhans-cell histiocytosis. Recently, as a result of our repeated misdiagnoses of various lymphoid neoplasms as histiocytic malignancies, it has even been suggested that the term malignant histiocytosis be abandoned (Wilson et al.). Until recently, diagnoses of histiocytic neoplasms were based partly on histopathologic criteria (growth of tumor in sinuses, or phagocytosis of erythrocytes) and partly on nonspecific cytochemical studies that have subsequently proven to be unreliable. Reviews of cases diagnosed as malignant histiocytoses have shown most are T cell lymphomas (Delsol et al.; Isaacson et al.; Stein et al.; Wilson et al.). These studies have used immunocytochemical panels as the major discriminant of cell lineage. In this regard the CD30 antibody (Ki-1/Ber H2) has been particularly useful in distinguishing large cell anaplastic lymphomas, mostly T in phenotype, from malignant histiocytoses, metastatic carcinoma, and malignant melanoma.

The terminologic inaccuracy of the histiocytic designation is further shown by the still commonly used terms histiocytic lymphoma and mixed lymphocytic-histiocytic lymphoma. These neoplasms have, with rare exceptions, been proven by multiparameter studies to contain various types of transformed lymphocytes, as we initially proposed (Lukes and Collins). Reed-Sternberg cells have also taken their turn in the histiocytic camp, but now also seem to be regarded as dysplastic lymphocytes instead.

The universally documented rarity of malignant histiocytoses, plus repeated misdiagnoses, have led to skepticism about the existence of this type of neoplasm. However, there are scattered case reports of well-documented cases (Franchino et al.; Hanson et al.; Monda et al.), and it is inconceivable that such a widespread and active system with diverse functions is not subject to malignancy.

We are unable to be more precise in recognizing these neoplasms because of their rarity (Lukes and colleagues have shown that considerably less than 1 percent of hematopoietic neoplasms are malignant histiocytoses), the failure to apply rigorous diagnostic criteria, the absence until recently of relatively specific markers for monocytes/macrophages, and finally, the complex biology of the mononuclear phagocyte system. Because there are functional subpopulations of this system, we should anticipate the same clinical and pathologic diversity of monocytic and histiocytic neoplasms that can now be demonstrated in lymphoid processes.

In this regard, there are four main types of tissue monocytes/macrophages; the number of marrow monocyte populations is unknown. These four types are usually found in specific microenvironments and

273

have immunophenotypic or structural features facilitating their recognition (Lennert; Wood et al.). Tissue macrophages are widely distributed as tingible body macrophages in nodes, pulmonary macrophages, and Kupffer cells, to name only a few of their sites. These phagocytic cells have a high content of hydrolytic enzymes and are readily shown to contain esterase, acid phosphatase, and chymotryptic activity. They do not mark with antibodies to CD1 or S-100. Mononuclear phagocyte system cells with dendritic morphology (and presumed antigen-presenting responsibilities) include follicular dendritic cells, interdigitating cells, and Langerhans cells. The latter are primarily found in squamous epithelium, contain Birbeck granules, and mark with S-100 and CD1. Interdigitating cells are found in such T cell areas as the paracortex of nodes and tonsil as well as the periarteriolar lymphoid sheaths of spleen. These nonphagocytic cells are very similar to Langerhans cells but lack Birbeck granules. Although there are numerous cell surface processes, no desmosomal junctions are present. S-100 reactivity is usually demonstrable, but CD1 is generally expected to be negative. Follicular dendritic cells are located specifically in germinal centers and characteristically have desmosomal cell junctions. S-100 and CD1 are not present, but Fc and complement receptors can be demonstrated.

Although our knowledge of this system and its diseases is still rudimentary, we can be confident that its malignant neoplasms will reflect the above functional and structural diversity. Our approach to these neoplasms must therefore be similar to that followed in this Fascicle for lymphoid processes. For each functional subpopulation of the mononuclear phagocyte system, we should expect to find one or more neoplasms. The diagnosis of neoplasia should be established by histopathologic demonstration of tumorous proliferations of dysplastic cells. Categorization of these neoplasms as monocyte/histiocyte type requires at this point detailed immunophenotypic and structural studies (Collins et al.; Risdall et al., 1979, 1980). We should also require for diagnosis that neoplastic cells do not mark with lineage-specific B and T cell markers as well as absence of immunoglobulin heavy chain and T β-gene rearrangement.

Differential diagnosis of malignant histiocytoses should be especially rigorous. True histiocytic neoplasms are most often confused with malignant lymphomas of transformed lymphocytes, especially those with particularly irregular nuclei or abundant cytoplasm. Anaplastic large cell lymphomas of the Ki-1 type and other T cell lymphomas frequently have been mistaken for malignant histiocytoses (Delsol et al.; Isaacson et al.; Stein et al.; Wilson et al.). Reactive histiocytes are prominent in malignant lymphomas, and activated histiocytes have been misinterpreted repeatedly as neoplastic. Finally, metastatic carcinoma composed of large cells with abundant cytoplasm may be easily confused with malignant histiocytosis, especially if there is apparent phagocytic activity. PIP for epithelial markers and electron microscopic demonstration of epithelial features will lead to the correct diagnosis.

Many mononuclear phagocyte system proliferations have been mistakenly accepted as malignant because the process was disseminated and associated with significant morbidity or mortality. An example of such a disorder confused with a neoplasm is the virus-associated hemo-phagocytic syndrome. In addition to virus-associated hemophagocytic syndromes, other benign histiocytic proliferations may be seen in storage diseases of all types and in infectious or noninfectious granulomatous disease.

Mononuclear phagocyte system neoplasms carry a leukemia designation if there is evidence that they have arisen from marrow sites. Those leukemias containing significant numbers of monocytes are included in this section. The myeloid leukemias are discussed in the next chapter, Myeloid Neoplasms. Although functional subpopulations of marrow monocytes exist, subclassification of monocytic leukemia in a manner analogous to that of lymphocytic leukemia (i.e., pre-B or T cell acute lymphocytic leukemia) is not possible at this time.

References

Chu, T., D'Angio, G.J., Favara, B., et al. Histiocytosis syndromes in children. Lancet 1:208-209, 1987.

Collins, R.D., Bennett, B., and Glick, A.D. Neoplasms of the Mononuclear Phagocytic System, pp. 1-33. In: The Reticuloendothelial System, Vol. 5. Herberman, R.B. and Friedman, H. (Eds.). New York: Plenum Press, 1983.

Delsol, G., Al Saati, T., Gatter, K.C., et al. Coexpression of epithelial membrane antigen (EMA), Ki-1, and interleukin-2 receptor by anaplastic large cell lymphomas. Diagnostic value in so-called malignant histiocytosis. Am. J. Pathol. 130:59-70, 1988.

Franchino, C., Reich, C., Distenfeld, A., Ubriaco, A., and Knowles, D.M. A clinicopathologically distinctive primary splenic histiocytic neoplasm. Demonstration of its histiocytic derivation by immunophenotypic and molecular genetic analysis. Am. J. Surg. Pathol. 12:398-404, 1988.

Hanson, C.A., Jaszcz, W., Kersey, J.H., et al. True histiocytic lymphoma: histopathologic, immunopheotypic and genotypic analysis. Br. J. Haematol. 73:187-198, 1989.

Isaacson, P.G., O'Connor, N.T., Spencer, J., et al. Malignant histiocytosis of the intestine: a T-cell lymphoma. Lancet 2:688-691, 1985.

Lennert, K. Malignant Lymphomas Other Than Hodgkin's Disease: Histology, Cytology, Ultrastructure, Immunology. New York: Springer-Verlag, 1978.

Lukes, R.J. and Collins, R.D. New approaches to the classification of the lymphomata. Br. J. Cancer 31(Suppl. 2):1-28, 1975.

_____, Taylor, C.R., and Parker, J.W. Multiparameter studies in malignant lymphoma based on studies in 1186 cases. Prog. Clin. Biol. Res. 132E:203-213, 1983.

Monda, L., Warnke, R., and Rosai, J. A primary lymph node malignancy with features suggestive of dendritic reticulum cell differentiation. A report of 4 cases. Am. J. Pathol. 122:562-572, 1986.

Risdall, R.J., McKenna, R.W., Nesbit, M.E., et al. Virus-associated hemophagocytic syndrome: a benign histiocytic proliferation distinct from malignant histiocytosis. Cancer 44:993-1002, 1979.

_____, Sibley, R.K., McKenna, R.W., Brunning, R.D., and Dehner, L.P. Malignant histiocytosis. Am. J. Surg. Pathol. 4:439-450, 1980.

Stein, H., Mason, D.Y., Gerdes, J., et al. The expression of the Hodgkin's disease associated antigen Ki-1 in reactive and neoplastic lymphoid tissue: evidence that Reed-Sternberg cells and histiocytic malignancies are derived from activated lymphoid cells. Blood 66:848-858, 1985.

Wilson, M.S., Weiss, L.M., Gatter, K.C., et al. Malignant histiocytosis. A reassessment of cases previously reported in 1975 based on paraffin section immunophenotyping studies. Cancer 66:530-536, 1990.

Wood, G.S., Turner, R.R., Shiurba, R.A., Eng, L., and Warnke, R.A. Human dendritic cells and macrophages. In situ immunophenotypic definition of subsets that exhibit specific morphologic and microenvironmental characteristics. Am. J. Pathol. 119:73-82, 1985.

ACUTE MYELOMONOCYTIC LEUKEMIA, FRENCH-AMERICAN-BRITISH CLASSIFICATION M-4

Definition. Acute myelomonocytic leukemia is a marrow-based neoplasm in which the cell of origin is a hematopoietic stem cell that is probably shared by both granulocytes and monocytes.

Clinical Features. Acute myelomonocytic leukemia accounts for approximately 20 to 30 percent of all acute myeloid leukemias in the United States.

Males and females are equally affected. The average age at onset is 55 years. Acute myelomonocytic leukemia is rare in children.

The most frequent presenting symptoms relate to bone marrow failure with anemia, thrombocytopenia and bleeding (40-50 percent of the patients), and infection (35 percent of the patients). Approximately 10 percent of the patients complain of bone and joint pain at the time of diagnosis. Gingival swelling and bleeding, headache, and weight loss are also occasionally noted. On initial physical examination, gingival hypertrophy is reported in 14 percent of the patients, splenomegaly in 40 percent, hepatomegaly in 50 percent, adenopathy in 35 percent, and skin infiltration in approximately 10 percent of the patients.

Leukocytosis is expected, with an average white blood cell count of 55,000/μL. Leukemic blasts comprise approximately 50 percent of the differential count. The mean hemoglobin level is 9.5 g/dL, with the mean platelet count of 113,000/μL. Elevated serum lysozyme is expected. Abnormal karyotypes are seen in the majority of the patients; the most common single abnormality reported is +8.

Several studies have indicated a slightly higher response rate in this variant compared with other subtypes of acute myeloid leukemia. Median duration of complete response is approximately 10 months. Central nervous system relapse has been reported in this variant.

Pathologic Features. For pathologic details, see Plate XLVI and Table 46. Marrow sections most often show completely cellular particles or biopsy with a homogeneous population of immature granulocytic and monocytic elements (plate XLVI-A). Monocyte precursors exceed 20 percent of

the total cell population, and numerous myeloblasts and promyelocytes are also present (Bennett et al.). Monocytic precursors have irregular nuclei, slightly eosinophilic cytoplasm, and numerous small pink granules on Wright's stained preparations. Granulocyte precursors may be recognized on Wright's stains by their larger azurophilic granules. Auer rods may be present. The immature cells stain diffusely positive with Sudan black and PAS stains (plate XLVI-G). Esterase stain demonstrates diffuse α-naphthyl acetate or butyrate positivity in monocytic precursors and chloroacetate esterase positivity in granulocyte precursors (plate XLVI-B). Electron microscopy demonstrates the characteristic granules, filaments, endoplasmic reticulum, and nuclei of monocytic and granulocytic cells (Glick). Abnormal erythroblasts with mitochondrial iron and/or cytoplasmic glycogen are occasionally present (Glick et al.).

References

Bennett, J.M., Catovsky, D., Daniel, M.T., et al. Proposals for the classification of the acute leukemias. A report of the French-American-British (FAB) co-operative group. Br. J. Haematol. 33:451-458, 1976.

Glick, A.D. Acute leukemia. Semin. Oncol. 3:229-241, 1976.

_____ , Paniker, K., Flexner, J.M., Graber, S.E., and Collins, R.D. Acute leukemia of adults. Am. J. Clin. Pathol. 73:459-470, 1980.

Additional References

Collins, R.D., Bennett, B., and Glick, A.D. Neoplasms of the Mononuclear Phagocyte System, pp. 1-33. In: The Reticuloendothelial System, Vol. 5. Herberman, R.B. and Friedman, H. (Eds.). New York: Plenum Press, 1983.

Hayhoe, F.G., Quaglino, D., and Doll, R. The Cytology and Cytochemistry of Acute Leukemias. Medical Research Council Special Report Series, No. 304, London: Her Majesty's Stationery Office, 1964.

Table 46

ACUTE MYELOMONOCYTIC LEUKEMIA

PATTERN
• Marrow — massive, diffuse, homogeneous infiltration • Spleen — infiltration of red pulp • Nodes — massive cortical and medullary infiltration with residual islands of lymphocytes

CYTOLOGY — NEOPLASTIC	MARKERS — NEOPLASTIC
• Immature granulocytic and monocytic elements present; Auer rods present • Immature monocytes are not easily recognized unless electron microscopy is done	• Cytochemistry: · Sudan black, peroxidase (+) >5 percent blasts · Combined esterase shows immature cells reacting with α-naphthyl and chloroacetate esterase · PAS, diffuse (+) • Flow: CD4 (+), CD2 (−) CD14 (ı)
INVOLVED SITES	**CLINICAL FEATURES**
• Marrow • Spleen • Nodes	• Most patients are 50-60 years of age; acute myelomonocytic leukemia is rare in children; incidence equal in both sexes • Marrow failure at presentation in most patients; bone and joint pain occurs in 10 percent of the patients • Hepatosplenomegaly occurs in 40-50 percent of the patients; 10 percent have skin infiltration, and 10 percent have gingival swelling
REACTIVE COMPONENTS	**DIFFERENTIAL DIAGNOSIS**
• Intermixed marrow elements	• Acute monocytic leukemia • Acute granulocytic leukemia • Non-Hodgkin's lymphoma

PLATE XLVI

A. ACUTE MYELOMONOCYTIC LEUKEMIA, MARROW
A mixture of blasts and differentiated cells is illustrated. A promyelocyte is present, as well as immature mononuclear cells showing nuclear folding. Wright's stain. X450.

B. ACUTE MYELOMONOCYTIC LEUKEMIA, MARROW
Most cells stain either brown with the α-naphthyl acetate or blue with chloroacetate esterase. This kind of bitypic staining is characteristic of acute myelomonocytic leukemia. Combined esterase stain. X180.

C. ACUTE MYELOID LEUKEMIA, MARROW
In this illustration, a collection of blasts with abundant cytoplasm contains fine granules, and an Auer rod is noted. Wright's stain. X560.

D. ACUTE MYELOID LEUKEMIA, MARROW
Blasts and a promyelocyte are present. In acute leukemia, there is often a variable degree of differentiation of neoplastic cells. Wright's stain. X560.

E. ACUTE MONOCYTIC LEUKEMIA (M-5A), MARROW
These blasts show no evidence of differentiation, and nuclei have minimal folding. Wright's stain. X450.

F. ACUTE MONOCYTIC LEUKEMIA (M-5B), MARROW
The predominant cells have folded nuclei and abundant cytoplasm with fine pink granules that appear to concentrate near the cell surface. Wright's stain. X450.

G. ACUTE MYELOMONOCYTIC LEUKEMIA, MARROW
In this illustration, heavy granulation is demonstrated in some cells, and more delicate staining is noted in others. Several Auer rods are seen. Sudan black B stain. X450.

H. ACUTE MONOCYTIC LEUKEMIA (M-5B), MARROW
Alpha-naphthyl acetate esterase positivity is typically diffuse and present in most cells in this type of leukemia. Nuclear folding is also evident. Combined esterase stain. X560.

PLATE XLVI

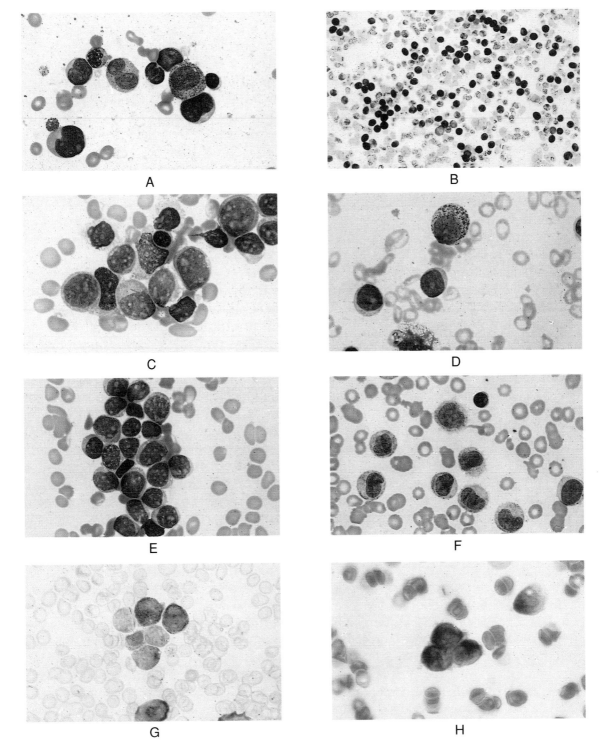

A

B

C

D

E

F

G

H

ACUTE MONOCYTIC LEUKEMIA, FRENCH-AMERICAN-BRITISH CLASSIFICATION M-5

Definition. Acute monocytic leukemia is a marrow-based neoplasm that is probably derived from stem cells. Monocytic differentiation predominates. Functional subpopulations of monocytes presumably exist but different types of monocytic leukemia have not been identified, in contrast to the situation with acute lymphocytic leukemia.

Clinical Features. Acute monocytic leukemia is rare in the United States. Males and females are equally affected. Two peaks of disease are seen, one in patients less than 10 years of age and the second in individuals more than 40 years of age (with a mean of 58 years).

Initial symptoms of the disease may be similar to those of other variants of acute leukemia, with bone marrow failure and resultant anemia, thrombocytopenia and bleeding (50 percent of the patients), and infection (38 percent of the patients). Patients may also present with symptoms and signs related to gingival infiltration and hypertrophy, which occurs in 30 to 40 percent of the newly diagnosed cases. Infiltration of the skin is reported in 15 to 30 percent of the patients.

Physical findings relate to the infiltration of the skin and/or gingiva. Additionally, significant splenomegaly is expected in approximately 50 percent of the patients, with hepatomegaly and lymphadenopathy reported in 40 to 60 percent of the patients.

This variant of acute leukemia is characterized by extreme leukocytosis at diagnosis, with mean white blood cell counts of 83,000/μL, and white blood cell counts in excess of 100,000/μL in 50 percent of all patients. The average percentage of monoblasts is 40 percent. The mean hemoglobin is 10.5 g/dL, with a mean platelet count of 89,000/μL. The highest levels of serum lysozyme are seen in this variant. Furthermore, approximately 20 percent of the cases are hypokalemic at presentation. Rearrangements of chromosome 11 have been reported.

The response to combination chemotherapy is similar to that of other variants of acute granulocytic leukemia, with complete remission attained in approximately 40 to 60 percent of the patients. The average duration of remission is less than 1 year. A relapse of disease may occur in the central nervous system.

Pathologic Features (Table 47). Marrows are diffusely involved and homogeneous in appearance. Neoplastic cells often show distinct nuclear folding and abundant cytoplasm. Most leukemic cells are monocyte precursors (Bennett et al.). Two main types of acute monocytic leukemia are recognized: (1) M-5A: poorly differentiated or blastic, characterized by large blasts (plate XLVI-E), with scattered monocyte-type granules on electron microscopy (fig. 89), but often negative cytochemical studies (Glick et al.); and (2) M-5B: differentiated monocytic leukemia composed of promonocytes, with characteristic Sudan black, PAS, and esterase positivity (plate XLVI-H). These more differentiated cells (plate XLVI-F) have a characteristic ultrastructure (fig. 90). Granulocytic components rarely comprise more than 10 percent of cells in either type of acute monocytic leukemia (Bennett et al.). Auer rods may be present.

Table 47

ACUTE MONOCYTIC LEUKEMIA,
FRENCH-AMERICAN-BRITISH CLASSIFICATION M-5A, M-5B

PATTERN
• Marrow — massive, homogeneous infiltrate • Skin — epidermal, dermal infiltrative process that may extend into subcutaneous tissue

CYTOLOGY — NEOPLASTIC	MARKERS — NEOPLASTIC

• M-5A: Immature cells with minimal nuclear folding, scant cytoplasm; electron microscopy shows scattered haloed granules, filament bundles
 	
• M-5B: Predominant cells have folded nuclei, abundant cytoplasm, fine pink granules; Auer rods may be present
	• Cytochemistry: Combined esterase, Sudan black, PAS may be negative or weakly reactive in M-5A, in contrast to distinct reactions in M-5B
	
	• Flow: HLA-DR (+)
	  CD11b, 11c (+)
	  CD13, 14 (+)
	  CD33 (+)
	  CD34 (±)

INVOLVED SITES	CLINICAL FEATURES
• Marrow • Skin	• Peak incidence bimodal: <10 years, >40 years; incidence equal in both sexes • Marrow failure common at presentation • Many patients present with skin nodules or gingival hypertrophy

REACTIVE COMPONENTS	DIFFERENTIAL DIAGNOSIS
• Intermixed normal marrow elements	• Acute myelomonocytic leukemia • Chronic myelomonocytic leukemia

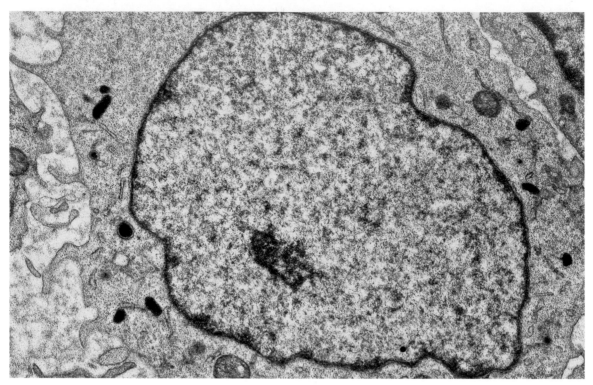

Figure 89
ACUTE MONOCYTIC LEUKEMIA (M-5A), MARROW
This electron micrograph reveals an early promonocyte with scattered haloed granules. X16,450.

References

Bennett, J.M., Catovsky, D., Daniel, M.T., et al. Proposals for the classification of the acute leukemias. A report of the French-American-British (FAB) co-operative group. Br. J. Haematol. 33:451-458, 1976.

Glick, A.D., Paniker, K., Flexner, J.M., Graber, S.E., and Collins, R.D. Acute leukemia of adults. Am. J. Clin. Pathol. 73:459-470, 1980.

Additional References

Cuttner, J., Conjalka, M.S., Reilly, M., et al. Association of monocytic leukemia in patients with extreme leukocytosis. Am. J. Med. 69:555-558, 1980.

Tobelem, G., Jacquillat, C., Chastang, C., et al. Acute monoblastic leukemia. Blood 55:71-76, 1980.

CHRONIC MYELOMONOCYTIC LEUKEMIA

Definition. Chronic myelomonocytic leukemia is a marrow-based neoplasm, probably arising from stem cells capable of monocytic and granulocytic differentiation.

Clinical Features. Chronic myelomonocytic leukemia is a relatively unusual disease that primarily affects the elderly. Most patients are 65 to 78 years of age and the disease is unusual under the age of 50. Males are affected slightly more often than females (1.2:1).

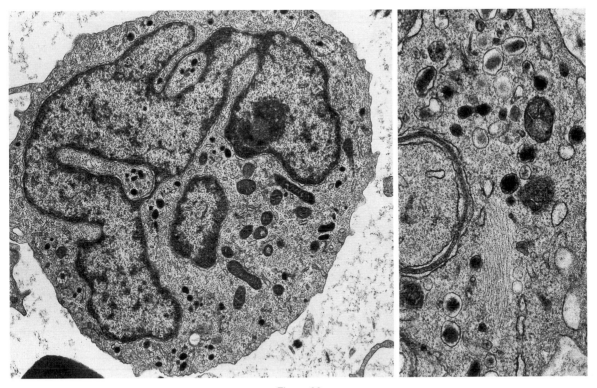

Figure 90
ACUTE MONOCYTIC LEUKEMIA M-5B, MARROW
On ultrastructural study, this leukemic promonocyte has numerous scattered granules, a folded nucleus, and microfilament bundles. X13,600. The latter are seen at higher magnification (right). X29,000. (Fig. 4 from Collins, R.D., Bennett, B., and Glick, A.D. Neoplasms of the Mononuclear Phagocyte System. In: The Reticuloendothelial System, Vol. 5. Herberman, R.B. and Friedman, H. [Eds.]. New York: Plenum Press, 1983.)

The disease is indolent in nature. Most patients complain of mild symptomatology for 6 to 12 months before the initial diagnosis. Weakness and malaise secondary to anemia may be the initial presentation, although infection or bruising may also occur. The diagnosis is often made at the time of a routine physical examination.

Physical findings at diagnosis are often relatively minor. Pallor is expected, with evidence of mild bruising. Mild hepatosplenomegaly is reported in approximately 35 percent of the patients, although the spleen size may increase with time. Mild lymphadenopathy may occur. Gingival hypertrophy is not seen.

Laboratory evaluation reveals a mild anemia in approximately 50 percent of the patients; thrombocytopenia (<100,000/µL) is reported in 60 percent. The white count may vary considerably, ranging from 3900 to 38,000/µL, and monocytosis is expected (>800/µL). The serum and urinary lysozyme levels, uric acid, and serum B_{12} are elevated in almost all of the patients. Leukocyte alkaline phosphatase is normal. The natural history of this disorder is slowly progressive, and the early use of combination chemotherapy is not warranted.

Pathologic Features (Table 48). The peripheral blood monocyte count is higher than 100,000/µL, with up to 30 percent myeloblasts and promyelocytes in the marrow (Bennett et al.). The bone marrow is hypercellular but is not as homogeneous in appearance as in acute leukemia. The increased number of promonocytes and monocytes present in the marrow and blood may not be recognized unless esterase stains are performed (figs. 91, 92). Muramidase levels in serum or urine may be elevated.

Reference

Bennett, J.M., Catovsky, D., Daniel, M.T., et al. Proposals for the classification of the acute leukemias. A report of the French-American-British (FAB) co-operative group. Br. J. Haematol. 33:451-458, 1976.

Additional References

Geary, C.G., Catovsky, D., Wiltshaw, E., et al. Chronic myelomonocytic leukaemia. Br. J. Haematol. 30:289-302, 1975.
Miescher, P.A. and Farquet, J.J. Chronic myelomonocytic leukemia in adults. Semin. Hematol. 11:129-139, 1974.
Zittoun, R. Annotation: subacute and chronic myelomonocytic leukaemia. Br. J. Haematol. 32:1-7, 1976.

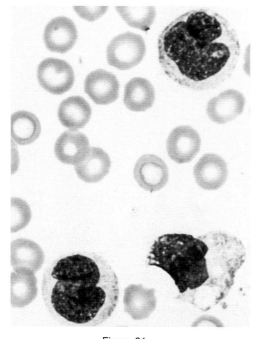

Figure 91
(Figures 91 and 92 are from the same patient)
CHRONIC MYELOMONOCYTIC LEUKEMIA,
PERIPHERAL BLOOD
Relatively differentiated monocytes with peripheral granules and folded nuclei are shown. Wright's stain. X1280. (Fig. 13 from Collins, R.D., Bennett, B., and Glick, A.D. Neoplasms of the Mononuclear Phagocyte System. In: The Reticuloendothelial System, Vol. 5. Herberman, R.B. and Friedman, H. [Eds.]. New York: Plenum Press, 1983.)

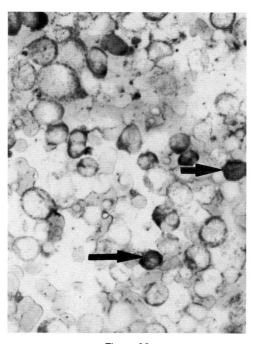

Figure 92
CHRONIC MYELOMONOCYTIC LEUKEMIA,
MARROW, COMBINED ESTERASE STAIN
Darkly staining monocytic precursors (arrows) are seen. The larger, more granular cells are granulocytic precursors, which are chloroacetate esterase positive. X320. (Fig. 14 from Collins, R.D., Bennett, B., and Glick, A.D. Neoplasms of the Mononuclear Phagocyte System. In: The Reticuloendothelial System, Vol. 5. Herberman, R.B. and Friedman, H. [Eds.]. New York: Plenum Press, 1983.)

Table 48

CHRONIC MYELOMONOCYTIC LEUKEMIA

PATTERN
• Marrow — hypercellular, polymorphous due to a mixture of hematopoietic elements, maturation of tumor cells

CYTOLOGY — NEOPLASTIC	MARKERS — NEOPLASTIC
• Differentiating granulocytes and monocytes present in approximately equal numbers	• Cytochemistry: Combined esterase shows marked increase in both granulocytic and monocytic elements • LAP normal • Ph[1] chromosome not present

INVOLVED SITES	CLINICAL FEATURES
• Marrow	• Elderly affected, with peak incidence between 60 and 70 years of age; incidence slightly greater in males • Insidious onset, often discovered incidentally • Pallor, bruising, hepatosplenomegaly

REACTIVE COMPONENTS	DIFFERENTIAL DIAGNOSIS
• Intermixed normal marrow elements	• Chronic myelogenous leukemia • Myelodysplastic syndromes

MACROPHAGE/HISTIOCYTE
TYPE NEOPLASMS

The characterization of these processes at a clinical and pathologic level is relatively crude and has been seriously hampered by their rarity. Furthermore, questions have been raised as to whether one of the diseases described below (histiocytic medullary reticulosis) is a histiocytic disorder or a T cell lymphoproliferative process (Robb-Smith). We include histiocytic medullary reticulosis under this category, awaiting further characterization of typical cases.

In our review of 1800 cases of non-Hodgkin's lymphoma evaluated by multiparameter techniques over a period of 12 years, only 15 cases of malignant neoplasms of genuine histiocytic type were found (Cramer and Lukes, unpublished). They presented morphologically in diffuse form in the paracortex, with varying combinations of the following three cell types: an immunoblast-like cell; a monocyte-macrophage type cell; and a spindle cell. In most cases, the monocyte-macrophage cell type was the most common and the spindle cell type was the least common, although a spindle cell component was always present. A neoplasm of true histiocyte type may be suspected from examination of hematoxylin and eosin stained sections on the basis of finding spindle cells with broad elongated cytoplasmic processes in association with the other cellular components mentioned above. Confirmation by immunoperoxidase or electron microscopy is necessary for a definitive diagnosis. Clinically, these patients were predominantly over the age of 50 years at presentation, although three

were younger than 30 years. Only eight patients had lymph node presentations, and two presented with a mediastinal mass; five patients had unusual sites of extranodal presentations in the spermatic cord, the uterine cervix, retromolar tissue, and multiple bone sites. Nine patients had disease of limited extent, with seven patients having clinical stage I and two patients having stage II disease. An enlarged liver was noted in only two patients, and none were observed with splenomegaly. B type systemic symptoms were uncommon at presentation. The number of reported cases of validated histiocytic neoplasms is small. Undoubtedly, a much larger population of acceptable cases must be studied before a clear picture of the clinical manifestations and the course of the disease will emerge.

Clinical Features. Very few patients with true histiocytic malignancies have been described. A male predominance has been reported, and the average age of onset is approximately 50 to 60 years. Patients in the second and third decades are also described.

Splenomegaly, peripheral lymphadenopathy, and skin lesions are the common causes of initial presentation. The skin lesions are described as multiple, rapidly growing, and bluish red in coloration.

Routine laboratory evaluation is normal in the majority of the patients, although mild anemia has been described. Bone marrow is rarely involved. Reports on prognosis and therapy cannot be evaluated because of the rareness of the disease and the inconsistently applied diagnostic criteria.

Pathologic Features (Table 49). Histologically, lymph nodes show extensive accumulations of neoplastic histiocytes characterized by abundant eosinophilic

Table 49

MACROPHAGE/HISTIOCYTE TYPE NEOPLASMS

PATTERN
• Macrophage/histiocyte type: diffuse growth, often with prominent sinus involvement

• Histiocytic medullary reticulosis
  • Sinuses infiltrated in nodes; lymphoid elements often depleted
  • Spleen – dramatic congestion and infiltration by three histiocytic types of Robb-Smith

CYTOLOGY — NEOPLASTIC	MARKERS — NEOPLASTIC
• Macrophage/histiocyte type: large cells with round nuclei, abundant cytoplasm; phagocytosis may be present • Histiocytic medullary reticulosis: mixture of three cell types — prohistiocytes; immunoblastic in appearance with large nuclei; pleomorphic histiocytes, and bland histiocytes with prominent erythrophagocytosis	• Cytochemistry: α-naphthyl-acetate esterase positivity, acid phosphatase positivity, PAS positivity • PIP: α_1-antichymotrypsin and α_1-antitrypsin positivity of immature and pleomorphic histiocytes; lysozyme positivity in bland histiocytes CD68 (KP-1) (+)

INVOLVED SITES	CLINICAL FEATURES

• Nodes
 	
• Spleen
 	
• Marrow
 	
• Skin
	• Macrophage/histiocyte type: very rare, usually presents with lymphadenopathy, splenomegaly, or skin lesions
	
	• Histiocytic medullary reticulosis
	  . Very rare; reported in all ages, with median age of 31 years; greater incidence in males
	  . Dramatic onset of hemolytic anemia, fever, weakness, and weight loss; may have peripheral adenopathy

REACTIVE COMPONENTS	DIFFERENTIAL DIAGNOSIS
• Eosinophils, plasma cells may be prominent • Depleted in histiocytic medullary reticulosis	• Malignant lymphoma, T cell type, including anaplastic large cell lymphoma, Ki-1 type • Viral-associated hemophagocytic syndrome

cytoplasm and atypical nuclei (plates XLVII-A,B). Most portions of the node are involved, sometimes isolating residual follicular centers or islands of small lymphocytes. Sinusal involvement may be a prominent feature of the growth pattern. Occasional focal sheet-like growth of the tumor causes the cells to appear more cohesive than in histiocytic medullary reticulosis (fig. 93) and may make malignant histiocytosis difficult to distinguish from large cell metastatic carcinoma. In some cases, infiltration of the nodal capsule and perinodal soft tissue is present. Vascular proliferation may be a prominent component in some cases. Reticulin fibers are prominent in malignant histiocytes, but their distribution is of uncertain diagnostic value (fig. 94).

Tumor cells are cytologically identical to the most atypical cells described in histiocytic medullary reticulosis, with thick nuclear membranes, an irregular chromatin pattern, and large irregular nucleoli. Phagocytic activity can occasionally be demonstrated, and consequently, cytochemical and ultrastructural studies are necessary to prove the neoplastic cells are

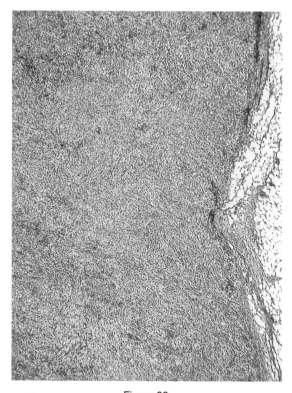

Figure 93
(Figures 93 and 94 and plate XLVII-A,B
are from the same patient)
MALIGNANT HISTIOCYTOSIS, MACROPHAGE CELL
TYPE PREDOMINATING, LYMPH NODE
This inguinal lymph node is diffusely involved by a cellular proliferation with a swirling pattern of cytoplasmic cells. X20.

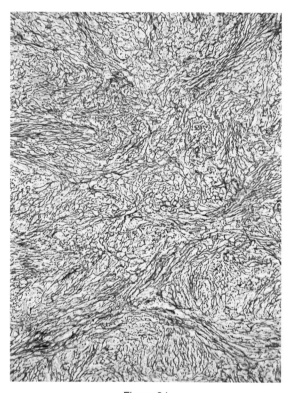

Figure 94
MALIGNANT HISTIOCYTOSIS, MACROPHAGE CELL
TYPE PREDOMINATING, LYMPH NODE
In this figure, the reticulin fibers are dramatically increased, forming a dense mesh in some areas and compact parallel masses elsewhere. Reticulin. X100.

of histiocytic origin. PAS and nonspecific esterase activity may be demonstrated in tumor imprints. Muramidase activity may be detected by immunoperoxidase methods but is useful only in more differentiated processes (Mendelsohn et al.). Some of these neoplasms also mark with antisera against α_1-antichymotrypsin. Ultrastructural examination is often required for confirmation, particularly in the more primitive neoplasms (fig. 95).

The pattern of infiltration of extranodal tissue appears similar in all malignant histiocytoses. Lung lesions may be present. The liver shows an extensive portal sinusal infiltrate with associated reactive changes in hepatocytes. The red pulp of the spleen and the bone marrow show a similar diffuse infiltration of neoplastic cells. Nodular accumulations of tumor cells are distinctly unusual, and the tumor is not confined in the marrow to areas adjacent to bony trabeculae. Skin lesions occur in approximately 10 percent of the cases and consist of a deep dermal infiltrate that spares the adnexa and epidermis. This is in contrast to the skin lesions of Letterer-Siwe disease in which the lesion involves the upper dermis with extension into epidermis and adnexa (Byrne and Rappaport).

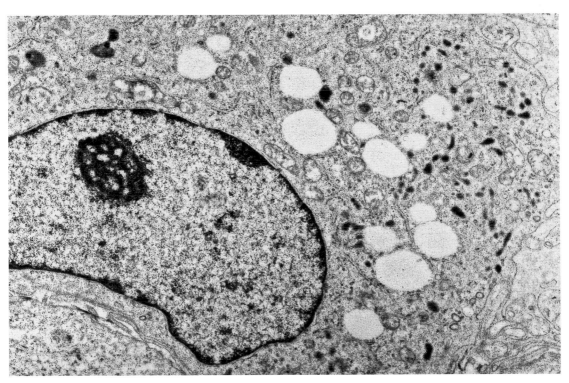

Figure 95
MALIGNANT HISTIOCYTOSIS, LYMPH NODE
This figure shows the ultrastructure of a neoplastic histiocyte. Numerous scattered monocytoid granules are demonstrated in the abundant cytoplasm. X13,800. (Fig. 19 from Collins, R.D., Bennett, B., and Glick, A.D. Neoplasms of the Mononuclear Phagocyte System. In: The Reticuloendothelial System, Vol. 5. Herberman, R.B. and Friedman, H. [Eds.]. New York: Plenum Press, 1983.)

Histiocytic Medullary Reticulosis

Definition. The term histiocytic medullary reticulosis was first used by Scott and Robb-Smith to describe a uniformly fatal neoplasm "characterized by a progressive cellular hyperplasia throughout the hematopoietic and lymphatic tissues." This name has been subsequently equated by many with malignant histiocytosis. We use histiocytic medullary reticulosis to refer to a specific subtype of malignant histiocytosis with identifying morphologic features related to the pattern of lymph node involvement and degree of cellular differentiation.

Clinical Features. Histiocytic medullary reticulosis is a rare disorder seen predominantly in males (2-3:1, M:F). The mean age is 31 years, although patients of all ages may be affected. Professor Robb-Smith reports having seen approximately one case a year since the original publication.

The most common mode of presentation is that of a wasting syndrome, with dramatic hemolytic anemia, fever, weakness, and weight loss, usually of relatively short duration. Peripheral lymphadenopathy is another common initial complaint. On physical examination, fever is common, and peripheral lymphadenopathy is seen in approximately 60 percent of the patients. Hepatosplenomegaly occurs in 75 to 95 percent of the cases and splenomegaly may be massive. Soft tissue masses and papulonodular lesions in the skin have also been noted with regularity.

Normochromic normocytic anemia is frequent and is thought to be secondary to erythrophagocytosis by histiocytes. Thrombocytopenia and leukopenia are found in 50 to 75 percent of the patients. Rarely, a leukemic phase of the disease may be seen, with elevated peripheral leukocyte counts secondary to histiocytosis. Hyperbilirubinemia is a prominent finding, often composed initially of indirect bilirubin.

The median survival in this disease is approximately 6 months. Combination chemotherapy, including doxorubicin, produced complete remission in a few patients, although many of the complete responders have experienced relapse within the central nervous system.

Pathologic Features (see Table 49). Histiocytic medullary reticulosis is characterized by the following cell types scattered in varying proportions in the node sinuses, red pulp of spleen, and marrow: (1) prohistiocyte or immunoblast-like cells; (2) a pleomorphic histiocyte exhibiting polypoid features and, occasionally, erythrophagocytosis; and (3) the bland or normal-appearing histiocytes in which dramatic erythrophagocytosis is routinely seen (plate XLVII-D). Lymph nodes characteristically show partial or complete filling of medullary and subcapsular sinuses with masses of noncohesive neoplastic cells (plate XLVII-C,D; fig. 96). Neoplastic cells vary greatly in cytologic features, with the most atypical cells showing irregular nuclear membranes with chromatin clumping, large and sometimes irregular nucleoli, and many mitotic figures. Other cells may be morphologically indistinguishable from benign histiocytes (Scott and Robb-Smith).

Differential Diagnosis. T cell proliferations, either clinically aggressive or overtly neoplastic, must be distinguished from histiocytic medullary reticulosis. These conditions may be associated with prominent histiocytosis and prominent erythrophagocytosis.

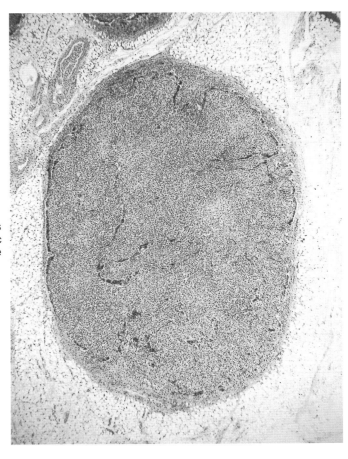

Figure 96
(Figure 96 and plate XLVII-C,D
are from the same patient)
HISTIOCYTIC MEDULLARY RETICULOSIS,
LYMPH NODE
This low magnification photomicrograph shows striking lymphocytic depletion and a dramatic accentuation of the sinuses due to packing of the sinuses by malignant histiocytes. X20.

Splenic Histiocyte Type

Franchino and colleagues described a single patient with a history of ulcerative colitis and splenomegaly. At splenectomy, multiple nodules of tumor were present, apparently arising in the red pulp. The tumor cells were large, with distinct cytoplasmic borders and abundant cytoplasm that was acidophilic and often vacuolated. Phagocytized erythrocytes, hemosiderin, and leukocytes were noted. Nucleoli were prominent. Binucleate and multinucleate tumor cells were present. By electron microscopy, cytoplasm was abundant and contained numerous mitochondria and phagolysosomes. Intercellular junctions and Birbeck granules were not present.

Tumor cells were shown to contain α_1-antitrypsin but were lysozyme negative. B and T cell restricted antigens were not present, nor was leukocyte-common antigen. The monocyte associated antigen CDw14 (Leu-M3) was expressed, as were myeloid/monocyte-associated antigens CD13 (My7) and CD33 (My9). The cells lacked CD15 (Leu-M1), S-100 protein, CD1, and CD30. DNA was germline, with no rearrangements of Ig heavy chain or T cell receptor β-chain.

On the basis of these studies, the authors concluded that this case might represent a neoplasm of tissue macrophage lineage.

291

PLATE XLVII

MALIGNANT HISTIOCYTOSIS, MACROPHAGE CELL PREDOMINATING, LYMPH NODE
(Plate XLVII-A,B and figures 93 and 94 are from the same patient)

These specimens are from an 18 year old male who presented with inguinal lymph node enlargement. A peribronchial mass was discovered soon afterward, and both lesions were biopsied prior to therapy. Labeled antibody stains for histiocyte enzymes (lysozyme, α_1-antichymotrypsin) were all positive in the tumor cells. Cells in tissue imprints of the second biopsy were also positive for the nonspecific esterase, α-naphthyl acetate esterase. A bone marrow biopsy revealed diffuse involvement by a blast-like cell without apparent monocytoid features. These cells unfortunately were not characterized further.

A. In this properly fixed lymph node specimen, the cytologic features are ideally portrayed with minimal distortion. Pale cytoplasmic macrophage-appearing cells dominate the proliferation. X600.

B. This imprint reveals a range in the morphologic appearance of the cellular population from monocytes to macrophages with a limited amount of cytoplasm. Wright's stain. X1000.

HISTIOCYTIC MEDULLARY RETICULOSIS, LYMPH NODE
(Plate XLVII-C,D and figure 96 are from the same patient)

This young black male presented with the dramatic onset of fever and anemia. An enlarged spleen was discovered early in the course of the disease. The initial lymph node biopsy material was technically not of optimal quality, and a definitive diagnosis was not made. A repeat biopsy fixed in Zenker's solution revealed the characteristic cytologic triad of prohistiocytes, bland histiocytes often with erythrophagocytosis, plus pleomorphic histiocytes. Most of the abnormal histiocytes were found in the lymph node sinuses. The patient responded briefly to chemotherapy but soon relapsed and died approximately 4 months after presentation.

C. At this magnification, accentuation and distortion of the sinuses by the histiocytic infiltration and lymphocytic depletion are evident. X80.

D. The three cell types described by Robb-Smith are apparent in this preparation. A histiocyte stuffed with red cells is apparent in the sinus. Other histiocytes have large nuclei with prominent nucleoli and closely resemble immunoblasts, while yet a third population has a pleomorphic and dysplastic appearance. Giemsa. X600.

PLATE XLVII

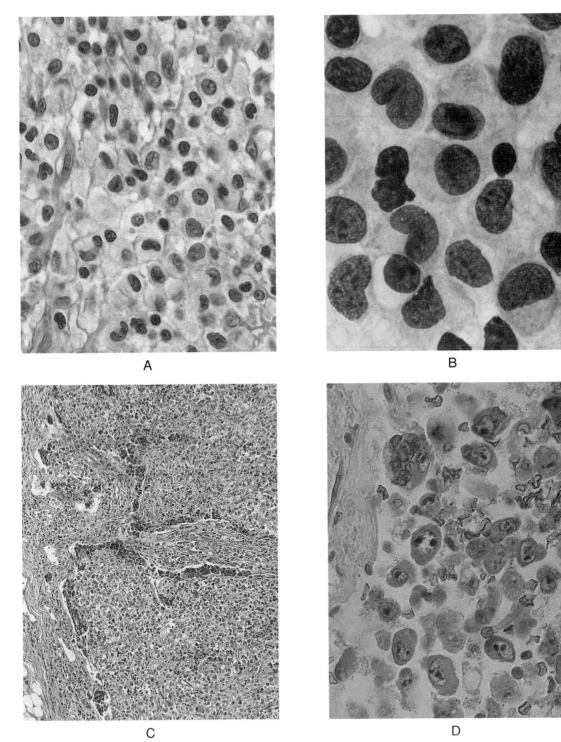

A

B

C

D

FOLLICULAR DENDRITIC CELL TYPE

There are very few descriptions of this neoplasm, the existence of which was predicted by Lennert in 1978. Monda and colleagues described four patients from 29 to 40 years of age presenting with painless cervical adenopathy. Tumor replaced the entire nodal parenchyma in some areas or had sharp boundaries from residual lymphoid tissue in others (Table 50). A nesting, whorling, or storiform pattern of growth was noted (fig. 97). Necrosis was not seen. Tumor cells were usually oval to spindle in shape (fig. 98), whereas some nuclei were highly atypical and multinucleated. PAS stains were negative. Mitotic activity was scant to moderate.

By immunocytochemistry, tumor cells marked with CD45 (LCA), dendritic reticulum cell antigen R4/23, and the C3b complement receptor (figs. 99, 100).

Electron microscopy showed scattered ribosomes, scant lysosomes, striking long and complex cytoplasmic extensions (fig. 101), as well as numerous desmosomes (fig. 102).

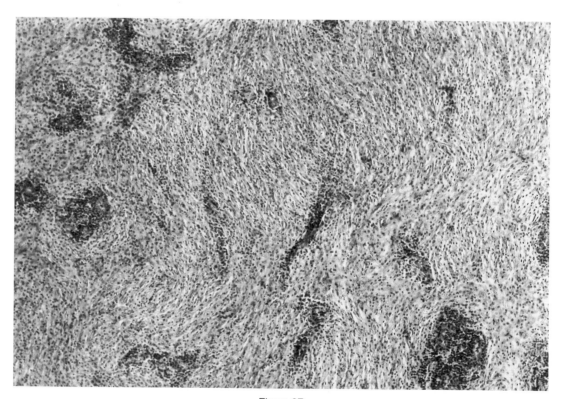

Figure 97
(Figures 97, 98, 101, and 102 are from the same patient)
FOLLICULAR DENDRITIC CELL TYPE
The lymph node structure is largely replaced by a monomorphic population of pale oval cells. The residual lymphoid tissue is limited to small follicles and perivascular collections of lymphocytes. (Fig. 3 from Monda, L., Warnke, R., and Rosai, J. A primary lymph node malignancy with features suggestive of dendritic reticulum cell differentiation. Am. J. Pathol. 122:562-572, 1986.)

Table 50

MALIGNANT HISTIOCYTOSIS, DENDRITIC TYPES

PATTERN
• Diffuse growth patterns, often sparing follicles — whorling pattern, occasionally storiform
• Lymph node sinuses may not be involved
• Necrosis may be present

CYTOLOGY — NEOPLASTIC	MARKERS — NEOPLASTIC
• **Follicular dendritic:** oval to spindle cells, some multinucleated; electron microscopy shows long cytoplasmic extensions with numerous desmosomes	• **Follicular dendritic** CD45 (+): tumor cells contain Fc receptor, complement receptor, dendritic antigen (R4/23); PAS (−)
• **Interdigitating:** large pleomorphic cells with pale cytoplasm; some cells multinucleated; electron microscopy shows interweaving cytoplasmic processes, no desmosomes or Birbeck granules	• **Interdigitating** CD45 (+): tumor cells contain HLA-DR, S-100 cytoplasmic protein, CD1 usually negative; lysozyme negative; α_1-antichymotrypsin (±)
• **Langerhans:** large cells with abundant cytoplasm, pleomorphic multilobated nuclei; electron microscopy shows Birbeck granules	• **Langerhans** CD45 (+): tumor cells contain HLA-DR, S-100 cytoplasmic protein; CD1 positive, tumor cells negative for lysozyme, α_1-antichymotrypsin

INVOLVED SITES	CLINICAL FEATURES
• Superficial nodes • Skin • Tonsil	• Very few patients reported; mostly adults with superficial adenopathy

REACTIVE COMPONENTS	DIFFERENTIAL DIAGNOSIS
• **Interdigitating:** neutrophil clumps described in one case • **Langerhans:** many eosinophils may be present	• Malignant lymphoma, B and T cell type, including anaplastic large cell lymphoma, Ki-1 type • Soft tissue sarcoma • Metastatic carcinoma

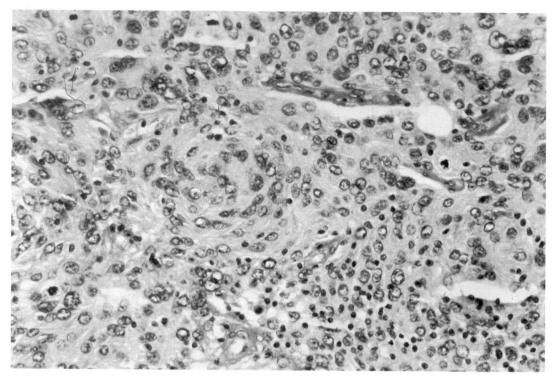

Figure 98
FOLLICULAR DENDRITIC CELL TYPE
The tumor cells are arranged in ill-defined whorls. The nuclear shape varies from round to oval. A sprinkling of mature lymphocytes is seen among the tumor cells. (Fig. 4 from Monda, L., Warnke, R., and Rosai, J. A primary lymph node malignancy with features suggestive of dendritic reticulum cell differentiation. Am. J. Pathol. 122:562-572, 1986.)

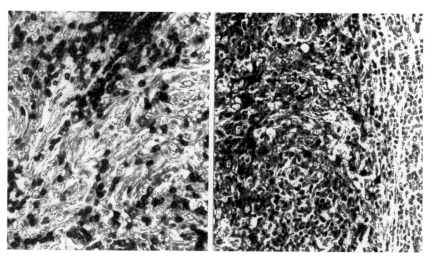

Figure 99
(Figures 99 and 100 are from the same patient)
FOLLICULAR DENDRITIC CELL TYPE
The tumor cells stain darkly for the dendritic reticulum cell antigen. Note the adjacent unstained lymphocytes. R4/23. X235. (Fig. 8C from Monda, L., Warnke, R., and Rosai, J. A primary lymph node malignancy with features suggestive of dendritic reticulum cell differentiation. Am. J. Pathol. 122:562-572, 1986.)

Weiss and colleagues reported four spindle cell neoplasms of unusual phenotype, and their cases 3 and 4 were presumed to be of dendritic cell origin on the basis of multiparameter studies. These patients were 45 and 66 years of age and both had superficial adenopathy. Their tumors had a prominent spindle growth pattern, and foci of necrosis were noted in one case. Electron microscopy showed complex cytoplasmic interdigitations with numerous desmosomes.

By immunocytochemistry, these cases were CD45 (LCA) negative, HLA-DR positive, and had receptors for C3b and C3d. Dendritic antigen R4/23 was positive in one of two cases, as was S-100 protein.

Four other patients were described in 1982 by van der Valk and associates. Data from their patients resembled those of the above cases, but immunocytochemicals tudies were less complete. Desmosomes were not demonstrated by electron microscopy.

INTERDIGITATING CELL TYPE

Only a handful of patients have been described with neoplasms shown to have arisen from interdigitating cells. One of the more completely studied cases was reported by Chan and Zaatari in a 67 year old man with fever and night sweats. Abdominal lymph nodes, spleen, liver, and lungs contained pleomorphic tumor in which nuclear lobation and convolutions were prominent (fig. 103). Some cells were multinucleated (see Table 50). There were multiple microabscesses in the tumor, with neutrophils in many tumor cells (fig. 104). Electron microscopy showed interweaving cytoplasmic processes, without junctional complexes or Birbeck granules (fig. 105).

Immunocytochemistry showed the tumor cells were reactive with antibodies against S-100 protein, CD1, and HLA (fig. 106). There was strong acid phosphatase positivity.

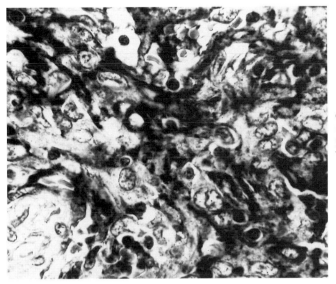

Figure 100
FOLLICULAR DENDRITIC CELL TYPE
This illustrates a strong staining for C3b receptor of the cell processes of the tumor cells. TO5. X640. (Fig. 8D from Monda, L., Warnke, R., and Rosai, J. A primary lymph node malignancy with features suggestive of dendritic reticulum cell differentiation. Am. J. Pathol. 122:562-572, 1986.)

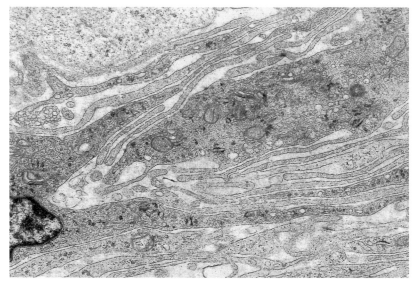

Figure 101
FOLLICULAR DENDRITIC CELL TYPE
Electron microscopy shows intertwined extremely elongated cell processes from several tumor cells. X12,130. (Fig. 10 from Monda, L., Warnke, R., and Rosai, J. A primary lymph node malignancy with features suggestive of dendritic reticulum cell differentiation. Am. J. Pathol. 122:562-572, 1986.)

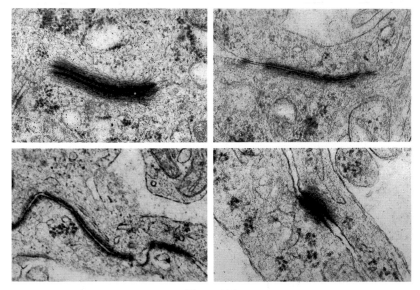

Figure 102
FOLLICULAR DENDRITIC CELL TYPE
Specialized cell junctions are present between tumor cells. They vary in length and complexity but most of the features are maculae adherents or desmosomes. X28,900. (Fig. 11 from Monda, L., Warnke, R., and Rosai, J. A primary lymph node malignancy with features suggestive of dendritic reticulum cell differentiation. Am. J. Pathol. 122:562-572, 1986.)

Weiss and associates reported 2 cases that also probably represent neoplasms of interdigitating cells. These patients were 34 and 60 years of age and had superficial adenopathy. A spindling growth pattern was noted, with the tumor cells having pale to slightly eosinophilic cytoplasm and oval nuclei. Multinucleation was present in one case. Electron microscopy on Case 1 showed spindle-shaped cells with occasional phagosomes and dense granules but with no Birbeck granules or desmosomes.

Immunophenotypic studies showed marking with leukocyte common antigen, several macrophage/myeloid markers, and strong expression of S-100 protein. Complement receptors and Langerhans marker Leu-6 were negative.

A final case was reported by Nakamura and colleagues in a 58 year old man with involvement of cervical nodes and small intestine. Growth pattern of the tumor was remarkable in that the follicles were preserved and a swirling pattern was not present. Tumor cells were large and pleomorphic. Electron microscopy showed prominent cytoplasmic processes with interdigitation. Immunophenotypic studies showed that the tumor cells contained cytoplasmic S-100 protein and HLA-DR.

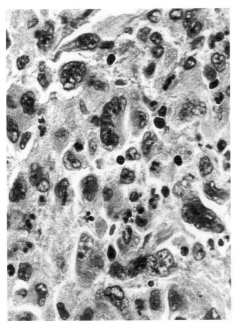

Figure 103
(Figures 103-106 are from the same patient)
INTERDIGITATING RETICULUM
CELL SARCOMA
The biopsy of the supraclavicular lymph node shows the large pleomorphic tumor cells with lobated nuclei and abundant eosinophilic cytoplasm. H&E. X350. (Fig. 1 from Chan, W.C. and Zaatari, G. Lymph node interdigitating reticulum cell sarcoma. Am. J. Clin. Pathol. 85:739-744, 1986.)

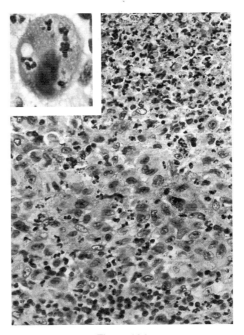

Figure 104
INTERDIGITATING RETICULUM
CELL SARCOMA
A ring of tumor cells, with scattered neutrophils, surrounds a microabscess. X100. A tumor cell with several intracytoplasmic neutrophils is illustrated (inset). H&E. X400. (Fig. 3 from Chan, W.C. and Zaatari, G. Lymph node interdigitating reticulum cell sarcoma. Am. J. Clin. Pathol. 85:739-744, 1986.)

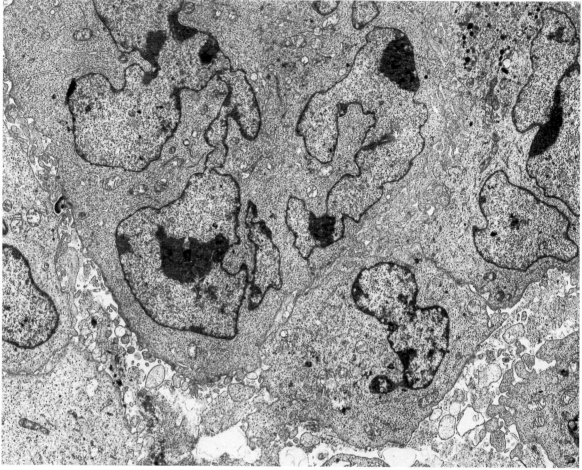

Figure 105
INTERDIGITATING RETICULUM CELL SARCOMA
Electron microscopy shows a large tumor cell with a multilobated nucleus. There are deep nuclear indentations, abundant cytoplasm, and prominent cytoplasmic processes interdigitating with the processes of adjacent smaller cells. Note the absence of Birbeck granules. Uranyl acetate, lead citrate. X7340. (Fig. 6 from Chan, W.C. and Zaatari, G. Lymph node interdigitating reticulum cell sarcoma. Am. J. Clin. Pathol. 85:739-744, 1986.)

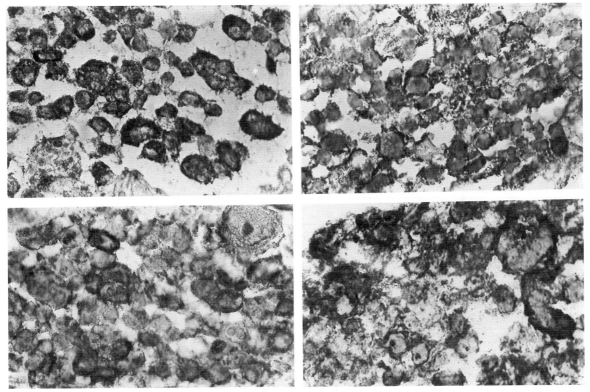

Figure 106
INTERDIGITATING RETICULUM CELL SARCOMA
Examples of immunohistochemistry demonstrate S-100 protein (upper left), CD1 (T6) antigens (lower left), CD4 (Leu-3a) antigens (upper right), and HLA-DR antigens (lower right). Immunoperoxidase. X340. (Fig. 5 from Chan, W.C. and Zaatari, G. Lymph node interdigitating reticulum cell sarcoma. Am. J. Clin. Pathol. 85:739-744, 1986.)

LANGERHANS CELL TYPE

Demonstration of the Birbeck granules by electron microscopy provides a reliable structural marker of this neoplasm.

Most histiocytoses involving cells containing Langerhans granules fall into the histiocytosis X group and are focal processes with a favorable prognosis. Imamura and associates apparently described the first case of a malignant process that differed in age of onset and cytologic features from Letterer-Siwe disease. A 9 year old female died after a 14 month illness that was characterized by a leukemic phase with a white count of 69,200/μL and 62 percent blasts, lymphadenopathy, and skin and lung involvement. Autopsy showed widespread tumor. Neoplastic cells had abundant cytoplasm and did not exhibit phagocytosis, and Langerhans granules were easily demonstrated in tumor cells by electron microscopy.

Differentiation of cases such as this from histiocytosis X is difficult, but the presence of 62 percent blasts in the peripheral blood and widespread tumefactions seem to establish this particular case as a malignant neoplasm of Langerhans granule-containing cells (see Table 50).

In 1984 Wood and associates described another case in a 71 year old man presenting with multiple papules on the head and trunk. Lesions were 1-10 mm in diameter, skin colored, or erythematous, with rolled borders and central ulceration. This patient had a progressive illness, ending in death by 6 months, with massive tumor involvement of lungs, liver, spleen, and nodes noted at autopsy. Tumor cells were large, with abundant eosinophilic cytoplasm. Nuclei were large and pleomorphic, some with extreme multilobation. Many eosinophils were present. Electron microscopy showed that most tumor cells contained Birbeck granules.

Tumor cells showed reactivity similar to that of normal Langerhans cells, namely HLA-DR, leukocyte common antigen, Ia, CD1, and CD4. There was also acid phosphatase and ATPase positivity with negative α-naphthyl butyrate esterase.

References

Byrne, G.E. and Rappaport, H. Malignant histiocytosis. Gann Monogr. Cancer Res. 15:145-162, 1973.

Chan, W.C. and Zaatari, G. Lymph node interdigitating reticulum cell sarcoma. Am. J. Clin. Pathol. 85:739-744, 1986.

Franchino, C., Reich, C., Distenfeld, A., Ubriaco, A., and Knowles, D.M. A clinicopathologically distinctive primary splenic histiocytic neoplasm. Demonstration of its histiocytic derivation by immunophenotypic and molecular genetic analysis. Am. J. Surg. Pathol. 12:398-404, 1988.

Imamura, M., Sakamoto, S., and Hanazono, H. Malignant histiocytosis: a case of generalized histiocytosis with infiltration of Langerhans' granule-containing histiocytes. Cancer 28:467-475, 1971.

Lennert, K. Malignant Lymphomas Other Than Hodgkin's Disease: Histology, Cytology, Ultrastructure, Immunology. New York: Springer-Verlag, 1978.

Mendelsohn, G., Eggleston, J.C., and Mann, R.B. Relationship of lysozyme (muramidase) to histiocytic differentiation in malignant histiocytosis. Cancer 45:273-279, 1980.

Monda, L., Warnke, R., and Rosai, J. A primary lymph node malignancy with features suggestive of dendritic reticulum cell differentiation. A report of 4 cases. Am. J. Pathol. 122:562-572, 1986.

Nakamura, S., Hara, K., Suchi, T., et al. Interdigitating cell sarcoma. A morphologic, immunohistologic, and enzyme-histochemical study. Cancer 61:562-568, 1988.

Robb-Smith, A.H.T. Before our time: half a century of histiocytic medullary reticulosis: a T-cell teaser? Histopathology 17:279-283, 1990.

Scott, R.B. and Robb-Smith, A.H.T. Histiocytic medullary reticulosis. Lancet 2:194-198, 1939.

van der Valk, P., Ruiter, D.J., den Ottolander, G.J., et al. Dendritic reticulum cell sarcoma? Four cases of a lymphoma probably derived from dendritic reticulum cells of the follicular compartment. Histopathology 6:269-287, 1982.

Weiss, L.M., Berry, G.J., Dorfman, R.F., et al. Spindle cell neoplasms of lymph nodes of probable reticulum cell lineage. True reticulum cell sarcoma? Am. J. Surg. Pathol. 14:405-414, 1990.

Wood, C., Wood, G.S., Deneau, D.G., et al. Malignant histiocytosis X. Report of a rapidly fatal case in an elderly man. Cancer 54:347-352, 1984.

Additional References

Greenberg, E., Cohen, D.M., Pease, G.L., and Kyle, R.A. Histiocytic medullary reticulosis. Mayo Clinic Proceedings 37:271-283, 1962.

Hanson, C.A., Jaszcz, W., Kersey, J.H., et al. True histiocytic lymphoma: histopathologic, immunophenotypic and genotypic analysis. Br. J. Haematol. 73:187-198, 1989.

Huhn, D. and Meister, P. Malignant histiocytosis. Cancer 42:1341-1349, 1978.

Jaffe, E.S. Malignant Histiocytosis and True Histiocytic Lymphomas, pp. 381-411. In: Major Problems in Pathology, Vol. 16. Surgical Pathology of the Lymph Nodes and Related Organs. Jaffe, E.S. and Bennington, J.L. (Eds.). Philadelphia: W.B. Saunders Company, 1985.

Lampert, I.A., Catovsky, D., and Bergier, N. Malignant histiocytosis. Br. J. Haematol. 40:65-77, 1978.

Pileri, S., Mazza, P., Rivano, M.T., et al. Malignant histiocytosis (true histiocytic lymphoma) clinicopathological study of 25 cases. Histopathology 9:905-920, 1985.

Rappaport, H. Tumors of the Hematopoietic System, pp. 49-90; 99-101. Fascicle 8, First Series. Atlas of Tumor Pathology. Washington: Armed Forces Institute of Pathology, 1966.

Turner, R.R., Wood, G.S., Beckstead, J.H., et al. Histiocytic malignancies: morphologic, immunologic, and enzymatic heterogeneity. Am. J. Surg. Pathol. 8:485-500, 1984.

Warnke, R.A., Kim, H., and Dorfman, R.F. Malignant histiocytosis (histiocytic medullary reticulosis). I. Clinicopathologic study of 29 cases. Cancer 35:215-230, 1975.

MYELOID NEOPLASMS

These neoplasms arise from a bone marrow myelopoietic stem cell, and the degree and type of differentiation determines the diagnosis (Fialkow et al.). Those diseases in which monocytic differentiation predominates are included in the mononuclear phagocyte system section, although the stem cell for mononuclear phagocytes is likely to be shared with other myelopoietic cells. Leukemias with neoplastic cells having both myeloid and lymphoid features are discussed in this section under the term hybrid leukemia.

The classification system in general use was devised by an international group and is known as the French-American-British classification (Bennett et al., 1976, 1985). In this system, lymphoid or myeloid differentiation is denoted by the use of L or M, respectively. Leukemias with no evidence of differentiation are designated M-0, whereas the granulocytic types are designated M-1 (myeloblastic without maturation), M-2 (myeloblastic with maturation), and M-3 (promyelocytic leukemia). M-4 is acute myelomonocytic leukemia, M-5 is monocytic leukemia, M-6 is erythroleukemia, and M-7 is megakaryocytic leukemia.

Several neoplasms of clinical and biologic importance are in this group. A great deal of information about the biology of myelopoiesis and lymphopoiesis has come from an analysis of the blast phases of chronic myelogenous leukemia. In addition, chronic myelogenous leukemia is a relatively frequent disease that poses significant therapeutic difficulties. Although rare, promyelocytic leukemia is of interest because of the major therapeutic implications of this diagnosis. The frequency of intravascular coagulation in this disease often requires anticoagulation on an emergency basis, in addition to chemotherapy directed against the leukemia.

References

Bennett, J.M., Catovsky, D., Daniel, M.T., et al. Proposals for the classification of the acute leukemias. A report of the French-American-British (FAB) co-operative group. Br. J. Haematol. 33:451-458, 1976.
_____ , J.M., Catovsky, D., Daniel, M.T., et al. Proposed revised criteria for the classification of acute myeloid leukemia. A report of the French-American-British cooperative group. Ann. Intern. Med. 103:626-629, 1985.
Fialkow, P.J., Singer, J.W., Raskind, W.H., et al. Clonal development, stem-cell differentiation, and clinical remissions in acute nonlymphocytic leukemia. N. Engl. J. Med. 317:468-473, 1987.

Additional References

Ahearn, M.J. Electron Microscopy as an Aid to the Diagnosis and Characterization of Acute Leukemia, pp. 87-129. In: The Acute Leukemias. Biologic, Diagnostic and Therapeutic Determinants. Stass, S.A. (Ed.). New York: Marcel Dekker, Inc., 1987.
Childs, C.C. and Stass, S.A. Characterization and Diagnosis of the Acute Leukemias, pp.1-26. In: The Acute Leukemias. Biologic, Diagnostic and Therapeutic Determinants. Stass, S.A. (Ed.). New York: Marcel Dekker, Inc., 1987.
Dalton, W., Jr. and Stass, S.A. A Morphologic and Cytochemical Approach to the Diagnosis of Acute Leukemia, pp. 27-86. In: The Acute Leukemias. Biologic, Diagnostic and Therapeutic Determinants. Stass, S.A. (Ed.). New York: Marcel Dekker, Inc., 1987.
Hayhoe, F.G., Quaglino, D., and Doll, R. The Cytology and Cytochemistry of Acute Leukemias. Medical Research Council Special Report Series, No. 304. London: Her Majesty's Stationery Office, 1964.
Neame, P.B., Soamboonsrup, P., Browman, G.P., et al. Classifying acute leukemia by immunophenotyping: a combined FAB-immunologic classification of AML. Blood 68:1355-1362, 1986.
Stanley, M., McKenna, R.W., Ellinger, G., and Brunning, R.D. Classification of 358 Cases of Acute Myeloid Leukemia by FAB Criteria, pp. 147-174. In: Chronic and Acute Leukemias in Adults. Bloomfield, C.D. (Ed.). Boston: Martinus Nijhoff Publishers, 1985.

Swerdlow, S.H., Glick, A.D., Cousar, J.B., and Collins, R.D. Acute leukemias of childhood. Hematol. Oncol. 3:99-131, 1985.

Yunis, J.J. and Brunning, R.D. Prognostic Significance of Chromosomal Abnormalities in Acute Leukaemias and Myelodysplastic Syndromes, pp. 597-620. In: Clinics in Haematology, Vol. 15. Gale, R.P. and Hoffbrand, A.V. (Eds.). London: W.B. Saunders Company, 1986.

HYBRID ACUTE LEUKEMIA

SYNONYMS AND RELATED TERMS: Mixed lineage leukemia, leukemia with lineage infidelity.

Definition. Hybrid leukemias are leukemias in which individual cells display markers of more than one cell line. This term is used to distinguish bilineal or biclonal leukemias in which leukemic cells are heterogeneous, with single cells displaying lymphoid phenotypes and others myeloid phenotypes. The existence of hybrid leukemias has become apparent recently through routine analyses of marrow or blood by flow cytometry with an extensive battery of monoclonal antibodies. Some cases may have inappropriately been diagnosed as hybrid for technical reasons (Greaves et al.).

Clinical Features. Both children and adults have been demonstrated to have hybrid leukemia, with an incidence estimated at 1 to 4 percent of the acute leukemias (Kristensen et al.; Neame et al.). Patients with hybrid leukemia may have a poorer prognosis than those whose disease has a more homogeneous differentiation. Some children with myeloid leukemia whose blasts expressed CD2 surface antigen failed standard myeloid induction therapy but subsequently achieved remission with acute lymphoblastic leukemia therapy (Mirro et al.). Patients with an acute lymphocytic leukemia carrying a phenotype of CD7 positivity and CD4 and CD8 negativity have shown an in vivo conversion from lymphoid to myeloid lineages. This CD7 positive, CD4 negative, CD8 negative phenotype was associated with a distinct clinical entity in which males under 35 years and over 65 years predominated (Kurtzberg et al.). There were frequent mediastinal or thymic masses with skin and central nervous system disease and high peripheral white counts. These patients responded poorly to conventional therapy for both lymphoid and myeloid leukemia. The differentiation of the leukemic cells in vitro along multiple lines indicated that this type of leukemia is derived from a very immature hematopoietic cell.

Chromosomal abnormalities in hybrid leukemias have not been consistent. Philadelphia chromosome has not been found in these cases.

Pathologic and Immunologic Features. Hybrid leukemias resemble other forms of acute leukemia in their growth patterns. Marrows are usually completely cellular and homogeneous in appearance on sections. The morphology of hybrid leukemic blasts has not been systematically evaluated. However, blasts have been described as having either myeloid or lymphoid appearances in Wright stain. Wright stain preparations have not been useful in the identification of phenotypic hybrid leukemias.

Hybrid leukemias are most easily recognized by integrating flow cytometry and cytochemical data. Some cases have had myeloid morphology, 20 to 30 percent Sudan black positive blasts with Auer rods and have also shown simultaneous expression of CD2, CD45, or TdT. The incidence of various "lymphoid" markers in cases predominantly myeloid in phenotype is as follows: TdT, 5 to 25 percent; CD19,

5 percent; CD10 (CALLA), 0 to 5 percent; CD2, 5 percent (many of these are acute promyelocytic leukemia); CD3, rare; and CD7, 10 to 25 percent.

Comment. There is extensive evidence that most if not all cases of acute leukemia are clonal processes. The phenotype of the leukemic cells may then be related to the level of hematopoietic development in which the malignant transformational event occurs (Gale and Bassat). Transformation at the level of a pluripotential stem cell might allow the production of leukemic cells in which both myeloid and lymphoid features were detectable. However, it also seems possible that a neoplasm of a pluripotential stem cell might have very restricted differentiation in a leukemic clone despite its pluripotential origin. Leukemias arising from multipotential or unipotential stem cells might be expected to have more restricted differentiation capacities such as those seen in acute promyelocytic leukemia.

References

Gale, R.P. and Ben Bassat, I. Hybrid acute leukaemia. Br. J. Haematol. 65:261-264, 1987.

Greaves, M.F., Chan, L.C., Furley, A.J.W., Watt, S.M., and Molgaard, H.V. Lineage promiscuity in hemopoietic differentiation and leukemia. Blood 67:1-11, 1986.

Kristensen, J.S., Ellegaard, J., Hansen, K.B., Clausen, N., and Hokland, P. First-line diagnosis based on immunological phenotyping in suspected acute leukemia: a prospective study. Leuk. Res. 12:773-782, 1988.

Kurtzberg, J., Waldmann, T.A., Davey, M.P., et al. CD7+, CD4-, CD8- acute leukemia: a syndrome of malignant pluripotent lymphohematopoietic cells. Blood 73:381-390, 1989.

Mirro, J., Zipf, T.F., Pui, C-H., et al. Acute mixed lineage leukemia: clinicopathologic correlations and prognostic significance. Blood 66:1115-1123, 1985.

Neame, P.B., Soamboonsrup, P., Browman, G., et al. Simultaneous or sequential expression of lymphoid and myeloid phenotypes in acute leukemia. Blood 65:142-148, 1985.

ACUTE MYELOID LEUKEMIAS, FRENCH-AMERICAN-BRITISH CLASSIFICATION M-1, M-2, M-7

Definition. Acute myeloid leukemias are bone marrow-derived neoplasms composed of blasts and cells differentiating into granulocytes. The cell of origin is a granulocytic precursor cell.

Clinical Features. Acute myeloid leukemias, including the M-1 and M-2 subtypes within the French-American-British classification system, constitute approximately 40 to 50 percent of all cases of acute leukemia in adults in the United States. Most patients are in their fourth or fifth decade, with males and females equally affected.

Patients first seek medical attention with symptoms or signs related to bone marrow failure. Thirty to 40 percent of the patients present with bleeding, whereas 30 percent have an infection. Bone or joint pain occurs in approximately 10 percent of the patients, and weight loss is described in 25 percent of the patients.

On physical examination, fever is present in 50 percent of the patients, evidence of a bleeding diathesis is seen in 30 percent, splenomegaly (which is usually slight) in 20 percent, hepatomegaly in 20 to 30 percent, and lymphadenopathy in approximately 20 percent.

The mean hemoglobin level is approximately 9 g/dL, with an average platelet count of 100,000/μL and an average white blood cell count of 33,000/μL at the time of diagnosis. The percentage of circulating myeloblasts is usually between 22 and 28 percent. Approximately 10 percent of the patients present with white counts in excess of 100,000/μL. With current techniques, approximately 60 percent of the patients may be shown to have a chromosomal abnormality in the leukemic cells. The most commonly described abnormalities include an 8;21 translocation and the loss of all or part of the long arm of chromosome 5 and/or 7.

With combination chemotherapy, including doxorubicin and cytosine arabinoside, approximately 60 to 70 percent of the patients will attain complete remission. The average duration of a complete response is approximately 1 year, and average survival is approximately 1.5 to 2 years. Bone marrow transplantation performed during complete remission from an HLA-matched donor may improve survival significantly. However, this therapeutic option remains experimental and is limited to individuals under the age of 30 or 35 who have such HLA-compatible donors.

Pathologic Features (Table 51). The marrow is diffusely infiltrated by blasts (plate XLVI-C,D; fig. 107) and promyelocytes (usually >30 percent of the total cells). Predominant cells are usually Sudan black or peroxidase positive. Auer rods may be present. PAS reaction shows a diffuse tinge with superimposed granules, and chloroacetate esterase reaction is positive in more mature cells. Rare (1-2 percent) monocytic cells, which are cells positive for α-naphthyl acetate esterase, are present. Electron microscopy shows blasts and cells with specific granulocytic lysosomal granules. In M-1 leukemia, the peroxidase or Sudan black reaction is positive in at least 3 percent of the cells, whereas in M-2 leukemia, over 50 percent of the cells are recognizable as myeloblasts or promyelocytes. Uncommon subvariants include M-2E (eosinophils predominate), M-2B (basophils predominate),

M-2G (dysplastic neutrophils predominate), and M-7 (megakaryoblasts predominate) (Boros and Bennett; Dalton and Stass). Immunophenotyping may be useful in classification, particularly in cases with indefinite cytochemical studies (Neame et al.).

References

Boros, L. and Bennett, J.M. The Acute Myeloid Leukemias. In: Leukemias. Goldman, J.M. and Preisler, H.D. (Eds.). London: Butterworths & Company, Ltd., 1984.

Dalton, W., Jr. and Stass, S.A. A Morphological and Cytochemical Approach to the Diagnosis of Acute Leukemia, pp. 27-86. In: The Acute Leukemias. Biologic, Diagnostic, and Therapeutic Determinants. Stass, S.A. (Ed.). New York: Marcel Dekker, Inc., 1987.

Neame, P.B., Soamboonsrup, P., Browman, R.M., et al. Classifying acute leukemia by immunotyping: a combined FAB-immunologic classification of AML. Blood 68:1355-1362, 1986.

Additional References

Bennett, J.M., Catovsky, D., Daniel, M.T., et al. Criteria for the diagnosis of acute leukemia of megakaryocyte lineage (M7). A report of the French-American-British Cooperative Group. Ann. Intern. Med. 103:460-462, 1985.

Bloomfield, C.D. and Brunning, R.D. FAB M7: acute megakaryoblastic leukemia—beyond morphology. Ann. Intern. Med. 103:450-452, 1985.

Burns, C., Armitage, J.O., Frey, A.L., et al. Analysis of the presenting features of adult acute leukemia: the French-American-British classification. Cancer 47:2460-2469, 1981.

Dick, F.R., Armitage, J.O., and Burns, C.P. Diagnostic concurrence in the subclassification of adult acute leukemia using French-American-British criteria. Cancer 49:916-920, 1982.

Mertelsmann, R.H, Tzvi Thaler, H.T., To, L., et al. Morphological classification, response to therapy, and survival in 263 adult patients with acute nonlymphoblastic leukemia. Blood 56:773-781, 1980.

Mirchandani, I. and Palutke, M. Acute megakaryoblastic leukemia. Cancer 50:2866-2872, 1982.

Reiffers, J., Raynal, F., and Broustet, A. Acute myeloblastic leukemia in elderly patients: treatment and prognostic factors. Cancer 45:2816-2820, 1980.

Rowley, J.D., Alimena G., Garson, O.M., et al. A collaborative study of the relationship of the morphological type of acute nonlymphocytic leukemia with patient age and karyotype. Blood 59:1013-1022, 1982.

Yunis, J.J., Bloomfield, C.D., and Ensrud, K. All patients with acute nonlymphocytic leukemia may have a chromosomal defect. N. Engl. J. Med. 305:135-139, 1981.

Table 51

ACUTE MYELOID LEUKEMIAS,
FRENCH-AMERICAN-BRITISH CLASSIFICATION M-1, M-2, M-7

PATTERN
• Marrow — diffusely and massively infiltrated; homogeneous appearance; moderate marrow fibrosis in M-7 (megakaryocytic type); older patients may have acute myeloid leukemia arising in <u>hypocellular</u> marrow
• Node — may show extensive infiltration with small islands of cortical lymphocytes
• Spleen — red pulp infiltration

CYTOLOGY — NEOPLASTIC	MARKERS — NEOPLASTIC

• Sections:
  · Medium sized neoplastic cells, slightly eccentric nuclei, usually single nucleolus, small amount of pale cytoplasm; numerous mononuclear and dysplastic megakaryocytes in megakaryocytic type (M-7)
• Smears:
  · Moderate cytoplasm, usually with distinct granulation; rare cases show eosinophilic, basophilic, or megakaryocytic differentiation
  · Auer rods often present
	• Cytochemistry: Combined esterase shows marked increase in both granulocytic and monocytic elements
	  · Sudan black, peroxidase (+) minority of cells in M-1, majority of cells in M-2
	  · PAS, diffuse (+)
	  · Chloroacetate esterase, positive in >5 percent blasts
	• Flow: HLA-DR (+)
	  CD33, 13, 15 (+)
	  CD34 (±)
	  CD14 (−)

INVOLVED SITES	CLINICAL FEATURES
• Marrow • Nodes • Spleen • Bone (chloroma)	• Most patients are 40-50 years of age; incidence equal in both sexes • Marrow failure-related symptoms common • Bone or joint pain occurs in approximately 10 percent of the patients

REACTIVE COMPONENTS	DIFFERENTIAL DIAGNOSIS
• Not apparently significant	• Myeloproliferative disorders • Leukemoid reaction • Acute lymphocytic leukemia • Acute myelomonocytic leukemia • Leukemic phase, malignant lymphoma • Chronic myelogenous leukemia, blast phase

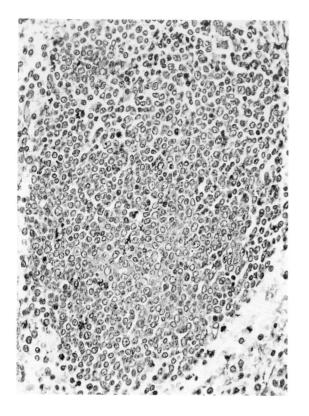

Figure 107
ACUTE MYELOID LEUKEMIA, MARROW PARTICLE
This marrow particle is completely cellular and infiltrated by a massive growth of leukemic cells. PAS. X280.

ACUTE PROMYELOCYTIC LEUKEMIA, FRENCH-AMERICAN-BRITISH CLASSIFICATION M-3

Definition. Acute promyelocytic leukemia is a bone marrow-derived neoplasm composed primarily of differentiated granulocytes at the promyelocytic stage of development.

Clinical Features. Acute promyelocytic leukemia accounts for approximately 5 percent of all the cases of acute myeloid leukemia in the United States. The disease occurs most frequently in the third decade of life, although it has been reported in children as well. Males and females are equally affected. The most common presenting symptom is bleeding, which occurs in approximately 50 percent of the patients. Weakness, fatigue, and infection may also occur. On physical examination, hemorrhages and petechiae are seen and are due to a bleeding diathesis. Splenomegaly is reported in 17 percent of the patients, hepatomegaly in 27 percent, and peripheral lymphadenopathy in 18 percent. The majority of the patients are leukopenic at diagnosis, with median leukocyte counts of 1800/µL (range of 1000-30,000/µL). Approximately 15 percent of the patients present with leukocytosis. The median hemoglobin level is 9.2 g/dL, with a median platelet count of 32,000/µL.

Seventy to 90 percent of the patients have a prolonged prothrombin time when diagnosed. The excessive bleeding seen in acute promyelocytic leukemia is more than that expected from thrombocytopenia alone. Bleeding is presumably secondary to disseminated intravascular coagulation, which is caused by the release of pro coagulant activity from the granular fraction of the promyelocytes. The risk of bleeding from disseminated intravascular coagulation is especially high at the initiation of chemotherapy due to tumor lysis and further release of procoagulant-containing granules. For this reason, most investigators recommend the use of prophylactic heparin therapy (10-20 units/kg) in addition to fresh frozen plasma, cryoprecipitate, and platelets. However, no randomized controlled trial of the efficacy of heparin in this setting has been performed.

A specific chromosomal structural rearrangement (15;17 translocation) has been reported in more than 50 percent of the acute promyelocytic leukemia patients studied.

With combination chemotherapy, including doxorubicin, complete remission may be obtained in approximately 60 percent of the patients. Some studies have indicated a prolonged duration of remission of approximately 2 years, although this finding has not been confirmed in all reports.

A microgranular variant of acute promyelocytic leukemia has been described (Golomb et al.; McKenna et al.) and is distinguished by an initial white blood cell count that is much higher (median of 83,000/mL) and has a shorter duration of complete remission (approximately 6 months). However, the two variants appear similar in all other clinical aspects.

Pathologic Features (Table 52). The marrow is solidly infiltrated by promyelocytes (plate XLVIII-A). In the hypergranular form, these young cells contain numerous large globular granules. Auer rods are numerous and often occur stacked in the cytoplasm (plate XLVIII-B–D). The cells in both types of promyelocytic leukemia are Sudan black and peroxidase positive; PAS reaction shows diffuse positivity, and chloroacetate esterase reaction is positive. Microgranular acute promyelocytic leukemia is often mistaken for monocytic leukemia because of the presence of nuclear folding and unusually small pink granules (plate XLVIII-E–H). Electron microscopy in hypergranular and microgranular cases demonstrates specific granulocytic granules that show the ultrastructural differences in the two types (figs. 108, 109). Microgranular cases often coexpress T cell markers CD2 and CD4, in addition to myeloid-associated markers CD13, 15, and 33.

References

Golomb, H.M., Rowley, J.D., Vardiman, J.W., Testa, J.R., and Butler, A. "Microgranular" acute promyelocytic leukemia. Blood 55:253-259, 1980.

McKenna, R.W., Parkin, J., Bloomfield, C.D., Sundberg, R.D., and Brunning, R.D. Acute promyelocytic leukaemia: a study of 39 cases with identification of a hyperbasophilic microgranular variant. Br. J. Haematol. 50:201-214, 1982.

Additional References

Drapkin, R.L., Gee, T.S., Dowling, M.D., et al. Prophylactic heparin therapy in acute promyelocytic leukemia. Cancer 41:2484-2490, 1978.

Gralnick, H.R. and Tan, H.K. Acute promyelocytic leukemia: a model for understanding the role of the malignant cell in hemostasis. Hum. Pathol. 5:661-673, 1974.

Tomonaga, M., Yoshida, Y., Tagawa, M., et al. Cytochemistry of acute promyelocytic leukemia (M3): leukemic promyelocytes exhibit heterogeneous patterns in cellular differentiation. Blood 66:350-357, 1985.

Table 52

ACUTE PROMYELOCYTIC LEUKEMIA, FRENCH-AMERICAN-BRITISH CLASSIFICATION M-3

PATTERN	
• Marrow — massive, homogeneous infiltration	
CYTOLOGY — NEOPLASTIC	**MARKERS — NEOPLASTIC**

• Most cases show prominent promyelocytic differentiation with large globular granules, numerous stacked Auer rods
 	
• Less common microgranular form has bilobed nuclei, small pink granules, basophilic cytoplasm
	• Cytochemistry: Sudan black, peroxidase, chloroacetate esterase strongly positive; PAS, diffuse positivity
	
	• Flow: HLA-DR (–)
	    CD33, 13, 15 (+)
	    CD2/CD4 (+), particularly microgranular form
	
	• 15;17 translocation in >50 percent of the cases

INVOLVED SITES	**CLINICAL FEATURES**
• Marrow	• A disease of the third decade, but has been described in children; incidence equal in both sexes • Bleeding diathesis 50 percent; leukopenia • Hepatosplenomegaly infrequent
REACTIVE COMPONENTS	**DIFFERENTIAL DIAGNOSIS**
• Not apparently significant	• Leukemoid reaction • Acute myelomonocytic leukemia • Acute monocytic leukemia

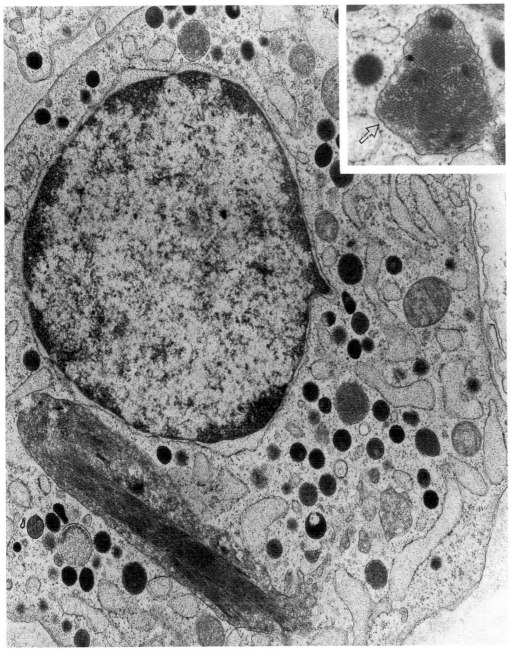

Figure 108
ACUTE PROMYELOCYTIC LEUKEMIA, MARROW
By electron micrography, a leukemic cell contains dilated rough endoplasmic reticulum, numerous electron-dense granules, and a large Auer rod. In cross-section, the Auer rod shows an internal tubular substructure in a hexagonal array (inset, arrow). The center to center distance between the two adjacent tubules is 250 Å. In contrast, the Auer rods seen in other types of acute granulocytic leukemia display an internal laminar periodicity of 60 to 100 Å and lack a tubular substructure. Uranyl acetate, lead citrate. X22,500. Inset X36,000.

PLATE XLVIII

A. ACUTE PROMYELOCYTIC LEUKEMIA, MARROW BIOPSY
A uniform proliferation of leukemic promyelocytes completely replaces this marrow. The cells have moderately irregular nuclear borders and abundant granular eosinophilic cytoplasm. H&E. X1280.

B. ACUTE PROMYELOCYTIC LEUKEMIA, MARROW BIOPSY
Most of these leukemic promyelocytes contain numerous large dark-staining granules that obscure the nuclear border. The nuclei of the promyelocytes with less granulation are irregular and have a monocytoid configuration. Wright's-Giemsa stain. X2000.

C. ACUTE PROMYELOCYTIC LEUKEMIA, HYPERGRANULAR TYPE, MARROW SMEAR
In addition to heavy cytoplasmic granulation, several of these cells contain multiple Auer rods in close approximation and frequently intertwined with one another. Many of the Auer rods have a needle-like configuration. Wright's-Giemsa stain. X2000.

D. ACUTE PROMYELOCYTIC LEUKEMIA, HYPERGRANULAR TYPE, MARROW SMEAR
Several leukemic promyelocytes contain large oval or elliptical inclusions that are Auer-like. Two cells have abundant coarse granules. Most of these cells have markedly irregular nuclear borders. Wright's-Giemsa stain. X2000.

E. ACUTE PROMYELOCYTIC LEUKEMIA, MICROGRANULAR TYPE, BLOOD SMEAR
There is a morphologic spectrum of leukemic cells. In this illustration, most cells show deep nuclear grooves, and the cytoplasm contains small granules. Wright's-Giemsa stain. X2000.

F. ACUTE PROMYELOCYTIC LEUKEMIA, MICROGRANULAR TYPE, MARROW SMEAR
The cells in this illustration exhibit similar cytoplasmic granules with less nuclear irregularity. Two of the leukemic promyelocytes contain multiple Auer rods. Wright's-Giemsa stain. X2000.

G. ACUTE PROMYELOCYTIC LEUKEMIA, BLOOD SMEAR
Cells with hyperchromatic convoluted nuclei and deeply basophilic cytoplasm with few or no visible granules predominate in these blood and marrow smears. Note the cytoplasmic projections on the cell in the center. These cells may resemble micromegakaryocytes. Acute promyelocytic leukemia cases in which these hyperbasophilic promyelocytes predominate are potentially the most difficult to recognize. Wright's-Giemsa stain. X2000.

H. ACUTE PROMYELOCYTIC LEUKEMIA, MARROW SMEAR
After induction chemotherapy, there was an incomplete response to therapy. Although fewer than 5 percent of the promyelocytes remained, occasional cells such as the one shown in the center of this field contained multiple Auer rods. Wright's-Giemsa stain. X2000.

PLATE XLVIII

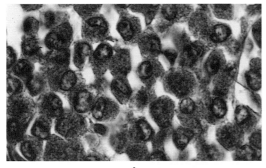

A

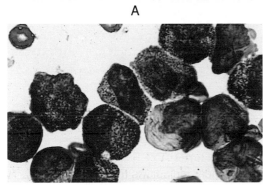

C

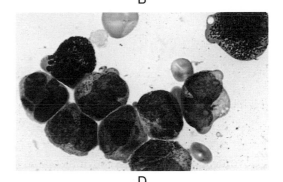

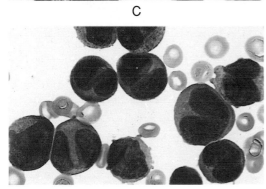

E

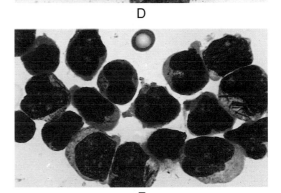

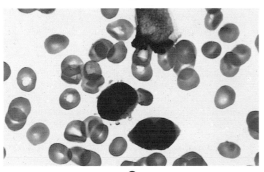

G

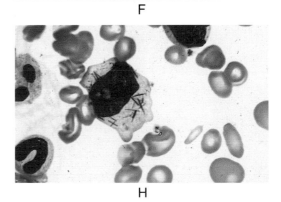

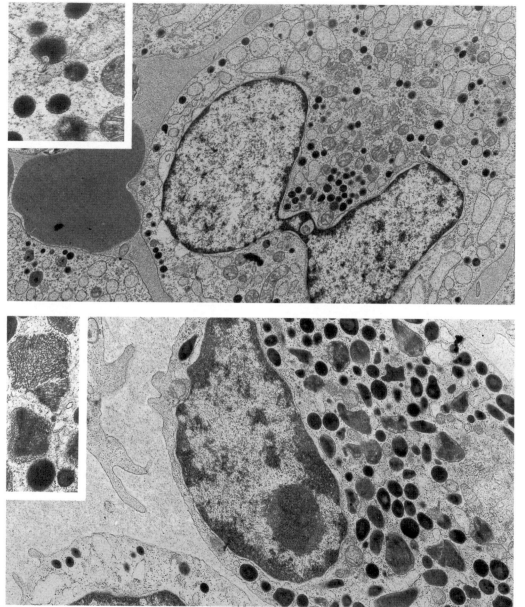

Figure 109
ACUTE PROMYELOCYTIC LEUKEMIA, MARROW

A. This electron micrograph illustrates a typical leukemic cell from a patient with microgranular acute promyelocytic leukemia. The cytoplasm contains numerous small granules, which at higher magnification (inset) contain a uniformly electron-dense amorphous material. The granules in the microgranular leukemic cells range in diameter from 100 to 400 nM, with a mean diameter of 250 nM. Uranyl acetate, lead citrate. X11,625. Inset X30,750. B. This micrograph illustrates a typical leukemic hypergranular promyelocyte. The cytoplasm is filled with large irregularly shaped granules, which at higher magnification (inset) often manifest a tubular substructure similar to that of the acute promyelocyte leukemic Auer rods. The granules in the hypergranular leukemic cells range in diameter from 120 to 1000 nM, with a mean diameter of 470 nM. Uranyl acetate, lead citrate. X11,625. Inset X29,250.

ERYTHROLEUKEMIA, FRENCH-AMERICAN-BRITISH CLASSIFICATION M-6

SYNONYMS AND RELATED TERMS: Di Guglielmo's syndrome; erythremic myelosis.

Definition. Erythroleukemia is a bone marrow-derived neoplasm of hematopoietic stem cells in which abnormal erythroid precursor cells predominate. Many cases of acute myeloid leukemia have an abnormal erythroid component, which often becomes less apparent over time.

Clinical Features. Erythroleukemia is rare in the United States. Males are affected twice as often as females, and the average age of onset is 48 years.

Initial symptoms in this disease relate to bone marrow failure, with anemia and fatigue, granulocytopenia and infection (in 60 percent of the patients), and thrombocytopenia with resultant bleeding (in 34 percent of the patients). Erythroleukemia may also occur as a terminal event of chronic myelogenous leukemia or polycythemia rubra vera. At diagnosis, hepatomegaly is observed in 43 percent of the patients, splenomegaly in 37 percent of the patients, and lymphadenopathy in 26 percent of the patients.

The average hemoglobin level at diagnosis is 7.9 g/dL, with a mean white blood cell count of 18,500/μL, including 12 percent blasts. The mean platelet count has been reported at 91,000/μL.

Complete remission has been achieved in 35 to 60 percent of the reported series, with improved response after the addition of doxorubicin to the chemotherapeutic regimen. Median survival is in the range of 8 to 12 months.

Pathologic Features (Table 53). The marrow and blood show excessive numbers of erythroid precursors (>50 percent) (plate XLIX-A,B) (Dalton and Stass). Abnormal forms with multilobated nuclei or increased nuclear cytoplasmic ratios are seen. These may show granular or diffuse PAS activity (plate XLIX-D,E) and often show diffuse α-naphthyl acetate esterase activity. Megaloblastic changes, nuclear atypia, and ringed sideroblasts may also be seen (plate XLIX-C) (Boros and Bennett). There is usually an associated proliferation of young granulocytic or monocytic cells with dysplasia or maturation arrest. Abnormal megakaryocytes and Auer rods may be present. Electron microscopy demonstrates glycogen clumps in erythroblasts, and ferruginous micelles may be seen in erythroid mitochondria. Erythroleukemia usually changes to a disease indistinguishable from acute myeloid leukemia or acute myelomonocytic leukemia.

References

Boros, L. and Bennett, J.M. The Acute Myeloid Leukemias. In: Leukemias. Goldman, J.M. and Preisler, H.D. (Eds.). London: Butterworths & Company, Ltd., 1984.

Dalton, W., Jr. and Stass, S.A. A Morphological and Cytochemical Approach to the Diagnosis of Acute Leukemia, pp. 27-86. In: The Acute Leukemias. Biologic, Diagnostic and Therapeutic Determinants. Stass, S.A. (Ed.). New York: Marcel Dekker, Inc., 1987.

Additional Reference

Roggli, V.L., Subach, J., and Saleem, A. Prognostic factors and treatment effects on survival in erythroleukemia: a retrospective study of 134 cases. Cancer 48:1101-1105, 1981.

PLATE XLIX
ERYTHROLEUKEMIA

A. MARROW PARTICLE

Marrow particle preparations are usually densely cellular in patients with erythroleukemia. This medium magnification photograph shows the more mature erythroid elements with deeply basophilic nuclei and pale cytoplasm in a mixture of hematopoietic cells. Contrast this with the homogeneity usually seen in other kinds of leukemia. PAS. X260.

B. MARROW SMEAR

In this illustration, a binucleated erythroblast and more differentiated erythroid elements are seen. Wright's stain. X520.

C. MARROW PARTICLE

Numerous ringed sideroblasts are present and are almost universally detected in erythroleukemia. Iron stain. X360.

D. MARROW SMEAR

This characteristic stippled positivity is usually demonstrated in immature erythroid elements. PAS. X800. (Fig. 17 from Glick, A.D., Paniker, K., Flexner, J.M., et al. Acute leukemia of adults. Am. J. Clin. Pathol. 73:459-470, 1980.)

E. MARROW SMEAR

Positivity in a globular fashion is noted in a differentiated erythroid cell. PAS. X360.

PLATE XLIX

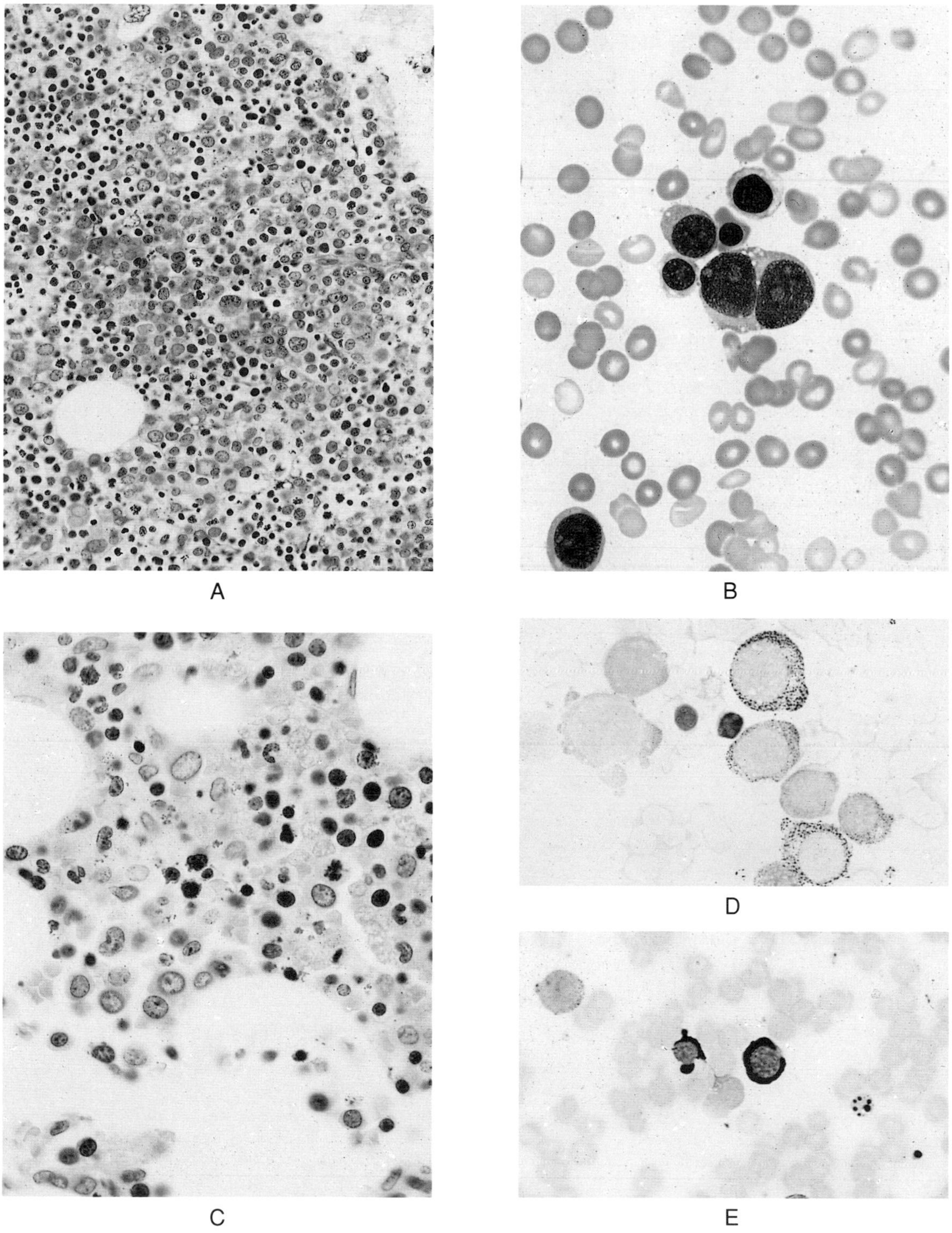

A

B

C

D

E

Table 53

ERYTHROLEUKEMIA,
FRENCH-AMERICAN-BRITISH CLASSIFICATION M-6

PATTERN	
• Marrow — massive, diffuse infiltration with heterogeneous appearance due to mixture of mature and immature erythroids with myeloid component	
CYTOLOGY — NEOPLASTIC	**MARKERS — NEOPLASTIC**
• Erythroid elements show capacity to differentiate, and myeloid elements will be present; megaloblastic changes, multilobation, binucleation usually seen in erythroids; Auer rods often present • Commonly evolves to acute myeloid or myelomonocytic leukemia	• Cytochemistry: Globular, granular, or diffuse PAS (+); immature cells often show globular (+); myeloid component of leukemia Sudan black, peroxidase (+) • Ringed sideroblasts always present
INVOLVED SITES	**CLINICAL FEATURES**
• Marrow	• Patients are usually 40-50 years of age; greater incidence in males • Marrow failure at presentation • May occur as terminal event in chronic myelogenous leukemia or polycythemia rubra vera
REACTIVE COMPONENTS	**DIFFERENTIAL DIAGNOSIS**
• Not apparently significant	• Acute myelomonocytic leukemia • Megaloblastic anemia

CHRONIC MYELOGENOUS LEUKEMIA

SYNONYMS AND RELATED TERMS: Chronic granulocytic leukemia; chronic panmyelosis.

Definition. Chronic myelogenous leukemia is a bone marrow-derived neoplasm composed principally of granulocytic cells in various stages of maturation. The cell of origin is a pluripotential stem cell that can differentiate into myeloid, mononuclear phagocytic or lymphoid cells (Fialkow et al.). For pathologic details, see Plate L and figures 110-118.

Clinical Features. Chronic myelogenous leukemia accounts for approximately 20 percent of all of the cases of leukemia in the United States and western Europe. Males are affected slightly more frequently than females. The disease is seen most commonly in the fourth decade, although the age range is wide. Some cases of chronic myelogenous leukemia are reported in children, but these are usually Philadelphia chromosome negative and may be a different disease.

The usual symptoms include fatigue, malaise, aching extremities, and fullness or discomfort in the left upper quadrant associated with splenomegaly. Fever, weight loss, and sweats may also be seen. Acute gouty arthritis, peripheral vascular insufficiency, and priapism may occur. On occasion, chronic myelogenous leukemia may be diagnosed in asymptomatic individuals following routine blood tests.

Splenomegaly, which is often massive, is found in the vast majority of the patients and is an expected occurrence at some time during the disease. Hepatomegaly is usually detected simultaneously with the onset of splenomegaly; lymphadenopathy is rare. Bone tenderness may be pronounced, and bleeding diathesis may be apparent with ecchymoses or bleeding from the mucous membranes.

Anemia is expected in all of the patients; the hemoglobin level is in the range of 9 to 12 g/dL. The platelet count may be quite variable, ranging from 25,000 to over 1,000,000/μL. The white blood cell count is elevated in all of the patients, ranging from 50,000 to 250,000/μL. All stages of myelocytes are seen in the peripheral blood. Approximately 90 percent of the patients have the Philadelphia chromosome, which most commonly consists of a translocation between chromosome 9 and 22. Other laboratory abnormalities include an elevation of serum uric acid, lactic dehydrogenase, and serum B_{12} levels. The leukocyte alkaline phosphatase is quite low.

With intermittent busulfan, hydroxyurea, or other oral chemotherapy, 80 to 90 percent of the patients will experience an improvement in all of the disease parameters and a return to a state of well-being. The Philadelphia chromosome is not eradicated by this therapy nor is the ultimate progression of disease altered. After approximately 1 to 4 years, patients are likely to develop increasing splenomegaly, bone marrow failure, fever, sweats, and weight loss. Chromosomal abnormalities in addition to the Philadelphia chromosome are often found at this time. The leukocyte alkaline phosphatase may become elevated, and the differential count in the marrow and peripheral blood shifts to a predominance of early myeloid precursors. This acute exacerbation, which occurs in 70 to 80 percent of the patients, most often resembles acute myeloid leukemia. However, the development of erythroleukemia, refractory anemia, red blood cell aplasia, and myelofibrosis have also been described. With further therapy for acute leukemia, survival is usually less than 6 months. Approximately 25 percent of the patients may develop an acute transformation that resembles acute lymphocytic leukemia with elevation of terminal deoxynucleotidyl transferase levels. These patients may respond to vincristine and prednisone, although survival is only approximately 1 year after this transformation.

Factors associated with a poorer prognosis at the time of diagnosis in chronic myelogenous leukemia include the absence of the Philadelphia chromosome, the presence of palpable splenomegaly, and bone marrow myeloblasts in excess of 5 percent. Patients in their sixties with processes resembling chronic myelogenous leukemia usually are Philadelphia chromosome negative and may relate to a myeloproliferative group of disorders.

Pathologic Features (Table 54). The most important diagnostic specimen in chronic myelogenous leukemia is the peripheral blood smear that shows marked neutrophilic leukocytosis, basophilia, and eosinophilia. The neutrophil series is represented by all stages of development from the myeloblast to the segmented neutrophil (plate L-A,B). The most numerous cells are myelocytes and segmented neutrophils, whereas myeloblasts do not generally exceed 2 percent of the total leukocytes. A variety of developmental abnormalities of the neutrophils may be noted, including hypogranulation, hyposegmentation, hypersegmentation, and abnormally small neutrophils. Mature and immature basophils (plate L-C) and eosinophils are commonly present. The platelets may be markedly increased in number and may be present in large clumps.

Marrow smears are very cellular due to an increase in neutrophils and precursors.

The percentages of promyelocytes and myelocytes is usually greater than in the peripheral blood. Myeloblasts do not usually exceed 2 to 3 percent, and the percentage of basophils and eosinophils may be less than in the peripheral blood. Megakaryocytes are generally abundant and may be markedly increased. Pseudo-Gaucher cells are found in the bone marrow smears in approximately 35 percent of the cases. In Romanowsky-stained smears, the cytoplasmic contents of these cells have a somewhat variable appearance, ranging from blue-pigmented globular and fibrillar accumulations to clear cord-like fibrillar inclusions.

Marrow biopsy sections are markedly hypercellular (fig. 110), although a few patients may have residual fatty tissue. Hypercellularity is principally due to an increase in all stages of granulocytes (fig. 111). When megakaryocytes are increased, they may occur in clusters and vary considerably in size (fig. 112).

Myelofibrosis is usually a late manifestation of chronic myelogenous leukemia but may occur at any stage of the disease. An increase in reticulin fibers has been reported in a relatively high percentage of the patients in the early stages (fig. 113). The fibrosis may initially be diffuse or focal, but the focal lesions progress to a diffuse pattern. There appears to be a progressive increase in the reticulin fibers with duration of the disease. The rapidity with which this occurs varies considerably from patient to patient. Collagen fibrosis may occur but is uncommon.

Infrequently, the evolution of the disease process in patients with Philadelphia chromosome positive chronic myelogenous leukemia is marked by the development of frank osteosclerosis. In these

Table 54

CHRONIC MYELOGENOUS LEUKEMIA

PATTERN
• Diffuse involvement of marrow • Involves red pulp in spleen, paracortical area of nodes • Blast transformation recognizable as nodules of immature cells

CYTOLOGY — NEOPLASTIC	MARKERS — NEOPLASTIC
• Full range of myeloid differentiation • Blast transformation — blasts may resemble myeloid or lymphoid cells	• Sudan black positive blasts and maturing cells; in blast transformation, blasts may show myeloid, monocytic, or lymphoid features • Philadelphia chromosome present in approximately 95 percent of cases. Breakpoint cluster region demonstrable by molecular genetics in 50 percent of Ph^1 (–) cases and useful in recognizing relapses

INVOLVED SITES	CLINICAL FEATURES
• Marrow • Spleen, nodes, soft tissue, skin in blast transformation; blast transformation may occur in these sites before it is demonstrable in marrow	• Indolent disease with leukocytosis and splenomegaly • Blast transformation occurs in 40 percent of the cases; may be manifested initially as lymphadenopathy, increasing splenomegaly, soft tissue infiltrates

REACTIVE COMPONENTS	DIFFERENTIAL DIAGNOSIS
• Scattered normal hematopoietic cells • Macrophages containing PAS positive material (pseudo-Gaucher cells)	• Leukemoid reaction • Chronic myelomonocytic leukemia • Chronic neutrophilic leukemia • Acute myeloid leukemia

PLATE L

A. CHRONIC MYELOGENOUS LEUKEMIA, PERIPHERAL BLOOD
(Plate L-A and B are from the same patient)

This 37 year old female had a history of abdominal fullness, and an enlarged spleen was noted. The hemoglobin was 11.2 g/dL, the leukocyte count was 112,000/μL, and the platelet count was 310,000/μL. The blood smear is characteristic of the chronic phase of chronic myelogenous leukemia. There is a continuous spectrum of neutrophil development from myeloblasts to segmented neutrophils, and several basophils are present. Wright's-Giemsa stain. X1200.

B. CHRONIC MYELOGENOUS LEUKEMIA, PERIPHERAL BLOOD
At a higher magnification, there is a myeloblast, a promyelocyte, metamyelocytes, and a segmented neutrophil. Two basophils and an eosinophil are also present. Platelets are abundant. Wright's-Giemsa stain. X2000.

C. CHRONIC MYELOGENOUS LEUKEMIA WITH BASOPHILIA, PERIPHERAL BLOOD
This patient, with a 32 month history of chronic myelogenous leukemia, had increasing fatigue and decreasing hemoglobin. The leukocyte count was 29,000/μL, and 69 percent of the leukocytes were basophils. Wright's-Giemsa stain. X2000.

D. CHRONIC MYELOGENOUS LEUKEMIA, ACCELERATED PHASE AND BASOPHILIA, PERIPHERAL BLOOD
This patient had a 29 month history of chronic myelogenous leukemia. Recently, he had developed increasing splenomegaly, decreasing hemoglobin, and increasing platelet count. The peripheral blood smear shows an increased number of immature neutrophils and an increased percentage of basophils. Two myeloblasts are present. Wright's-Giemsa stain. X2000.

E. CHRONIC MYELOGENOUS LEUKEMIA, BLAST CRISIS, BONE MARROW
Some of the blasts in this patient with myeloid blast crisis have prominent nucleoli. There is evidence of maturation of the leukemic blasts to promyelocytes. Wright's-Giemsa stain. X1200.

F. CHRONIC MYELOGENOUS LEUKEMIA, MEGAKARYOBLASTIC CRISIS, BONE MARROW
This marrow smear from a patient in megakaryoblastic crisis contains blasts with a slightly condensed nuclear chromatin and relatively indistinct nucleoli. Wright's-Giemsa stain. X2000.

G. CHRONIC MYELOGENOUS LEUKEMIA, LYMPHOID BLAST TRANSFORMATION, BONE MARROW
The blasts from this marrow reacted with the antibody to CD10 (CALLA) and contained intracytoplasmic μ-heavy chain (not shown), a characteristic of pre-B cells. Wright's-Giemsa stain. X1000.

H. CHRONIC MYELOGENOUS LEUKEMIA, LYMPHOID BLAST TRANSFORMATION, BONE MARROW
In another example of lymphoid blast transformation, the blasts contain numerous cytoplasmic vacuoles and resemble lymphoblasts of the L3 type. The blasts were TdT positive and reacted with antibody to CD10 (CALLA) (not shown). Wright's-Giemsa stain. X1000.

PLATE L

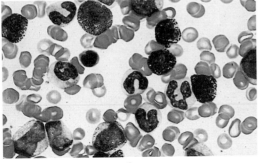

A

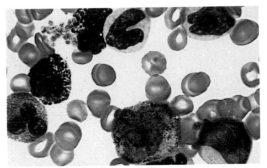

B

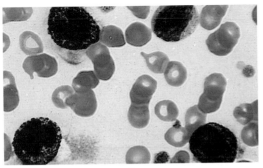

C

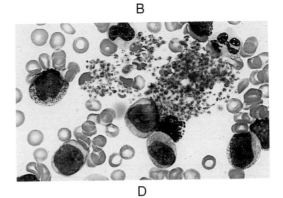

D

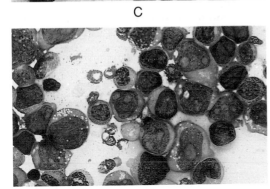

E

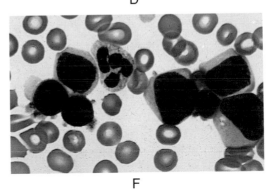

F

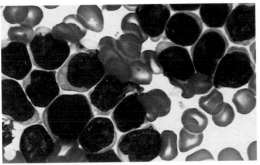

G

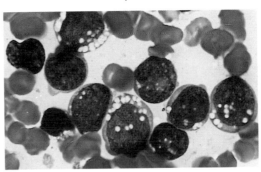

H

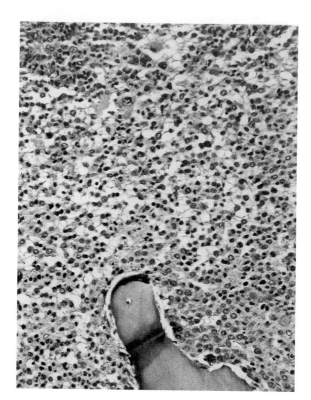

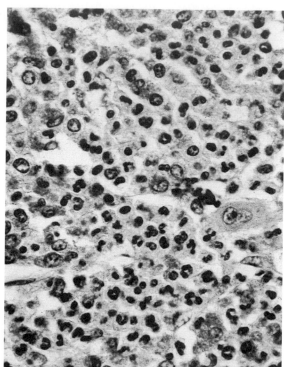

Figure 110
(Figures 110 and 111 are from the same patient)
CHRONIC MYELOGENOUS LEUKEMIA,
MARROW BIOPSY
The marrow is markedly hypercellular in this recently diagnosed patient. H&E. X90.

Figure 111
CHRONIC MYELOGENOUS LEUKEMIA,
MARROW BIOPSY
A higher magnification of the specimen reveals mostly segmented granulocytes. H&E. X350.

instances, the marrow may be virtually indistinguishable from that seen during advanced stages of agnogenic myeloid metaplasia (fig. 114).

Variants. Eosinophilic (Marinone et al.) and basophilic (Parkin et al.) variants of chronic myelogenous leukemia have been reported. These cases are usually accompanied by an increase of neutrophils in all stages of development and therefore should be viewed as examples of chronic myelogenous leukemia with marked eosinophilia or basophilia. The Philadelphia chromosome has been detected in the hematopoietic cells of some of these patients.

Blast Transformation of Chronic Myelogenous Leukemia

Transformation of chronic myelogenous leukemia, clinically and morphologically, may occur in a subacute form or overt blast crisis. The subacute type of transformation is marked by clinical and hematologic deterioration, but the blasts do not replace the marrow and remain in the minority. This type of evolution is characterized by several possible hematologic alterations, including increasing basophilia (plate L-D), myelofibrosis, marked eosinophilia, and progressive abnormalities of

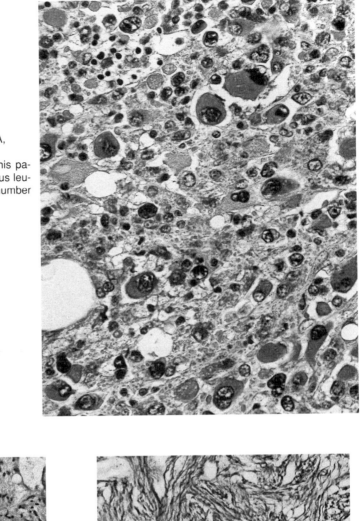

Figure 112
CHRONIC MYELOGENOUS LEUKEMIA,
MARROW BIOPSY
The marrow is markedly hypercellular in this patient with newly diagnosed chronic myelogenous leukemia. The megakaryocytes are increased in number and are dysplastic. H&E. X400.

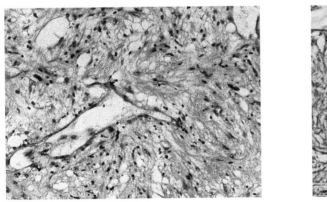

A

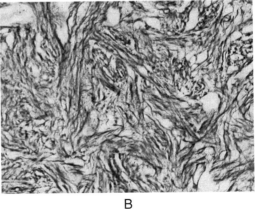

B

Figure 113
CHRONIC MYELOGENOUS LEUKEMIA, MARROW BIOPSY
A. The marrow space is almost completely replaced by dense fibrous connective tissue in this 61 year old male with a 42 month history of chronic myelogenous leukemia. The hematologic values included a hemoglobin of 13.9 g/dL, a white blood cell count of 83,000/μL, and a platelet count of 48,000/μL. H&E. X100. B. There is a marked increase in dense reticulin fibers that form a pattern of intertwining bundles. Wilder's reticulin stain. X250.

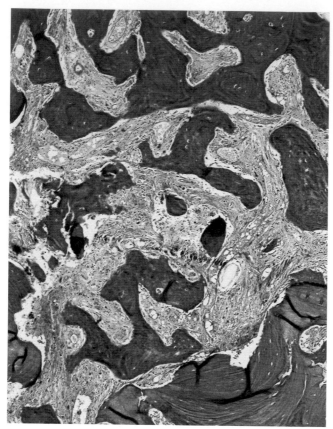

Figure 114
CHRONIC MYELOGENOUS LEUKEMIA,
MARROW BIOPSY
This biopsy shows extensive osteosclerosis in a
29 year old female with a 9 month history of chronic
myelogenous leukemia. She had recently manifested
progressive anemia, thrombocytopenia, and increasing basophilia. X100.

neutrophil, megakaryocyte, and erythroid development.

Blast crisis is characterized by a preponderance of blasts (usually more than 30 percent in blood/marrow smears) and has the clinical and hematologic features of acute leukemia. Blast crisis may be classified as myeloid or lymphoid based on the cytologic, cytochemical, biochemical, and immunologic characteristics of the leukemic cells. In approximately 65 percent of the cases of blast transformation, the differentiation pattern is myeloid; in the remaining 35 percent, the pattern is lymphoid.

In the most common type of myeloid blast crisis, the blasts have the cytologic and cytochemical features of the blasts in acute myeloblastic leukemia (plate L-E). Auer rods may be found but are less common than in de novo acute myeloblastic leukemia. Less frequently, the proliferating blasts in myeloid blast crisis have the features of megakaryoblasts, erythroblasts, or monoblasts. The megakaryocytic variant may be recognized by the evidence of differentiation of the blasts to micromegakaryocytes (plate L-F). In some instances, the blasts may show no evidence of differentiation. The evidence of megakaryoblastic differentiation in these cases is based on the ultrastructural demonstration of platelet peroxidase (fig. 115). In most lymphoid blast crises, the leukemic cells

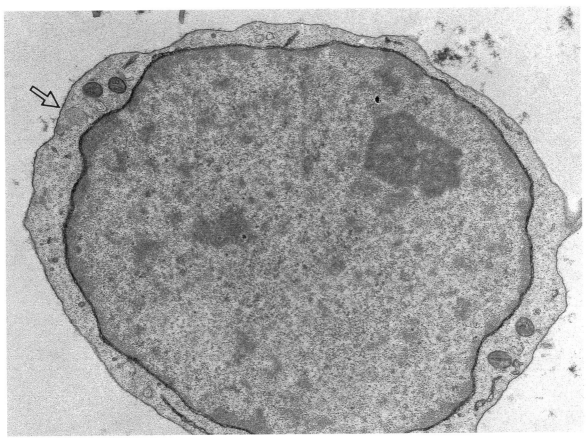

Figure 115
CHRONIC MYELOGENOUS LEUKEMIA, MEGAKARYOBLASTIC CRISIS,
PLATELET PEROXIDASE PREPARATION

A leukemic cell from a patient in blast crisis was reacted for platelet peroxidase and contains a dense reaction product in the cisterna of the nuclear envelope and rough endoplasmic reticulum. A cytoplasmic granule (arrow) is platelet peroxidase negative. These ultracytochemical results are diagnostic of a megakaryoblast. Lead citrate. X15,000.

have the morphologic features of lympho-blasts (plate L-G,H), as observed in the L1 and L2 types of acute lymphocytic leukemia.

In a few cases of chronic myelogenous leukemia in transformation, the blast crisis occurs as focal lesions in the bone marrow (figs. 116, 117) or in an extramedullary site (fig. 118). Extramedullary blast trans-formation may occur in several sites, including the spleen and lymph nodes, where it may precede evidence of blast transformation in the marrow by several months. The blasts in the extramedullary focus may have myeloid or lymphoid characteristics. Cytogenetic studies of these blasts frequently show clonal chromosome evolution.

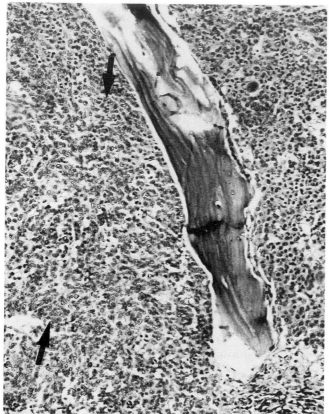

Figure 116
(Figures 116 and 117 are from the same patient)
CHRONIC MYELOGENOUS LEUKEMIA,
FOCAL BLAST CRISIS, BIOPSY
This 42 year old male presented with splenomegaly, a leukocyte count of 68,000/µL, and focal blast transformation. The peripheral blood smear findings were diagnostic of chronic phase of chronic myelogenous leukemia. The bone marrow aspirate contained 3 percent lymphoid-appearing blast cells. The bone trabeculum is bordered on one side (arrow) by a focus of blasts (see fig. 117). H&E. X100.

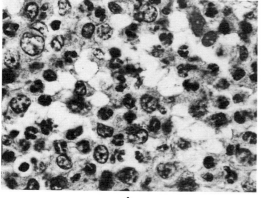

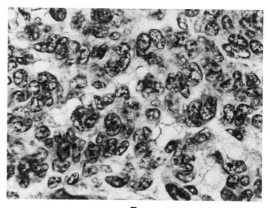

A

B

Figure 117
CHRONIC MYELOGENOUS LEUKEMIA, FOCAL BLAST CRISIS, MARROW
A. At a higher magnification, most of this marrow shows the usual maturation to neutrophils seen in the chronic phase of chronic myelogenous leukemia. X400. B. The marrow bordering the other aspect of the bony trabeculum is completely replaced by blast cells. H&E. X400.

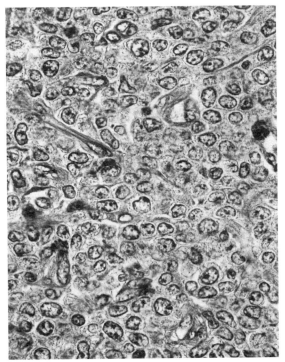

Figure 118
CHRONIC MYELOGENOUS LEUKEMIA,
EXTRAMEDULLARY BLAST CRISIS, LYMPH NODE
A 22 year old male with a 14 month history of chronic myelogenous leukemia developed an extramedullary blast crisis that manifested as lymphadenopathy. The bone marrow aspirate contained 3 percent myeloblasts, and the marrow cells contained the Philadelphia chromosome. The lymph node architecture was totally effaced by an infiltration of blast forms that do not have differentiating features. Chromosome analysis of the lymph node tissue reveals an additional Philadelphia chromosomal abnormality in the blasts. X400.

Philadelphia Chromosome Negative Chronic Myelogenous Leukemia

In approximately 5 to 10 percent of the cases of chronic myelogenous leukemia, the Philadelphia chromosome will not be found. The blood from some of these patients shows a higher percentage of blasts and monocytoid cells and a more severe degree of thrombocytopenia than blood from Philadelphia chromosome positive patients. At least 50 percent of these patients have the genetic abnormalities of chronic myelogenous leukemia, as shown by genetic analysis of the breakpoint cluster region.

Chronic Myelogenous Leukemia in Childhood

Chronic myelogenous leukemia occurs in children but comprises less than 5 percent of the cases of leukemia in this age group. It occurs in two forms: adult and juvenile. The adult type is Philadelphia chromosome positive and is characterized by all of the clinical and hematologic features of adult chronic myelogenous leukemia described above. The juvenile form occurs in a somewhat younger age group and lacks the Philadelphia chromosome. An important diagnostic feature of the juvenile type is a high level of fetal hemoglobin, usually ranging from 40 to 50 percent. Other laboratory findings characteristic of the juvenile type include decreased levels of hemoglobin A_2, reduced erythrocyte carbonic anhydrase, decreased titer of I antigen, and displacement of the oxygen dissociation curve to the left. The juvenile form of chronic myelogenous leukemia is marked by a more rapid clinical course than the adult type.

References

Fialkow, P.J., Jacobson, R.J., and Papayannopoulou, T. Chronic myelocytic leukemia: clonal origin in a stem cell common to the granulocyte, erythrocyte, platelet and monocyte/macrophage. Am. J. Med. 63:125-130, 1977.

Marinone, G., Rossi, G., and Verzura, P. Eosinophilic blast crisis in a case of chronic myeloid leukaemia. Br. J. Haematol. 55:251-256, 1983.

Parkin, J.L., McKenna, R.W., and Brunning, R.D. Philadelphia chromosome-positive blastic leukaemia. Br. J. Haematol. 52:663-677, 1982.

Additional References

Boggs, D.R. Editorial: hematopoietic stem cell theory in relation to possible lymphoblastic conversion of chronic myeloid leukemia. Blood 44:449-453, 1974.

Cervantes, F. and Rozman, C. A multivariate analysis of prognostic factors in chronic myeloid leukemia. Blood 60:1298-1304, 1982.

Ezdinli, E.Z., Sokal, J.E., Crosswhite, L., and Sandberg, A.A. Philadelphia-chromosome-positive and -negative chronic myelocytic leukemia. Ann. Intern. Med. 72:175-182, 1970.

Goldman, J.M. and Lu, D. New approaches in chronic granulocytic leukemia. Semin. Hematol. 19:241-256, 1982.

Kardinal, C.G., Batemen, J.R., and Weiner, J. Chronic granulocytic leukemia. Arch. Intern. Med. 136:305-313, 1976.

Peterson, L.C., Bloomfield, C.D., and Brunning, R.D. Blast crisis as an initial or terminal manifestation of chronic myeloid leukemia. Am. J. Med 60:209-220, 1976.

Rosenthal, S., Canellos, G.P., Whang-Peng, J., and Gralnick, H.R. Blast crisis of chronic granulocytic leukemia. Am. J. Med. 63:542-547, 1977.

Shaw, M.T., Bottomley, R.H., Grozea, P.N., and Nordquist, R.E. Heterogeneity of morphological, cytochemical and cytogenetic features in the blastic phase of chronic granulocytic leukemia. Cancer 35:199-207, 1975.

GRANULOCYTIC SARCOMA

SYNONYMS AND RELATED TERMS: Chloroma.

Definition. Granulocytic sarcomas presumably arise in the peripheral tissue from precursor cells that are able to differentiate into granulocytic elements; ultimately, there is spread to the marrow. The peripheral lesions are similar in appearance, whether the patients have an underlying marrow neoplasm or develop a peripheral granulocytic process de novo. The term chloroma reflects the evanescent light-green tinge to the cut surface of the mass.

Clinical Features. Granulocytic sarcoma is a rare tumor. Males and females are equally affected. Although traditionally thought to be more common in children or young adults, recent series have reported a mean age of onset of 48 years, with a range of 2 to 81 years.

Approximately 50 percent of the case reports are in patients with known myeloproliferative syndromes, including chronic myelogenous leukemia, polycythemia rubra vera, and hypereosinophilic syndrome. Most of these cases are associated with the onset of blast crisis of the myeloproliferative syndrome. Another 30 percent of patients have no known underlying disease at the time granulocytic sarcoma is diagnosed. Ninety percent of these patients will develop acute leukemia 1 to 49 months later (mean of 10 months). The remaining 20 percent of the patients have known acute myeloid leukemia at the time of onset of the granulocytic sarcoma.

The majority of granulocytic tumors occur in the subperiosteal region of the bone, most commonly in the skull, sternum, ribs, or proximal portions of long bones. The tumor is thought to arise in the marrow and traverse the Haversian canal to reach the subperiosteum. Tumor collections may occur in soft tissue areas as well, most commonly in the head and neck region. Other sites affected are the lymph nodes, skin, and gastrointestinal and reproductive tracts.

The course and prognosis of granulocytic sarcoma are similar to those of the underlying acute myeloid leukemia. In patients who have a negative bone marrow, overt acute myeloid leukemia will usually develop, sometimes after several years. The localized tumor is radiosensitive, although local radiation will not alter the natural expected evolution to acute leukemia.

Pathologic Features. Granulocytic sarcomas are characteristically greenish in the gross specimen. This color fades on exposure to air and is due to the presence of myeloperoxidase.

In approximately 35 percent of these cases, there is overt granulocytic differentiation, and eosinophilic myelocytes or megakaroycytic elements are detected (fig. 119). The remainder may be very difficult to recognize on histopathologic sections alone (Neiman et al.). A diffuse infiltrative growth pattern with interspersed macrophages may produce a picture similar to Burkitt's lymphoma. Neoplastic cells are of medium size, with slightly eccentric nuclei, usually single central nucleoli, and a small amount of pale cytoplasm.

Chloroacetate esterase, paraffin immunoperoxidase with Leu-M1, cytochemistry on smears and tissue, or electron microscopy are required for diagnosis in these difficult cases. These techniques are particularly useful when the suspected diagnosis of granulocytic neoplasm is followed by a negative bone marrow.

Reference

Neiman, R.S., Barcos, M., Berard, C., et al. Granulocytic sarcoma: a clinicopathologic study of 61 biopsied cases. Cancer 48:1426-1437, 1981.

Additional References

Muss, H.B. and Moloney, W.C. Chloroma and other myeloblastic tumors. Blood 42:721-728, 1973.
Wiernik, H. and Serpick, A.A. Granulocytic sarcoma (chloroma). Blood 35:361-369, 1970.

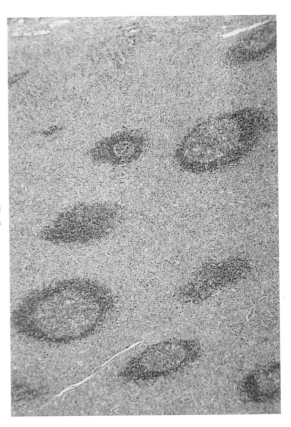

Figure 119
MYELOID LEUKEMIA, LYMPH NODE
This low magnification photomicrograph shows the typical patterns of leukemic involvement, with sheets of tumor cells isolating follicular centers and islands of residual lymphocytes.

MASTOCYTOSIS

Definition. Mastocytosis is a local or systemic proliferation of mast cells. Clearly malignant forms may occur either as localized tumors (mast cell sarcoma) or malignant systemic mastocytosis with leukemia. The cell of origin is probably a hematopoietic stem cell in the systemic form.

Clinical Features. Mastocytosis may be divided into benign and malignant categories. In the benign form, clinical symptoms and signs may either be limited to the skin or reflect systemic mast cell disease. Malignant mastocytosis is extremely rare; it may occur de novo or develop in the course of benign mast cell disease.

Cutaneous mastocytosis (urticaria pigmentosa) usually occurs in childhood and spontaneously disappears in most patients by the age of 20. When the disease begins later in life, it is less likely to undergo spontaneous remission. The skin lesions are small, multiple, red-brown hyperpigmented macules and, occasionally, papules, which are most often scattered about the trunk. Although they may occur anywhere, the palms, soles, and mucous membranes are usually spared. The lesions are often pruritic, especially after a warm shower. Flushing of the skin may occur, especially after local trauma. Darier's sign (urticaria after trauma) and dermatographism (whealing on uninvolved skin) may be seen.

Benign systemic mastocytosis occurs most often in adult males. Although many organ systems may be involved, approximately 50 percent of the patients with proven disease have no symptoms, an additional 30 percent have very minor symptoms, and less than 15 percent have major symptoms or signs of disease. Bone involvement occurs in 10 to 40 percent of the cases. The pelvis, ribs, vertebrae, skull, and long bones are most commonly affected. The lesions may be discrete or generalized, with osteosclerosis or osteoporosis observed on x-ray. Nonspecific deep aching bone pain may result. Patients may have upper abdominal pain from gastritis or peptic ulcer disease, and diarrhea may also occur. These symptoms are due to the release of histamine from mast cells. The resultant increase in gastric acid production causes ulcer disease, and inactivation of pancreatic lipase may produce malabsorption and diarrhea. Liver involvement may be manifest by hepatomegaly or elevated alkaline phosphatase. Liver failure is rare. Splenomegaly and flushing after abdominal trauma are the results of splenic involvement. A rare, pure splenic variety of the disease has been described in which all of the symptoms and signs disappeared after splenectomy.

Neuropsychiatric problems are encountered in approximately 12 percent of the patients. These symptoms include a decreased attention span, fatigue, malaise, and personality changes. The etiology of these symptoms is unknown. Systemic symptoms of mast cell disease may also occur, consisting of pruritus, flushing, tachycardia, and syncope. All of the symptoms and signs of systemic mast cell disease may be potentiated by agents that cause degranulation of mast cells, such as aspirin, codeine, alcohol, and vinca alkaloids. Antihistamines have been used to treat various manifestations of the disease. Cimetidine has recently been reported as beneficial in the amelioration of gastrointestinal symptomatology. In addition, sodium cromoglycate given orally has produced significant improvement in the pruritus, flushing, diarrhea, abdominal pain, and disorders of cognitive function that may occur.

Approximately 15 percent of the patients with systemic mastocytosis may experience an evolution to malignant disease (Brunning et al.). Malignant mastocytosis rarely occurs in children; most patients are adult males in the sixth and seventh decades. Skin lesions are rare. Anemia and eosinophilia are expected in the majority. No effective therapy is yet known, and survival is short. The majority of the patients die within 1 year of the time of diagnosis.

Pathologic Features (Table 55). Benign mastocytosis may take the form of mastocytoma, cutaneous mastocytosis, or benign systemic mastocytosis. Mature mast cells are noted in all three types, with typical cytochemical reactions. The marrow in benign systemic mastocytosis becomes fibrotic (plate LI-A,B) and shows either thickened bony trabeculae (plate LI-C) or osteoporosis. Splenic infiltrates are usually perivascular (plate LI-D) or peritrabecular. Nodal involvement may be distinctive due to interfollicular localization of the infiltrate (fig. 120).

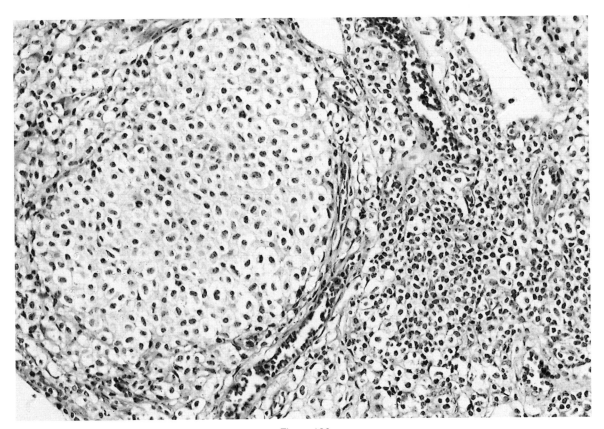

Figure 120
MASTOCYTOSIS, LYMPH NODE
In this figure, the lymph node is distorted by a nodular proliferation of pale cytoplasmic cells in the cortex of the lymph node. This is the typical pattern of nodal involvement in mastocytosis. X180.

Table 55

MASTOCYTOSIS

PATTERN
• Skin — dermal nodules • Marrow — diffuse infiltrate of fibro-eosinophilic nodules • Node — cortical infiltration often surrounding follicular centers • Spleen — perivascular infiltrates

CYTOLOGY — NEOPLASTIC	MARKERS — NEOPLASTIC
• Bland-appearing cells; folded nuclei, abundant cytoplasm • Malignant types may have hypogranular cells, with mast cell feature apparent only by electron microscopy	• Cytochemistry: Napthol-AS-D chloroacetate esterase markedly (+); granules metachromatic with Giemsa and toluidine blue (in malignant mastocytosis, toluidine blue (+) reaction is maximal at pH 5.0 to 6.0, in contrast to benign types)

INVOLVED SITES	CLINICAL FEATURES
• Skin • Marrow, infrequent bone lesions • Nodes • Spleen	• Cutaneous mastocytosis: Multiple red-brown hyperpigmented macules that show whealing reaction after trauma • Systemic mastocytosis: Most common in adult males; may be asymptomatic or have pruritus, flushing, tachycardia, and syncope; bone lesions occur in 10-40 percent of the cases • Rare progression to malignant disease

REACTIVE COMPONENTS	DIFFERENTIAL DIAGNOSIS
• Eosinophils prominent • Reactive fibroblasts	• Hairy cell leukemia

Rarely, malignant mastocytosis may be localized as tumor masses in soft tissue or spleen. Most patients have a systemic proliferation of immature cells. The organs chiefly affected are the marrow, spleen, liver, and nodes. Connective tissue deposition often accompanies the infiltration (Lennert and Parwaresch). The neoplastic mast cells may show various dysplastic features; chief among these is the hypogranulation in the most immature cells. Electron microscopy is required for confirmation in benign or malignant mastocytosis if cytochemical reactions are equivocal (figs. 121, 122).

References

Brunning, R.D., McKenna, R.W., Rosai, J., Parkin, J.L., and Risdall, R. Systemic mastocytosis. Extracutaneous manifestations. Am. J. Surg. Pathol. 7:425-438, 1983.

Lennert, K. and Parwaresch, M.R. Mast cells and mast cell neoplasia. Histopathology 3:349-365, 1979.

Additional References

Demis, D.J. The mastocytosis syndrome. Ann. Intern. Med. 59:194-206, 1963.

Hirschowitz, B.I. and Groarke, J.F. Effect of cimetidine on gastric hypersecretion and diarrhea in systemic mastocytosis. Ann. Intern. Med. 90:769-771, 1979.

Roberts, L.J., Jr. and Oates, J.A. Disorders of Vasodilator Hormones: The Carcinoid Syndrome and Mastocytosis, pp. 1363-1378. In: Williams Textbook of Endocrinology, 7th ed. Williams, R.H., et al. (Eds.). Philadelphia: W.B. Saunders Company, 1985.

Soter, N.A., Austen, K.F., and Wasserman, S.I. Oral disodium cromoglycate in the treatment of systemic mastocytosis. N. Engl. J. Med. 301:465-469, 1979.

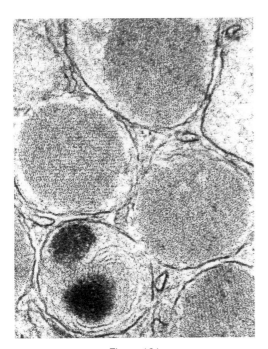

Figure 121
MASTOCYTOSIS, MARROW
Some mast cell granules on electron microscopy have a lower-density lattice-like matrix. X102,900.

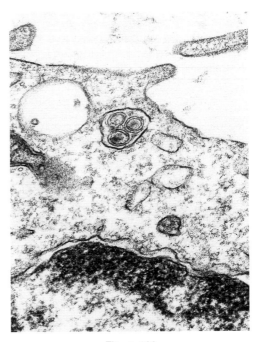

Figure 122
MASTOCYTOSIS, MARROW
This figure demonstrates the electron microscopy of mast cells from a patient with mastocytosis dying in hypotensive crisis. Most mast cells appear degranulated. On the left side of this photograph, one membrane-bound structure appears empty, and the second contains only scroll-like structures. Toluidine blue stains in this case at autopsy were negative for granules. X78,400.

PLATE LI
MASTOCYTOSIS

A. MARROW
(Plate LI-A and B are from the same patient)

An eosinophilic fibrohistiocytic lesion is shown adjacent to a lymphocytic nodule. Mast cell infiltrates in the marrow are often associated with a swirling cellular connective tissue deposition and an eosinophilic infiltrate. PAS. X140.

B. MARROW

Numerous mast cells with maroon-staining granules are demonstrated within the fibroblastic-appearing nodule. Giemsa. X140.

C. BONE

Marked osteosclerosis may occur in mastocytosis. The interanastomosing bony trabeculae exhibit extensive remodeling of the basophilic cores with chiefly lamellar pale-staining bone on the surfaces. Some marrow spaces are filled with a highly vascular fibrous tissue associated with predominantly spindle-shaped mast cells. Giemsa. X55.

D. SPLEEN

Striking perivascular fibrotic zones extend throughout the white pulp. Numerous mast cells would be evident at higher magnification with metachromatic stains. X20.

PLATE LI

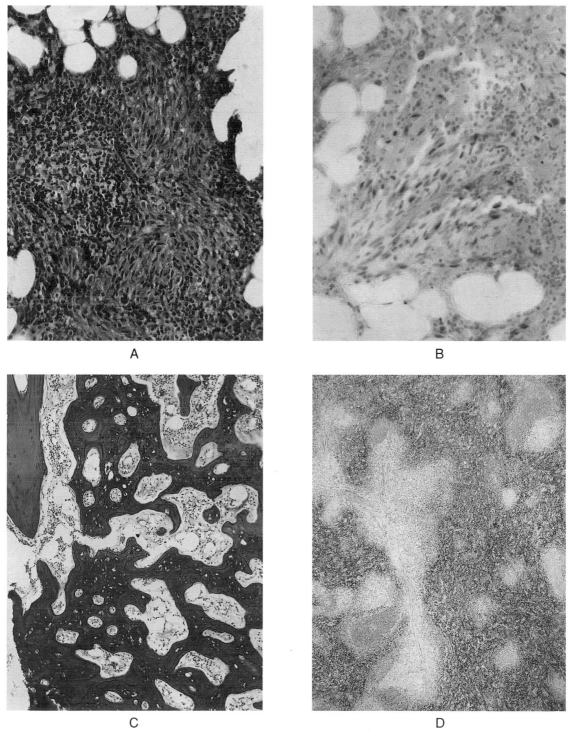

A

B

C

D

BENIGN HEMATOPOIETIC DISORDERS THAT RESEMBLE NEOPLASMS OR MAY DEVELOP INTO NEOPLASMS

Several reactive conditions affecting the marrow or soft tissues may be clinically or pathologically confused with leukemias, lymphomas, or histiocytoses. Some of these disorders are noteworthy because they evolve into neoplasms, whereas others are life-threatening illnesses due to alterations of immunity or marrow function. Confusion may arise from discrepancies between clinical features and pathologic diagnosis. Some patients with benign illnesses have mistakenly been diagnosed by pathologists as having malignant processes; conversely, some patients with correct pathologic diagnoses of reactive states have life-threatening illnesses. Furthermore, difficulties in patient management are significantly increased if there is an evolution of the reactive process to a lymphoma or leukemia. Overall, the complexities in this area are due to the imprecise diagnostic criteria for many entities at a clinical and pathologic level, a lack of understanding of the causal or pathogenetic mechanisms, and the frequent evolution of diagnostic status from reactive to neoplastic.

These disorders are grouped according to their usual natural history (Tables 56-58) and then briefly considered individually. This section does not provide coverage of all of the hematopoietic reactive processes but focuses on the problem areas described above.

FOLLICULAR HYPERPLASIA

Definition. This term refers to an increase in the number of follicular centers, usually associated with an increase in size as well. Several etiologic factors may be associated with hyperplasia.

Clinical Features. Both children and adults are affected. Adenopathy may be isolated (cervical, inguinal common) or regional. No local abnormalities may be apparent in tissues draining into the nodes. Some patients have associated infections (including syphilis), rheumatoid arthritis (Motulsky et al.; Nosanchuk and Schnitzer), or drug reactions, and rare patients with isolated immunodeficiencies develop reactive follicular hyperplasia.

Pathologic and Immunologic Features. There is architectural distortion by an increase in number and usually size of follicular centers. Follicles generally remain well separated and are located principally in the nodal cortex. Variations in follicular size and shape, apparent follicle fusion, and loss of mantle zone may all be seen in reactive states (Butler). Follicular center cells typically show the normal ratio of cleaved and noncleaved cells, with interspersed macrophages containing nuclear debris. "Zoning" of follicular centers with polar arrangements of darker-staining cells is diagnostic of reactive follicles. Interfollicular plasma cells are usually present, and there may be hyperplasia of parafollicular B cells in reactive states such as toxoplasmosis or Sjögren's syndrome. B cells are polytypic by all methods studied, with rare exceptions.

Differential Diagnosis. Follicular center cell lymphomas of small or large cleaved cells are usually considered as the diagnostic alternative to follicular hyperplasia

Table 56

PRELYMPHOMATOUS CONDITIONS AND LYMPHOPROLIFERATIVE STATES CONFUSED WITH LYMPHOMAS, LISTED IN RELATION TO EXPECTED CLINICAL COURSE*

Course May Be Benign

- Reactive follicular hyperplasia
- Rheumatoid arthritis
- Hashimoto's thyroiditis
- Reactive adenitis associated with vaccinations, infectious mononucleosis, and herpes zoster
- Dilantin adenopathy; drug hypersensitivity adenopathy
- Pseudolymphomas of skin, stomach, or lung
- Angiofollicular hyperplasia (Castleman's disease)
- Gluten-sensitive enteropathy

Illness May Be Progressive and Recurrent, Associated With Serious Abnormalities in Immune Function, or Develop Into Overt Malignant Lymphoma

- Immunoblastic lymphadenopathy and other abnormal immune reactions
- Angiofollicular hyperplasia (Castleman's disease)
- Sjögren's syndrome
- Plasma cell infiltration of the intestine, α-chain disease
- Pseudolymphomas of lung, skin, or eye
- Systemic lupus erythematosus/histiocytic necrotizing lymphadenitis
- Abnormal follicular hyperplasia associated with HIV infection
- X-linked immunodeficiency
- Immunosuppressed transplant patients with polymorphic B cell proliferations
- Lymphomatoid papulosis

---

* Some disorders are found in both groups, indicating that not all cases in each group will have the same natural history.

Table 57

PRELEUKEMIC CONDITIONS AND MYELOPROLIFERATIVE DISORDERS CONFUSED WITH LEUKEMIAS, LISTED IN RELATION TO EXPECTED CLINICAL COURSE*

Course May Be Benign

- Leukemoid reactions
- Marrow injury with maturation arrest
- Megaloblastic anemias
- Sideroblastic anemias

Illness May Be Progressive and Recurrent or Associated With Serious Abnormalities in Marrow Function

- Leukemoid reactions
- Sideroblastic anemias
- Myelodysplastic syndromes
- Myeloproliferative disorders
    Agnogenic myeloid metaplasia
    Polycythemia
    Essential thrombocythemia
- Marrow injury, various types, including previous chemotherapy
- Down's syndrome

* Some disorders are found in both groups, indicating that not all cases in each group will have the same natural history.

Table 58

MONONUCLEAR PHAGOCYTIC PROLIFERATIONS CONFUSED WITH MALIGNANT HISTIOCYTOSES, LISTED IN RELATION TO EXPECTED CLINICAL COURSE*

Course May Be Benign

- Histiocytosis X, local
- Storage diseases
- Viral-associated hemophagocytic syndrome
- Sinus histiocytosis with massive adenopathy

Illness May Be Progressive and Recurrent or Associated With Serious Abnormalities in Immune Function

- Histiocytosis X, disseminated
- Viral-associated hemophagocytic syndrome
- Familial hemophagocytic reticulosis

* Some disorders are found in both groups, indicating that not all cases in each group will have the same natural history; premalignant conditions involving the mononuclear phagocyte system are not recognized.

(Dorfman and Warnke). Factors indicating benignancy are the overall preservation of architecture with follicles predominantly in the nodal cortex, heterogeneity in appearance and phenotype of follicular center cells, and the absence of infiltration of interfollicular areas, subcapsular sinus, or capsule by cleaved cells (well-prepared material is required for this evaluation).

References

Butler, J.J. Non-neoplastic lesions of lymph nodes of man to be differentiated from lymphomas. Natl. Cancer Inst. Monogr. 32:233-255, 1969.

Dorfman, R.F. and Warnke, R. Lymphadenopathy simulating the malignant lymphomas. Hum. Pathol. 5:519-550, 1974.

Motulsky, A.G., Weinberg, S., Saphir, O., and Rosenberg, E. Lymph nodes in rheumatoid arthritis. Arch. Intern. Med. 90:660-676, 1952.

Nosanchuk, J.S. and Schnitzer, B. Follicular hyperplasia in lymph nodes from patients with rheumatoid arthritis. Cancer 29:243-254, 1969.

ANGIOFOLLICULAR HYPERPLASIA

SYNONYMS AND RELATED TERMS: Castleman's disease.

Definition. This is a localized or multicentric disease of uncertain cause, usually affecting the mediastinal or axillary nodes. The hyaline vascular form shows vascular proliferation, absent sinuses, and variable numbers of plasma cells, whereas the plasma cell variant is recognized by sheets of plasma cells in interfollicular areas in association with follicular changes (Castleman et al.; Keller et al.).

Clinical Features. Patients typically have large (up to 7 cm) asymptomatic mediastinal masses that do not progress or recur after excision. Extranodal masses have been described (fig. 123). Multicentric processes may be progressive. Patients with multicentric lesions have anemia, polyclonal hyperglobulinemia, thrombocytopenia, and marrow plasmacytosis and may have a progressive course complicated by malignant lymphoma or Kaposi's sarcoma (Frizzera et al.; Miller et al.). Plasmacytomas rarely develop as a complication of angiofollicular hyperplasia.

Pathologic and Immunologic Features. Follicular centers are increased but often vary in size and appearance. Small reactive follicular centers may be present, but a typical case contains increased follicular centers with central arterioles and whorls of mantle lymphocytes (fig. 124). Sinuses are usually absent. There is a marked increase in interfollicular plasma cells in the plasma cell variant. Foci of pale cytoplasmic cells ("plasmacytoid T cells") may be present (plate LII). Plasma cells are usually polytypic in angiofollicular hyperplasia, but rare cases show monotypism. "Plasmacytoid T cells" apparently express several myelomonocytic markers.

Differential Diagnosis. In the multicentric or progressive form, sheet-like growths of large transformed lymphocytes indicate the presence of a malignant lymphoma. Follicular structures are distributed throughout the node in angiofollicular hyperplasia, in contrast to the usual appearance of follicular hyperplasia with follicles principally located in the cortex.

The small cleaved cell type of follicular lymphomas shows an abnormal crowding of follicles, usually with extension through the entire nodal pulp and capsule. Homogeneity of follicular center cells is an important feature, often without macrophages or mitoses.

With plasmacytoid lymphocytic lymphoma, follicles may be small but usually do not show the vascular pattern seen in

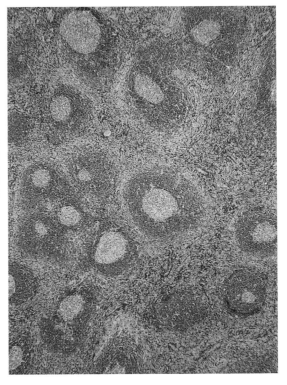

Figure 123
ANGIOFOLLICULAR HYPERPLASIA, CHEST WALL MASS
   In this extranodal specimen, the nodules of lymphoid tissue contain reactive follicles of varying size. The follicular centers are single and round to oval. The lymphoid follicles are separated by hyaline vascular tissue of varying width, but the thick hyalinized follicular vessels frequently described in this lesion are not apparent. X20.

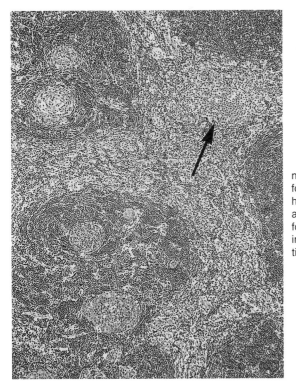

Figure 124
(Figure 124 and plate LII are from the same patient)
ANGIOFOLLICULAR HYPERPLASIA, LYMPH NODE
   In this figure, nodal architecture is distorted by lymphocytic nodules that vary in size and include several small reactive follicular centers. These lymphoid nodules are separated by highly vascular connective tissue. In this hyaline vascular variant, the follicular vessels may not be striking. A small cellular focus (arrow) containing pale cytoplasmic cells is noted in the intensely vascular internodular tissue associated with several tingible body macrophages. X80.

PLATE LII
ANGIOFOLLICULAR HYPERPLASIA, LYMPH NODE
(Plate LII and figure 124 are from the same patient)

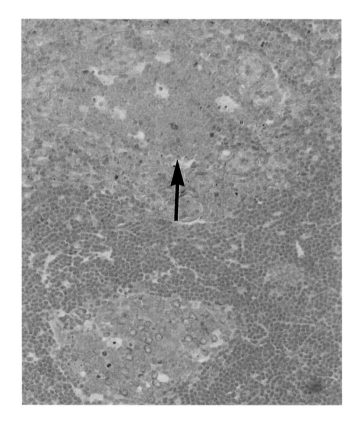

The features of this reactive follicular center are compared with a small nest of cytoplasmic cells (arrow) adjacent to a postcapillary venule. These pale cells are probably a special type of monocyte. Giemsa. X200.

angiofollicular hyperplasia. The architecture of the node is usually obscured by a lymphocytic and plasmacytic infiltrate that is best seen with MGP and Giemsa stains. Sheets of plasma cells are usually not present. PIP is almost universally monotypic.

References

Castleman, B., Iverson, L., and Menendez, V.P. Localized mediastinal lymph-node hyperplasia resembling thymoma. Cancer 9:822-830, 1956.

Frizzera, G., Banks, P.M., Massarelli, G., and Rosai, J. A systemic lymphoproliferative disorder with morphologic features of Castleman's disease. Am. J. Surg. Pathol. 7:211-231, 1983.

Keller, A.R., Hochholzer, L., and Castleman, B. Hyaline vascular and plasma-cell types of giant lymph node hyperplasia of the mediastinum and other locations. Cancer 29:670-683, 1972.

Miller, R.T., Mukai, K., Banks, P.M., and Frizzera, G. Systemic lymphoproliferative disorder with morphologic features of Castleman's disease. Arch. Pathol. Lab. Med. 108:626-630, 1984.

LYMPHOPROLIFERATIVE PROCESSES (PSEUDOLYMPHOMAS) OF THE GUT, SKIN, LUNG, AND EYE

Lymphoproliferative disorders often produce disease by affecting various organs and glands that are not traditionally considered, in part or in whole, lymphoid tissues (e.g., stomach, skin, lung, eye) (fig. 125). The pathogenesis of these lymphoproliferative disorders presumably varies among the different tissues affected, and several pathogenetic factors are probably operative within a single site. The importance of these processes lies in their frequency, their mimicking of lymphomas (hence the term pseudolymphomas), and their association with the development of malignant lymphoma. An estimated 10 to 25 percent of all malignant lymphomas arise from immunologic reactions or chronic stimulation in nonlymphoid sites (Brooks and Enterline; Wolf and Spjut). This is an interesting problem, but this discussion focuses on the differentiation of these lymphoproliferative processes from malignant lymphomas and the establishment of general diagnostic guidelines for all lymphoproliferative processes that mimic lymphomas rather than on each tissue or organ in turn.

In general, the histopathologic and immunologic criteria used to differentiate malignant lymphomas of the nodes from reactive states are applicable here (Burke). A conservative approach is advocated, and lymphomas should not be diagnosed unless there is convincing histopathologic or immunologic evidence. There are exceptions to all rules in this area, and generalizations are thereby fallible in specific cases.

The features that strongly favor malignancy are: (1) mass lesions exhibiting invasive and destructive features; (2) monomorphic aggregates or sheets of transformed lymphocytes (note that histologically malignant processes such as lymphomatoid papulosis may have benign clinical courses); (3) dysplastic cytologic features; (4) nodal involvement; (5) monomorphic small lymphocytic infiltrates, particularly if they are monotypic (Knowles and Jakobiec); (6) lymphoid neoplasms with plasmacytic differentiation, if monotypic CIg is demonstrated (Astarita et al.); (7) monotypism demonstrated by immunologic studies, abnormal immunologic phenotype, or karyotypic abnormalities (note that all clonal lymphoid processes do not progress to overt malignancy); and (8) clonal gene rearrangements.

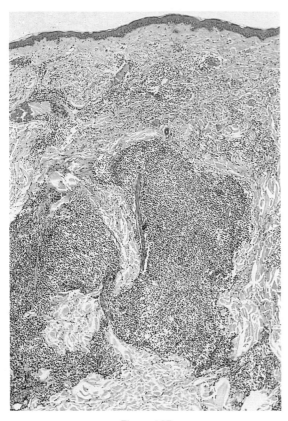

Figure 125
PSEUDOLYMPHOMA, SKIN
Distributed throughout all levels of the dermis except for the most superficial portions are lymphoid nodules of varying size and configuration, often situated around vessels. Close inspection of the lymphoid nodules reveals follicular centers containing tingible body macrophages and a mixture of cleaved and noncleaved cells that marked with CDw75/LN1 (not shown). This case illustrates how extensive infiltrates may be benign (there was no evidence of disease elsewhere on staging, and the subsequent clinical course has not revealed evidence of lymphoma). H&E. X95.

Finally, it should be pointed out that, in many cases, neoplastic processes and benign processes may coexist in the same biopsy sample for reasons discussed above. Demonstrating benign areas, therefore, does not prove that adjacent processes are also benign. There is clear evidence that some malignant lymphomas may be initially detected as very small foci in the midst of an otherwise reactive process.

Most lymphomas may be recognized by these guidelines. In the following sections, special attention is paid to Hashimoto's thyroiditis and Sjögren's syndrome because of the frequency with which these processes evolve into malignant lymphomas.

References

Astarita, R.W., Minckler, D., Taylor, C.R., Levine, A., and Lukes, R.J. Orbital and adnexal lymphomas. Am. J. Clin. Pathol. 73:615-621, 1980.

Brooks, J.J. and Enterline, H.T. Gastric pseudolymphoma. Its three subtypes and relation to lymphoma. Cancer 51:476-486, 1983.

Burke, J.S. The Diagnosis of Extranodal Lymphomas and Lymphoid Hyperplasias ("Pseudolymphomas") Other Than Those Involving the Lung, pp. 298-328. In: Major Problems in Pathology, Vol. 16. Surgical Pathology of the Lymph Nodes and Related Organs. Jaffe, E.S. and Bennington, J.L. (Eds.). Philadelphia: W.B. Saunders Company, 1985.

Knowles, D.M., Jr. and Jakobiec, F.A. Ocular adnexal lymphoid neoplasms. Hum. Pathol. 13:148-162, 1982.

Wolf, J.A. and Spjut, H.J. Focal lymphoid hyperplasia of the stomach preceding gastric lymphoma. Cancer 48:2518-2523, 1981.

Additional References

Colby, T.V. and Carrington, C.B. Pulmonary lymphomas. Hum. Pathol. 14:884-887, 1983.

Feoli, F., Carbone, A., Dina, M.A., et al. Pseudolymphoma of the lung: lymphoid subsets in the lung mass and in peripheral blood. Cancer 48:2218-2222, 1981.

Jakobiec, F.A., Iwamoto, T., and Knowles, D.M., Jr. Ocular adnexal lymphoid tumors. Arch. Ophthalmol. 100:84-98, 1982.

Julsrud, P.R., Brown, L.R., Li, C.Y., Rosenow, E.C., III, and Crowe, J.K. Pulmonary processes of mature-appearing lymphocytes: pseudolymphoma, well-differentiated lymphocytic lymphoma, and lymphocytic interstitial pneumonitis. Radiology 127:289-296, 1978.

Katzenstein, A.L. Surgical pathology of non-neoplastic lung disease. Maj. Prob. Pathol. 13:359-379, 1982.

Koss, M.N., Nichols, P.W., and Hochholzer, L. Pulmonary lymphomas and lymphomatoid granulomatosis. Semin. Res. Med. 9:325-333, 1988.

Kradin, R.L. and Mark, E.J. Benign lymphoid disorders of the lung, with a theory regarding their development. Hum. Pathol. 14:857-867, 1983.

Molenaar, W.M., Schwarze, E.W., and Lennert, K. An immunological study of germinal centres in four ophthalmic immunocytomas. Virchows Arch. [Pathol. Anat.] 399:141-148, 1983.

Morgan, G. and Harry, J. Lymphocytic tumours of indeterminate nature: a 5-year follow-up of 98 conjunctival and orbital lesions. Br. J. Ophthalmol. 62:381-383, 1978.

Ranchod, M., Lewin, K., Jr., and Dorfman, R.F. Lymphoid hyperplasia of the gastrointestinal tract. Am. J. Surg. Pathol. 2:383-400, 1978.

Saraga, P., Hurlimann, J., and Ozzello, L. Lymphomas and pseudolymphomas of the alimentary tract. Hum. Pathol. 12:713-723, 1981.

SJÖGREN'S SYNDROME

Definition. Two of the following three conditions must be present to diagnose Sjögren's syndrome: keratoconjunctivitis sicca; xerostomia; or rheumatoid arthritis/systemic lupus erythematosus.

Clinical Features. This syndrome usually affects women in their fifth to eighth decades. In addition to parotid swelling, patients may have adenopathy (usually cervical and rarely generalized) or develop extraglandular infiltrates (e.g., in the lung) (Kassan and Gardy). Polyclonal hypergammaglobulinemia and elevated rheumatoid factor are usually present. Patients with Sjögren's syndrome have an increased risk of developing immunoblastic lymphoma B and plasmacytoid lymphocytic lymphomas (Anderson and Talal; Levine et al.).

Pathologic and Immunologic Features. Salivary glands may show a pattern of myoepithelial sialadenitis alone, myoepithelial sialadenitis with small circumscribed proliferation areas, or myoepithelial sialadenitis with extensive confluent proliferation areas. Proliferation areas are pale staining and contain immunoblasts, medium sized lymphoid cells, and plasmacytoid cells. Affected nodes usually have partial architectural distortion, varying degrees of follicular hyperplasia, and foci of parafollicular B (monocytoid B) cells. Extranodal infiltrates may be overtly lymphomatous or contain varying mixtures of small and transformed lymphocytes and plasma cells. Immunologically, sialadenitis alone is polytypic, whereas sialadenitis with small proliferation areas may be monotypic or polytypic. Sialadenitis with extensive proliferation areas is always monotypic (Schmid et al.).

Differential Diagnosis. Features indicating the presence of malignant lymphoma include sialadenitis with small proliferation areas that are monotypic or sialadenitis with extensive proliferation areas. Other lymphomas are recognized by monomorphic aggregates of immunoblasts or as plasmacytoid lymphocytic processes. The latter type is often underdiagnosed.

References

Anderson, L.G. and Talal, N. The spectrum of benign to malignant lymphoproliferation in Sjögren's syndrome. Clin. Exp. Immunol. 9:199-221, 1971.

Kassan, S.S. and Gardy, M. Sjögren's syndrome. Am. J. Med. 64:1037-1046, 1978.

Levine, A.M., Taylor, C.R., Schneider, D.R., et al. Immunoblastic sarcoma of T-cell versus B-cell origin. I. Clinical features. Blood 58:52-61, 1981.

Schmid, U., Helbron, D., and Lennert, K. Development of malignant lymphoma in myoepithelial sialadenitis (Sjögren's syndrome). Virchows Arch. [Pathol. Anat.] 395:11-43, 1982.

Additional References

Kassan, S.S., Thomas, T.L., Moutsopoulos, H.M., et al. Increased risk of lymphoma in sicca syndrome. Ann. Intern. Med. 89:888-892, 1978.

Kelly, D.R., Spiegel, J.C., and Maves, M. Benign lymphoepithelial lesions of the salivary glands. Arch. Otolaryngol. 101:71-75, 1975.

Lucas, R.B. and Thackray, A.C. The So-Called "Benign Lymphoepithelial Lesions," pp. 952-953. In: Systemic Pathology, 2nd ed. Symmers, W.St.C. (Ed.). Edinburgh: Churchill Livingstone, 1976.

Moutsopoulos, H.M., Chused, T.M., Mann, L., et al. Sjögren's syndrome (Sicca syndrome). Ann. Intern. Med. 92(2 part 1):212-226, 1980.

Talal, N. and Schnitzer, B. Lymphadenopathy and Sjögren's syndrome. Clin. Rheum. Dis. 3:421-433, 1977.

von Gumberz, C. and Seifert, G. Immunoglobulin-containing plasma cells in chronic parotitis and malignant lymphomas of the parotid gland. Virchows Arch. [Pathol. Anat.] 389:79-92, 1980.

Zulman, J., Jaffe, R., and Talal, N. Evidence that the malignant lymphoma of Sjögren's syndrome is a monoclonal B-cell neoplasm. N. Engl. J. Med. 299:1215-1220, 1978.

HASHIMOTO'S THYROIDITIS

Definition. This is an autoimmune disease that principally involves the thyroid and is associated with lymphocytic infiltrates and acinar atrophy.

Clinical Features. Most patients with symptomatic Hashimoto's thyroiditis are females in their seventies. It is noteworthy that 75 to 100 percent of the thyroid lymphomas are in patients with Hashimoto's thyroiditis (Burke et al.; Maurer et al.), but the frequency of lymphomas in patients with Hashimoto's thyroiditis is 1 percent or less.

Pathologic and Immunologic Features. Affected thyroid glands show hyperplastic follicular centers in portions or in all of the thyroid. Hyperplastic follicles contain mixtures of follicular center cells, as described in the section on follicular hyperplasia. Thyroid acini may be small and may have abundant acidophilic cytoplasm and dense hyaline fibrosis. Malignant lymphomas of the thyroid almost always contain areas of Hashimoto's thyroiditis and are diagnosed by monomorphous aggregates of cleaved or noncleaved cells, the former often in follicular patterns. Immunoblasts with plasmacytic derivatives predominate in immunoblastic lymphoma B.

Follicular center cells are polytypic in Hashimoto's thyroiditis and monotypic in malignant lymphoma.

Differential Diagnosis. Malignant lymphomas arising in Hashimoto's thyroiditis usually produce mass lesions, with massive infiltration of the thyroid or extension into adjacent strap muscles. In most of these patients, the problem is not in the recognition that a neoplasm is present but in properly classifying the neoplasm. Those thyroid glands with a lymphocytic infiltrate are most likely lymphomatous, either follicular small cleaved cell type, large noncleaved cell type, or immunoblastic lymphoma B. Most "undifferentiated" tumors in this circumstance prove to be lymphoma.

References

Burke, J.S., Butler, J.J., and Fuller, L.M. Malignant lymphomas of the thyroid. Cancer 39:1587-1602, 1977.

Maurer, R., Taylor, C.R., Terry, R., and Lukes, R.J. Non-Hodgkin lymphomas of the thyroid. Virchows Arch. [Pathol. Anat.] 383:293-317, 1979.

Additional References

Compagno, J. and Oertel, J.E. Malignant lymphoma and other lymphoproliferative disorders of the thyroid gland. Am. J. Clin. Pathol. 74:1-11, 1980.

Heimann, R., Vannineuse, A., De Sloover, C., and Dor, P. Malignant lymphomas and undifferentiated small cell carcinoma of the thyroid. Histopathology 2:201-213, 1978.

SYSTEMIC LUPUS ERYTHEMATOSUS AND HISTIOCYTIC NECROTIZING LYMPHADENITIS

Definition. Systemic lupus is an autoimmune disease in which adenopathy may be prominent. Histiocytic necrotizing lymphadenitis was initially described in Japan but is now reported worldwide. It is a disease of unknown cause and in some cases, has a clinical and pathologic similarity to lupus.

Clinical Features. The adenopathy seen in systemic lupus is usually cervical, but is occasionally generalized. Adenopathy is often the presenting manifestation. In histiocytic necrotizing lymphadenitis, young women are usually affected and have persistent cervical adenopathy, fever, and leukopenia in some cases (Turner et al.).

Pathologic and Immunologic Features. Nodes in lupus show follicular hyperplasia, interfollicular expansion with plasma cells, and immunoblasts (Fox and Rosahn). Sharply circumscribed areas of necrosis may be present, but granulocytes are absent in these areas. In addition, perivascular collagenization or vasculitis may be seen. Hematoxylin bodies are occasionally present. Follicles are not hyperplastic in histiocytic necrotizing lymphadenitis. Large discrete areas of necrosis are usually present, notable for the absence of granulocytes (Feller et al.; Pileri et al.). No specific immunopathologic markers are recognized.

Differential Diagnosis. Patients with systemic lupus erythematosus rarely develop immunoblastic lymphoma, B cell type, but the likelihood of malignant lymphoma developing in either systemic lupus erythematosus or histiocytic necrotizing lymphadenitis is low. Poorly prepared sections in patients with histiocytic necrotizing lymphadenitis may be misinterpreted as malignant lymphoma because of architectural distortion, scattered immunoblasts, and the presence of necrosis.

References

Feller, A.C., Lennert, K., Stein, H., Bruhn, H.D., and Wuthe, H.H. Immunohistology and aetiology of histiocytic necrotizing lymphadenitis. Histopathology 7:825-839, 1983.

Fox, R.A. and Rosahn, P.D. The lymph nodes in disseminated lupus erythematosus. Am. J. Pathol. 19:73-79, 1943.
Pileri, S., Kikuchi, M., Helbron, D., and Lennert, K. Histiocytic necrotizing lymphadenitis without granulocytic infiltration. Virchows Arch. [Pathol. Anat.] 395:257-271, 1982.
Turner, R.R., Martin, J., and Dorfman, R.F. Necrotizing lymphadenitis. Am. J. Surg. Pathol. 7:115-123, 1983.

Additional Reference

Case records of the Massachusetts General Hospital. Weekly clinicopathological exercises. Case 42-1979. N. Engl. J. Med. 301:881-887, 1979.

PERSISTENT GENERALIZED ADENOPATHY AND AIDS

Definition. Persistent generalized adenopathy is defined as persistent lymphadenopathy in two or more sites for 3 months or longer in the absence of infections or drug intake known to be associated with adenopathy. Biopsied nodes show reactive changes.

Acquired immunodeficiency syndrome (AIDS) is defined as a reliably diagnosed indicator disease (e.g., unusual infection or common infection shown to be unusually virulent, Kaposi's sarcoma in patients under 60 years, central nervous system lymphoma) or, in the presence of laboratory evidence for HIV infection, various infections, neoplasms, or neurologic and wasting syndromes.

Clinical Features. Homosexual men, intravenous drug abusers, some transfused patients, and hemophiliacs are particularly at risk. Persistent generalized adenopathy is part of the AIDS-related complex, but the actual incidence of conversion of persistent adenopathy to AIDS is unknown. Patients usually have superficial adenopathy (cervical or axillary nodes are commonly involved), as well as adenopathy in unusual sites (epitrochlear, popliteal). Extranodal sites are often involved when lymphomas develop (Levine et al.). Parotid enlargement is a striking AIDS-related clinical finding (plate LIII-D).

Pathologic and Immunologic Features. AIDS is characterized by a marked decrease in cellularity with absent germinal centers, lymphocyte depletion, and an increase in small branching vessels. T helper cells are reduced in the paracortex, mantle, and follicular centers, while T suppressor cells are increased. Immunologic studies by frozen section immunoperoxidase show that the small irregular lymphocytes infiltrating follicular centers mark as T cells, and masses of round lymphocytes extending into follicular centers mark as B cells.

The morphologic changes in lymphoid tissue in both AIDS-related complex and AIDS are diverse and variable. The most important and diagnostically challenging aspects for pathologists are the changes found in lymph node biopsies in patients with the persistent generalized lymphadenopathy syndrome, which is a major manifestation of AIDS-related complex. Node biopsies in the persistent generalized lymphadenopathy syndrome consistently show a distinctive follicular center proliferation and alteration. The following four types of follicular changes are found in most cases of persistent generalized lymphadenopathy syndrome in association with variable interfollicular abnormalities: (1) intense follicular center cell proliferation with diminished or absent lymphocytic mantles; (2) lymphocytic infiltration of the peripheral areas of follicular centers, resulting in an appearance of ragged margins and linear small lymphocytic infiltrates; (3) islets or masses of small lymphocytes in the follicular centers; and (4) disruption of follicular centers by extensive infiltrates of small lymphocytes and hemorrhage (plate LIII; figs. 126-129) (Brynes et al.; Guarda et al.; Ioachim et al.; Meyer et al.).

In the interfollicular areas, broad zones of parafollicular cells may be prominent; plasma cells are usually numerous, whereas macrophages are less frequent. Benign vascular proliferation may be striking in patients who have Kaposi's sarcoma in other areas.

The latter interfollicular features may be prominent but are variable. However, our experience shows that patients will almost always be HIV positive if at least three of the follicular alterations are encountered.

Lymphocyte depletion of the lymph nodes with minor degrees of small-vessel proliferation appears to represent the nodal changes in patients with AIDS (fig. 130). Two neoplasms, Kaposi's sarcoma and immunoblastic lymphoma B, are also commonly found in these patients (plates LIV, LV) (Levine et al.; Ziegler et al.).

Differential Diagnosis. Features indicating the presence of malignant lymphoma are monomorphic aggregates or sheets of transformed lymphocytes (this process may be focal). Kaposi's sarcoma is indicated by capsular hypervascularity with slit-like spaces, mitoses, and fragmentation or red cells.

Malignant lymphoma should not be diagnosed unless monomorphic aggregates of transformed lymphocytes are detected. In exuberant follicular hyperplasia, follicles may be very large, although they are usually not back to back in distribution, and the lymphocytic population is not homogeneous. With few exceptions, the lymphomas developing in AIDS patients have been high grade B cell types, diffuse small noncleaved cell, Burkitt's or non-Burkitt's variants, or immunoblastic lymphoma B. Extranodal presentations are frequent in sites such as the central nervous system (plate LV), rectal-anal, and soft tissues. Most patients presenting at this time with central nervous system lymphomas have related HIV infections. These neoplasms are associated with rapidly progressive disease, and response to therapy is poor.

Kaposi's sarcoma may be very difficult to recognize in its early stages. The primary changes may appear in the capsular area. Hypervascularity in that area with slit-like endothelial spaces and mitotic activity strongly indicate Kaposi's sarcoma (plate LIV-A).

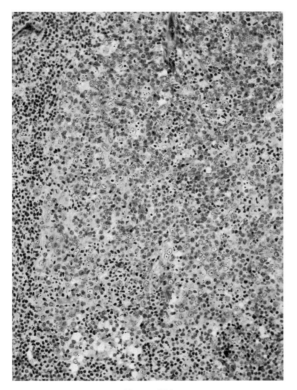

Figure 126
PERSISTENT GENERALIZED ADENOPATHY,
LYMPH NODE

The margin of this follicular center is irregular and ill defined as a result of lymphocytic infiltrates. Small lymphocytes also extend in small clusters or linear array deep into the center of the follicle. X160. (Fig. 4B from Meyer, P.R., Yanagihara, E.T., Parker, J.W., and Lukes, R.J. A distinctive follicular hyperplasia in the acquired immune deficiency syndrome (AIDS) and the AIDS related complex. Hematol. Oncol. 2:319-347, 1984.)

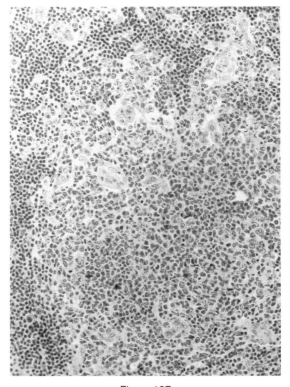

Figure 127
PERSISTENT GENERALIZED ADENOPATHY,
LYMPH NODE

In this figure, exaggerated lymphocytic infiltration of a follicular center markedly alters its margin. X150. (Fig. 4A from Meyer, P.R., Yanagihara, E.T., Parker, J.W., and Lukes, R.J. A distinctive follicular hyperplasia in the acquired immune deficiency syndrome (AIDS) and the AIDS related complex. Hematol. Oncol. 2:319-347, 1984.)

PLATE LIII

A. PERSISTENT GENERALIZED ADENOPATHY, LYMPH NODE
(Plate LIII-A and B are from the same patient)

This low magnification photomicrograph shows exuberant follicular hyperplasia of the lymph node, with prominent parafollicular cell proliferation in the region of the lymph node sinuses. X40. (Fig. 1 from Meyer, P.R., Yanagihara, E.T., Parker, J.W., and Lukes, R.J. A distinctive follicular hyperplasia in the acquired immune deficiency syndrome (AIDS) and the AIDS related complex. Hematol. Oncol. 2:319-347, 1984.)

B. PERSISTENT GENERALIZED ADENOPATHY, LYMPH NODE

The edge of a hyperplastic follicular center at the top and the adjacent parafollicular cell hyperplasia are shown at a higher magnification. X160.

C. PERSISTENT GENERALIZED ADENOPATHY, LYMPH NODE

A hyperplastic follicular center at the top of this illustration exhibits a diminished lymphocytic mantle zone associated with marked plasmacytosis in the adjacent interfollicular area. MGP. X160.

D. AIDS-RELATED COMPLEX, PAROTID GLAND

A cyst containing acidophilic material is shown at the top in a parotid gland distorted by intense lymphoid proliferation. The follicular centers exhibit all of the proliferative and infiltrative features noted in persistent generalized lymphadenopathy. Parotid glands are often dramatically enlarged in patients with persistent generalized lymphadenopathy. In this patient, HIV was cultured from saliva and identified in parotid tissue by electron microscopy. H&E. X32.

PLATE LIII

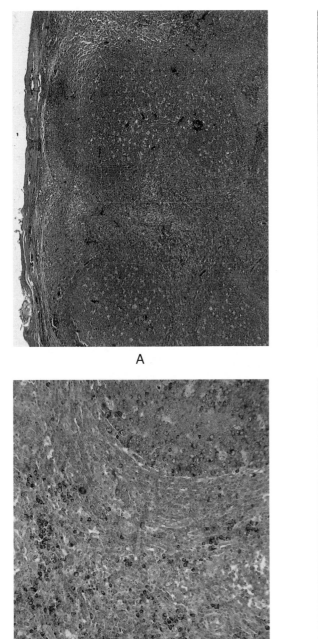

A

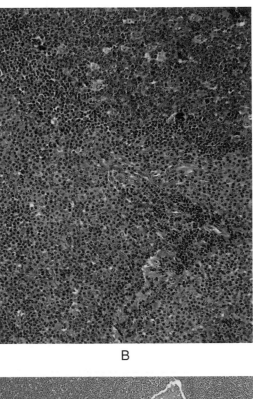

B

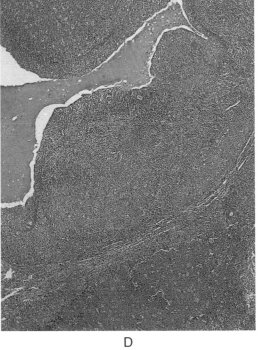

C

D

PLATE LIV

A. AIDS AND KAPOSI'S SARCOMA, LYMPH NODE
(Plate LIV-A and figure 130 are from the same patient)

This small lymph node exhibits lymphocyte depletion and Kaposi's sarcoma in the perinodal tissue with extension through the capsule. X60.

B. AIDS AND IMMUNOBLASTIC LYMPHOMA B, LYMPH NODE
(Plate LIV-B and C are from the same patient)

In this illustration, the lymphomatous infiltrate widely expands the perinodal tissue and extends around the node. X25.

C. AIDS AND IMMUNOBLASTIC LYMPHOMA B, LYMPH NODE

The infiltration of the perinodal tissues is comprised of transformed lymphocytes with slight plasmacytoid features, fulfilling the criteria for the diagnosis of immunoblastic lymphoma B. X600.

PLATE LIV

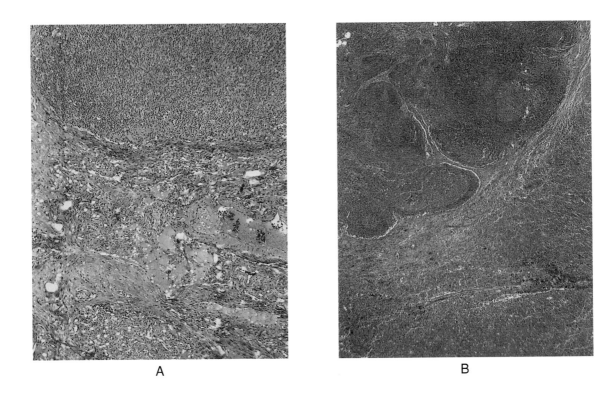

A

B

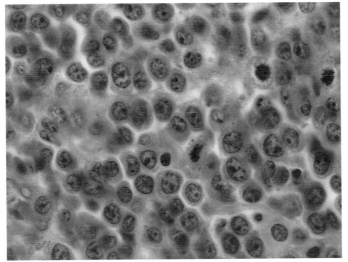

C

PLATE LV
AIDS AND IMMUNOBLASTIC LYMPHOMA B, CENTRAL NERVOUS SYSTEM
(Plate LV is from the same patient)

A. This adult male presented with evidence of a frontal lobe lesion. Two types of cellular infiltrates are apparent: diffuse and perivascular with extension into relatively uninvolved adjacent parenchyma. The perivascular growth with more solid masses is typical of central nervous system lymphomas. X80.

B. The lymphomatous cells in perivascular areas are transformed lymphocytes with plasmacytoid features. X600.

C. There is intense pyroninophilia of the tumor cells in this illustration. MGP. X400.

D. Amphophilia of the cytoplasm is demonstrated. Giemsa. X400.

PLATE LV

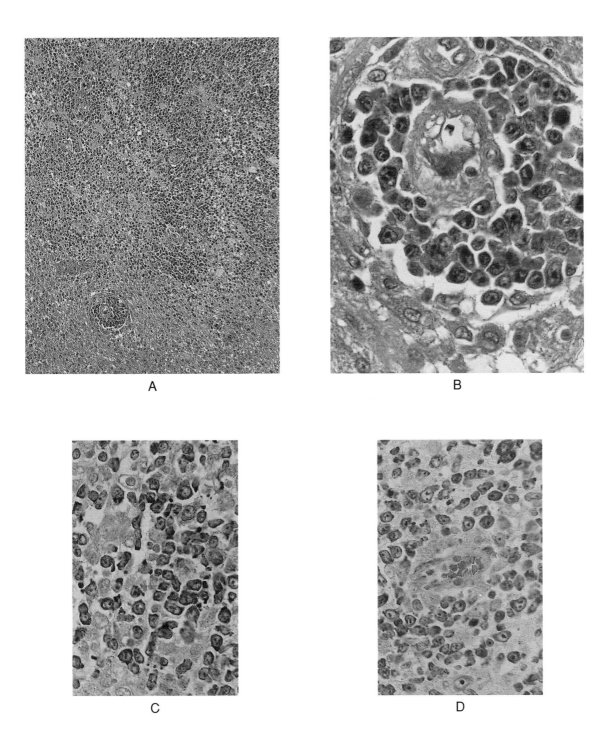

A

B

C

D

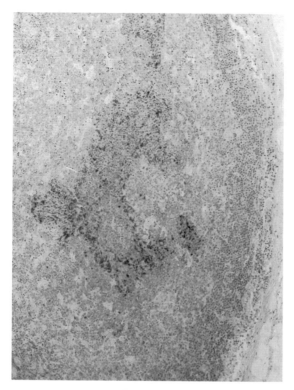

Figure 128
PERSISTENT GENERALIZED ADENOPATHY,
LYMPH NODE

This figure shows a focus of lymphocytic infiltration of the follicular center that produces a clearly defined islet of small lymphocytes. X80. (Fig. 4C from Meyer, P.R., Yanagihara, E.T., Parker, J.W., and Lukes, R.J. A distinctive follicular hyperplasia in the acquired immune deficiency syndrome (AIDS) and the AIDS related complex. Hematol. Oncol. 2:319-347, 1984.)

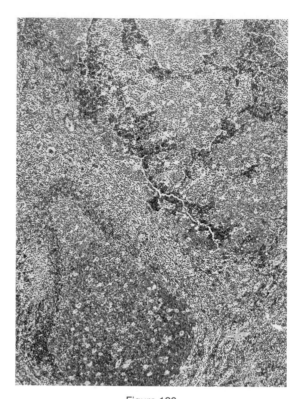

Figure 129
PERSISTENT GENERALIZED ADENOPATHY,
LYMPH NODE

An intact hyperplastic follicular center is shown adjacent to a follicular center disrupted by extensive lymphocytic infiltration and hemorrhage. X60. (Fig. 4D from Meyer, P.R., Yanagihara, E.T., Parker, J.W., and Lukes, R.J. A distinctive follicular hyperplasia in the acquired immune deficiency syndrome (AIDS) and the AIDS related complex. Hematol. Oncol. 2:319-347, 1984.)

References

Brynes, R.K., Chan, W.C., Spira, T.J., Ewing, E.P., Jr., and Chandler, F.W. Value of lymph node biopsy in unexplained lymphadenopathy in homosexual men. J.A.M.A. 250:1313-1317, 1983.

Guarda, L.A., Butler, J.J., Mansell, P., et al. Lymphadenopathy in homosexual men. Morbid anatomy with clinical and immunologic correlations. Am. J. Clin. Pathol. 79:559-568, 1983.

Ioachim, H.L., Lerner, C.W., and Tapper, M.L. The lymphoid lesions associated with the acquired immunodeficiency syndrome. Am. J. Surg. Pathol. 7:543-553, 1983.

Levine, A.M., Meyer, P.R., Begandy, M.K., et al. Development of B-cell lymphoma in homosexual men. Ann. Intern. Med. 100:7-13, 1984.

Meyer, P.R., Yanagihara, E.T., Parker, J.W., and Lukes, R.J. A distinctive follicular hyperplasia in the acquired immune deficiency syndrome (AIDS) and the AIDS related complex. Hematol. Oncol. 2:319-347, 1984.

Ziegler, J.L., Drew, W.L., Miner, R.C., et al. Outbreak of Burkitt's-like lymphoma in homosexual men. Lancet 2:631-633, 1982.

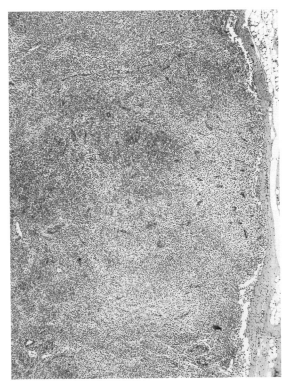

Figure 130
(Figure 130 and plate LIV-A are from the same patient)
AIDS, LYMPH NODE
Lymphocyte depletion and vascular proliferation resembling immunoblastic lymphadenopathy are shown in this figure. No reactive follicles are found. X25. (Fig. 2 from Meyer, P.R., Yanagihara, E.T., Parker, J.W., and Lukes, R.J. A distinctive follicular hyperplasia in the acquired immune deficiency syndrome (AIDS) and the AIDS related complex. Hematol. Oncol. 2:319-347, 1984.)

IMMUNOBLASTIC REACTIONS IN INFECTIOUS MONONUCLEOSIS, VACCINATIONS, AND HERPES

Definition. In these diseases, there may be a severe exaggerated immune response producing an extreme immunoblastic proliferation closely simulating malignant lymphoma. These exaggerated proliferations may represent normal responses to these viral antigens.

Clinical Features. Infectious mononucleosis may produce fever, tonsillitis, cervical adenopathy, mild hepatitis, and splenomegaly in adolescents or young adults. In herpes zoster, adenopathy may precede the development of typical zoster lesions. Adenopathy is found in the lymphatic drainage of vaccination sites.

Pathologic and Immunologic Features. Interfollicular areas are usually mottled in appearance due to interspersed small and transformed lymphocytes; homogeneous clusters or sheets of transformed cells are less common. Downey-type cells are seen in the peripheral blood and node sinuses in infectious mononucleosis (fig. 131) but are not present in postvaccinal adenopathy. Atypical lymphocytes in the peripheral blood in infectious mononucleosis are T cytotoxic cells.

In all of these cases, there is often a marked immunoblastic proliferation that usually distorts, but does not obliterate, nodal architecture (plate LVI) (Childs et al.; Gowing; Hartsock). The partial preservation of architecture, even in the presence of a dramatic number of immunoblasts, is an indicator of this type of reactive process (plate LVII). Nevertheless, many pathologists have seen cases in which reactive changes of this type closely resembled malignant lymphoma. The presence of transformed lymphocytes in the sinuses provides additional support for a benign diagnosis.

Differential Diagnosis. Biopsies of enlarged cervical nodes or tonsillar masses in teenagers or young adults should not be interpreted as malignant lymphomas if there is partial architectural preservation, even if large aggregates of immunoblasts are present. Serologic reactions for infectious mononucleosis should be obtained

361

PLATE LVI

A. IMMUNOBLASTS IN INTERFOLLICULAR TISSUE, LYMPH NODE
Several immunoblasts mixed with small lymphocytes are shown at high magnification. The immunoblasts have distinct dice-like nucleoli, finely dispersed chromatin, and detectable cytoplasm. X600.

B. IMMUNOBLASTS IN INTERFOLLICULAR TISSUE, LYMPH NODE
The immunoblasts have intensely pyroninophilic cytoplasm. MGP. X600.

C. REACTIVE FOLLICULAR HYPERPLASIA, TONSIL
The mixed composition of this reactive follicular center is shown. There are several tingible body macrophages, a few large noncleaved follicular center cells, and a predominance of cleaved follicular center cells. Note the resemblance of the large noncleaved cells to the immunoblasts in Plate LVIII-A and B. X600.

D. POSTVACCINAL ADENITIS
(Plate LVI-D and E are from the same patient)
In this illustration, most of the nodal architecture is altered by a pale-staining cellular proliferation in the paracortex separating reactive follicles. X10.

E. POSTVACCINAL ADENITIS
Immunoblasts of medium and large type are noted at the edge of the residual lymphocytic mantles at the top of this illustration. Numerous mitoses are present. X400.

PLATE LVI

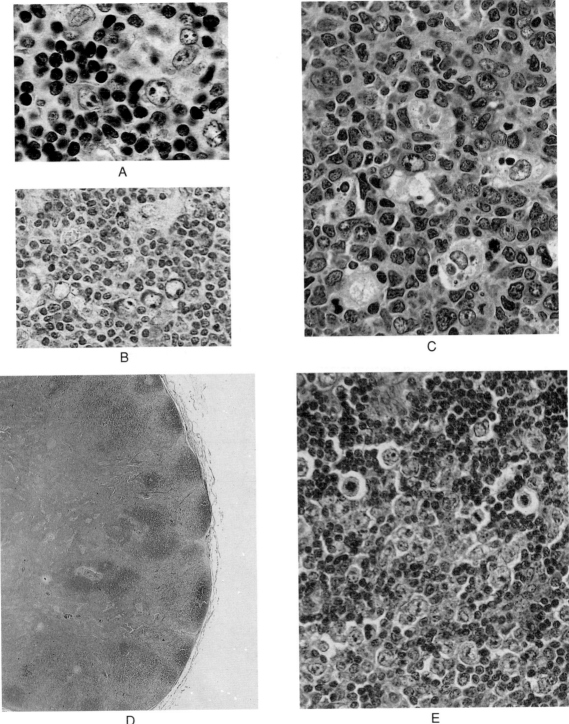

PLATE LVII
INFECTIOUS MONONUCLEOSIS, LYMPH NODE
(Plate LVII-A–D are from the same patient)

A. An extreme degree of immunoblastic proliferation almost completely replaces the lymph node architecture, leaving a few isolated uninvolved areas of lymphoid tissue in this 42 year old physician. X20.

B. The cellular proliferation is composed predominantly of medium and large immunoblasts with intermingled small lymphocytes and scattered eosinophils. The immunoblasts have prominent amphophilic cytoplasm and round to oval nuclei, usually with two or three small dice-like nucleoli. Occasionally, the nucleoli are large and centrally situated. This proliferation illustrates that immunoblastic reactions, when severe, may closely simulate immunoblastic lymphoma. X400.

C and D. The immunoblasts are strikingly pyroninophilic, as shown in the MGP stain (C) and are amphophilic in the Giemsa stain (D). X600.

E. Note the mixture of cells, including medium and large immunoblasts (arrow) and a multinucleated cell. H&E. X400. (Fig. 4 from Tindle, B.H., Parker, J.W., and Lukes, R.J. "Reed-Sternberg cells" in infectious mononucleosis? Am. J. Clin. Pathol. 58:607-617, 1972.)

F. This illustration shows a Reed-Sternberg-like cell in a lymph node from a patient with infectious mononucleosis. H&E. X600. (Fig. 8 from Tindle, B.H., Parker, J.W., and Lukes, R.J. "Reed-Sternberg cells" in infectious mononucleosis? Am. J. Clin. Pathol. 58:607-617, 1972.)

PLATE LVII

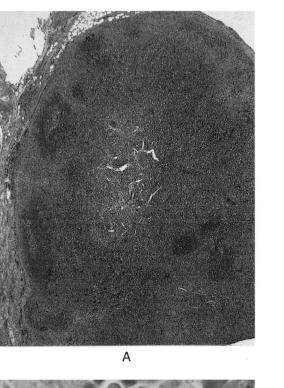

A

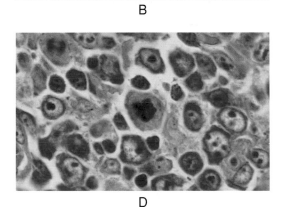

B

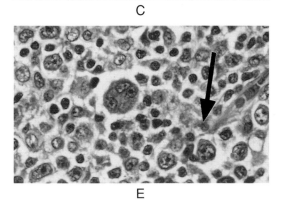

C

D

E

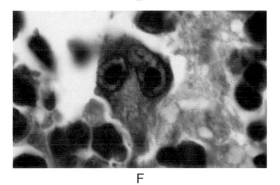

F

PLATE LVIII
DISSEMINATED HERPES, LYMPH NODE
(Plate LVIII is from the same patient)

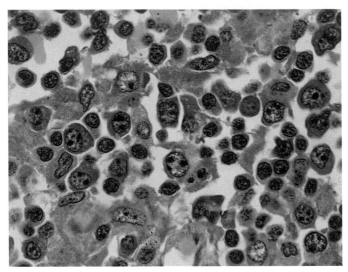

A. This 28 year old female with unexplained high fever (106°F) and enlarged lymph nodes exhibited necrotizing lymphadenitis and a severe immunoblastic reaction. The patient appeared moribund but responded to high doses of corticosteroids. The proliferation was dominated by immunoblasts and plasmacytoid immunoblasts in a large area of the lymph node. Plastic sections. X600. (Courtesy of Dr. Richard Ellis, San Pedro, CA.)

B. In these areas of immunoblastic proliferation, many cells contain large acidophilic inclusions surrounded by pale zones, with displacement of small nucleoli against the nuclear membranes. The inclusions were not pyroninophilic. Immunoperoxidase-labeled antibodies identified the nuclear inclusions as herpes; herpetic infection was confirmed in sequential studies of her serum. She remains well 3 years later. Plastic sections. X1000. (Courtesy of Dr. Richard Ellis, San Pedro, CA.)

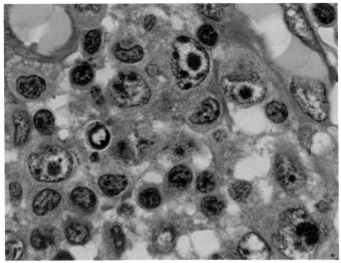

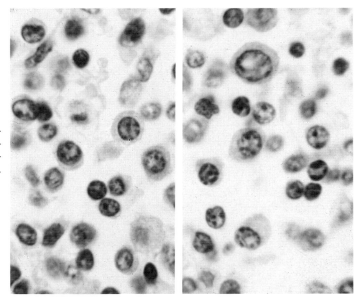

Figure 131
INFECTIOUS MONONUCLEOSIS,
LYMPH NODE
These pale, cytoplasmic, medium sized lymphocytes with central nuclei resemble the Downey cells seen in the peripheral blood. The largest cell on the right is an immunoblast. H&E. X1200.

routinely in these cases before final diagnoses are made. In extreme cases, adenitis in viral infections may closely simulate immunoblastic lymphoma, B cell type (plates LVII, LVIII). Architectural preservation in such cases may be difficult to find. Polyclonality on PIP or the presence of transformed lymphocytes in sinuses is further evidence of an immunoblastic reaction.

In the past, Hodgkin's disease has been misdiagnosed in these immunoblastic reactions due to architectural distortion and the presence of Reed-Sternberg-like cells that are often more apparent around areas of necrosis (plate LVII-E,F) (Tindle et al.). However, the architectural distortion in immunoblastic reactions is not typical of Hodgkin's disease, and the immunoblastic proliferation is also not typical.

References

Childs, C.C., Parham, D.M., and Berard, C.W. Infectious mononucleosis. Am. J. Surg. Pathol. 11:122-132, 1987.

Gowing, N.F. Infectious mononucleosis. Pathol. Annu. 10:1-20, 1975.

Hartsock, R.J. Postvaccinal lymphadenitis. Hyperplasia of lymphoid tissue that simulates malignant lymphoma. Cancer 21:632-649, 1968.

Tindle, B.H., Parker, J.W., and Lukes, R.J. "Reed-Sternberg cells" in infectious mononucleosis? Am. J. Clin. Pathol. 58:607-617, 1972.

Additional References

Patterson, S.D., Larson, E.B., and Corey, L. Atypical generalized zoster with lymphadenitis mimicking lymphoma. N. Engl. J. Med. 302:848-851, 1980.

Salvador, A.H., Harrison, E.G., Jr., and Kyle, R.A. Lymphadenopathy due to infectious mononucleosis: its confusion with malignant lymphoma. Cancer 27:1029-1040, 1971.

DRUG REACTIONS

Definition. Reactions to various drugs may produce an exaggerated and abnormal reaction with variable degrees of follicular and paracortical participation. A striking immunoblastic and vascular component is often present. Adenopathy usually subsides rapidly after the drugs are discontinued. Hydantoins have the reputation of producing clinically significant adenopathy but are probably an infrequent cause of adenopathy.

Clinical Features. Most patients develop tender cervical or generalized adenopathy 1 to 6 weeks after starting drugs and have fever, eosinophilia, and various skin lesions. Adenopathy usually regresses after the drugs are stopped and the evolution into lymphoma is very unusual (Saltzstein and Ackerman; Symmers). Penicillin, sulfa drugs, and carbamazebine are also reported to produce lymphadenopathic reactions.

Pathologic and Immunologic Features. Variable hyperplasia of follicular centers is noted, along with immunoblastic proliferation in interfollicular areas (Dorfman and Warnke). Foci of necrosis are occasionally present, as are neutrophilia, eosinophilia, and plasmacytosis.

Differential Diagnosis. Hodgkin's disease may be suggested by partial architectural distortion, the presence of plasma cells and eosinophils in the interfollicular area, and the presence of Reed-Sternberg-like cells, which is reported in the literature but is rarely seen in practice.

References

Dorfman, R.F. and Warnke, R. Lymphadenopathy simulating the malignant lymphomas. Hum. Pathol. 5:519-550, 1974.

Saltzstein, S.I. and Ackerman, L.V. Lymphadenopathy induced by anticonvulsant drugs and mimicking clinically and pathologically malignant lymphomas. Cancer 12:164-182, 1959.

Symmers, W.St.C. Drug-Induced Lymphoma-Like Lymphadenopathies and Their Relation to Lymphomas, pp. 696-701. In: Systemic Pathology, 2nd ed. Symmers, W.St.C. (Ed.). Edinburgh: Churchill Livingstone, 1976.

Additional References

Gams, R.A., Neal, J.A., and Conrad, F.G. Hydantoin-induced pseudolymphoma. Ann. Intern. Med. 69:557-568, 1968.

Greene, D.A. Localized cervical lymphadenopathy induced by diphenylhydantoin sodium. Arch. Otolaryngol. 101:446-448, 1975.

Li, F.P., Willard, D.R., Goodman, R., and Vawter, G. Malignant lymphoma after diphenylhydantoin (dilantin) therapy. Cancer 36:1359-1362, 1975.

Matzner, Y. and Polliack, A. Lymphoproliferative disorders in four patients receiving chronic diphenylhydantoin therapy: etiologic correlation or chance association? Isr. J. Med. Sci. 14:865-869, 1978.

ABNORMAL IMMUNE REACTIONS, INCLUDING IMMUNOBLASTIC LYMPHADENOPATHY

Sometimes pathologists are confronted with unusual nodal proliferations that are difficult to classify because the lesions are not clearly lymphomatous and yet exceed the known manifestation of the most exaggerated immune reactions. Immunoblastic lymphadenopathy, with its marked immunoblastic and plasmacytic reaction associated with arborizing vascular proliferation, prominent acidophilic interstitial material, and overall nodal hypocellularity, appears to be the prototypic example of a disorder intermediate between severe normal immune reaction and malignant lymphoma (Lukes and Tindle). Angioimmunoblastic lymphadenopathy with dysproteinemia (another abnormal reaction) may possess follicular centers, often lacks acidophilic interstitial material, and seems to encompass a broader group (Frizzera et al.).

The unusual character of these two disorders has stimulated proposals of their T cell lymphomatous nature, an issue that will not be resolved until a sizable group of well-characterized cases has been studied by gene rearrangement analysis coupled with clinical follow-up.

Meanwhile, we have continued to see numerous cases with an apparently expanding array of morphologic expressions, including severe immunoblastic and vascular proliferation, usually without a follicular component. For this group, we have used the term abnormal immune reaction because we suspect patients are unable to react normally and are vulnerable to the development of immunoblastic lymphomas. The evolution to immunoblastic lymphoma may be diagnosed by finding monomorphous areas of immunoblasts that are one high magnification field in diameter (fig. 132) or by demonstrating monotypism by immunologic studies.

Definition. Abnormal immune reactions refer to the clinical and pathologic evidence of an extreme or unusual immune response, usually to unknown stimulants. Immunoblastic lymphadenopathy is a type of abnormal immune reaction in which the nodal architecture is completely effaced. Angioimmunoblastic lymphadenopathy with dysproteinemia is a somewhat broader group than immunoblastic lymphadenopathy because of the inclusion of cases with partial architectural preservation.

Clinical Features. There is often a dramatic onset of symptoms with generalized lymphadenopathy in 80 percent of the patients. B symptoms, splenomegaly, hepatomegaly, and Coombs' positive hemolytic anemia are common. Hypersen-

sitivity to therapeutic agents may be implicated as the initial event in 35 percent of the cases. Response to steroid therapy is dramatic in some cases, and relapses are also dramatic upon cessation of therapy. These diseases rapidly evolve to immunoblastic lymphoma of B cells in 10 to 20 percent of the cases and to T cell neoplasms in an unknown percentage. Immunoblastic lymphadenopathy is usually a rapidly progressive and fatal disease with a median survival of 1 year.

Pathologic and Immunologic Features. Immunoblastic lymphadenopathy is a diffuse process affecting the entire node and is associated with the absence of follicles and overall decreased cellularity. Necrosis is infrequent. The chief microscopic features are arborizing small vessel proliferation with PAS positive thickened walls, numerous immunoblasts, plasmacytoid immunoblasts and plasma cells, decreased lymphocytes, and deposits of granular acidophilic interstitial material widely separating the cells (plate LIX). In angioimmunoblastic lymphadenopathy, some of these features may be seen, but nodal architecture may be partially preserved and acidophilic material lacking (plate LX-A,B).

Karyotypic and clonal abnormalities have been described in some cases (Lipford et al.). B immunoblasts and plasma cells are polyclonal, whereas T cells vary considerably in distribution pattern and type.

Differential Diagnosis. *Hodgkin's disease, mixed cellularity and diffuse fibrosis.* Hodgkin's disease may be suggested by the depleted appearance of some cases of abnormal immune reaction, in addition to the polymorphic cellular infiltrate that is often rich in eosinophils. In contrast to

PLATE LIX
IMMUNOBLASTIC LYMPHADENOPATHY, LYMPH NODE
(Plate LIX-A–C are from the same patient)

A. In this illustration, the nodal architecture is markedly distorted, with obliteration of the sinuses and absence of follicular centers. The node appears less cellular than normal and of heterogeneous composition. Numerous curling, branching, thick-walled small vessels are present. Ultrastructural studies of the interstitial material and deposits in vessel walls have revealed organelles and cellular debris, indicating cell destruction. X50.

B. Pale-staining interstitial background material is seen in this illustration. The small vessel walls are thickened, and the vascular lumina are compressed. X150.

C. Small branching vessels are distributed in a mixed cellular infiltration containing scattered plasma cells and immunoblasts that are separated by the pale-staining interstitial material. PAS. X400.

D. This lymph node is diffusely involved by a loosely distributed, somewhat hypocellular population in which there is a prominent component of PAS positive thick-walled small vessels, some of which are branching. The cells are separated by abundant pale amorphous interstitial material. At this intermediate magnification, the cellular population appears to be of mixed composition, including small and transformed lymphocytes. PAS. X295.

PLATE LIX

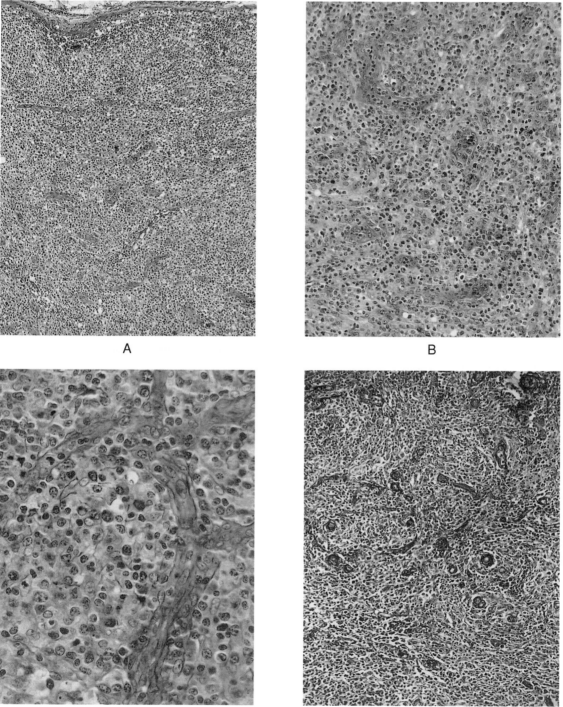

A

B

C

D

PLATE LX

A. ABNORMAL IMMUNE REACTION RESEMBLING IMMUNOBLASTIC LYMPHADENOPATHY, LYMPH NODE
(Plate LX-A and B are from the same patient)

In this illustration, there is a diffuse proliferation throughout the node with a residual reactive follicle. Several vessels with slightly thickened walls are noted. The cellular proliferation is heterogeneous. This process differs from immunoblastic lymphadenopathy by having follicles. Furthermore, the vascular proliferation is less prominent and lacks arborization. X80.

B. ABNORMAL IMMUNE REACTION RESEMBLING IMMUNOBLASTIC LYMPHADENOPATHY, LYMPH NODE

An extraordinary degree of plasma cell proliferation and plasmacytoid immunoblasts is dramatically demonstrated on Giemsa stain. No monomorphous areas of immunoblasts were found, and the paraffin immunoperoxidase was polytypic. Giemsa. X800.

C. ABNORMAL IMMUNE REACTION EVOLVING TO IMMUNOBLASTIC LYMPHOMA B, LYMPH NODE
(Plate LX-C and D are from the same patient)

There is a diffuse proliferation in which scattered immunoblasts and plasma cells are distributed. The immunoblasts are abnormal, as evidenced by large polypoid forms. They also have single central prominent nucleoli, and the cytoplasm is amphophilic. The development of such cytologic atypia in immunoblasts suggests immunoblastic lymphoma B. H&E. X400.

D. ABNORMAL IMMUNE REACTION EVOLVING TO IMMUNOBLASTIC LYMPHOMA B, LYMPH NODE

On paraffin immunoperoxidase, a monotypic κ-population was demonstrated in the scattered large cells. Although monomorphous areas of immunoblasts were not seen, the monotypism indicates a neoplastic process. X400.

PLATE LX

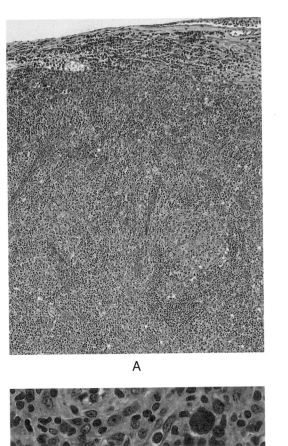

A

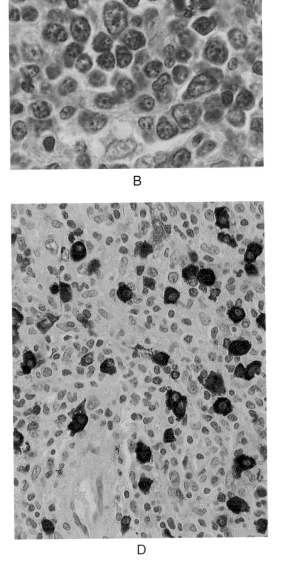

B

C

D

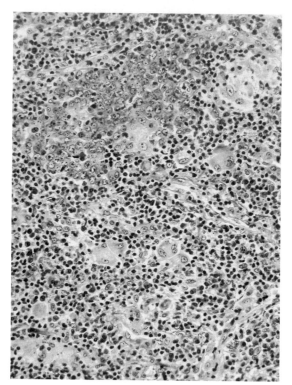

Figure 132
LUNG, ABNORMAL IMMUNE REACTION, WITH
FOCUS OF IMMUNOBLASTIC LYMPHOMA B
A large lung lesion in an elderly female is shown in this figure. There is marked plasmacytic proliferation that is polytypic. A small monomorphic collection of plasmacytoid immunoblasts is found in an area at the top, indicating evolution to immunoblastic lymphoma B. Recuts to determine monotypism by paraffin immunoperoxidase did not reveal the focus. X200.

Hodgkin's disease, immunoblastic lymphadenopathy often has a dramatic clinical onset. The predominant immunoblastic proliferation also sets immunoblastic lymphadenopathy apart, and PIP fails to show CD15 (Leu-M1) positivity in immunoblastic lymphadenopathy. The most useful differential feature may be the even effacement of nodal architecture expected in immunoblastic lymphadenopathy, in contrast to the irregularly consolidated appearance in most cases of Hodgkin's disease.

Lymphocyte depletion of AIDS. The lymphocyte depletion and vascular proliferation seen in some cases of AIDS may resemble immunoblastic lymphadenopathy. In the latter, immunoblastic proliferation and eosinophil infiltration are usually prominent; clinical features may also be helpful.

T cell lymphomas; IBL-like T cell malignant lymphoma of the Japanese. Some T cell lymphomas are associated with a pattern of hypervascularity and nodal effacement similar to immunoblastic lymphadenopathy. The large cells in these processes usually lack the amphophilic cytoplasm of B immunoblasts. The presence of aggregates of dysplastic large cells provides additional evidence of malignancy.

Immunoblastic lymphoma, B cell type. Immunoblastic lymphoma, B cell type should be diagnosed when there are clearly defined aggregates of immunoblasts producing discrete masses or sheets of cells (plate LX-C,D; fig. 132). Monotypism in the large cell population may be accepted as evidence of malignancy. These changes may be focal and difficult to find except in well-prepared material. Rebiopsy is indicated in doubtful cases; the lymphomatous processes usually evolve quickly, and second biopsies often show unequivocal changes due to lymphoma.

References

Frizzera, G., Moran, E.M., and Rappaport, H. Angioimmunoblastic lymphadenopathy with dysproteinaemia. Lancet 1:1070-1073, 1974.
Lipford, E.H., Smith, H.R., Pittaluga, S., et al. Clonality of angioimmunoblastic lymphadenopathy and implications for its evolution to malignant lymphoma. J. Clin. Invest. 79:637-642, 1987.

Lukes, R.J. and Tindle, B.H. Immunoblastic lymphadenopathy. A hyperimmune entity resembling Hodgkin's disease. N. Engl. J. Med. 292:1-8, 1975.

Additional References

Boros, L., Bhaskar, A.G., and D'Souza, J.P. Monoclonal evolution of angioimmunoblastic lymphadenopathy. Am. J. Clin. Pathol. 75:856-860, 1981.

Frizzera, G., Moran, E.M., and Rappaport, H. Angio-immunoblastic lymphadenopathy. Diagnosis and clinical course. Am. J. Med. 59:803-818, 1975.

Lukes, R.J. and Tindle, B.H. Immunoblastic lymphadenopathy: a prelymphomatous state of immunoblastic sarcoma. Recent Results Cancer Res. 64:241-246, 1978.

Nathwani, B.N., Rappaport, H., Moran, E.M., Pangalis, G.A., and Kim, H. Malignant lymphoma arising in angioimmunoblastic lymphadenopathy. Cancer 41:578-606, 1978.

Nathwani, B.N., Rappaport, H., Moran, E.M., Pangalis, G.A., and Kim, H. Evolution of immunoblastic lymphoma in angioimmunoblastic lymphadenopathy. Recent Results Cancer Res. 64:235-240, 1978.

GLUTEN-SENSITIVE ENTEROPATHY

Definition. Gluten-sensitive enteropathy is characterized by diarrhea and malabsorption induced by the presence of gluten in the diet.

Clinical Features. Adults are usually affected with diarrhea and malabsorption; symptoms promptly remit after removal of gluten from the diet. Complicating malignant lymphomas are usually found in the bowel, causing symptoms by bleeding, obstruction, or perforation. Malignant lymphomas may be diagnosed concurrently or after many years of enteropathy; their onset is usually insidious.

Pathologic and Immunologic Features. Small bowel biopsy shows villus atrophy and hyperplasia of the crypts with numerous lymphocytes and plasma cells in the lamina propria. Plasma cell infiltration may be massive. There are variable numbers of immunoblasts, some with plasmacytoid features. Plasma cells are initially polytypic.

Differential Diagnosis. *Malignant lymphoma, immunoblastic lymphoma, B and T cell.* The development of malignant lymphoma is usually insidious but may be heralded by obstructive symptoms or perforation. Most malignancies developing in this setting are now thought to have B cell or T cell features. Reports of malignant histiocytosis were probably due to the presence of large numbers of reactive histiocytes intermixed in these lymphomas (Isaacson et al., 1979, 1982, 1985). Carcinomas of the small intestine also occur at a greatly increased frequency (Swinson et al.).

References

Isaacson, P., Wright, D.H., Judd, M.A., and Mepham, B.L. Primary gastrointestinal lymphomas. Cancer 43:1805-1819, 1979.

_____, Jones, D.B., Sworn, M.J., and Wright, D.H. Malignant histiocytosis of the intestine. J. Clin. Pathol. 35:510-516, 1982.

_____, O'Connor, N.T., Spencer, J., et al. Malignant histiocytosis of the intestine. Lancet 2:688-691, 1985.

Swinson, C.M., Slavin, G., Coles, E.C., and Booth, C.C. Coeliac disease and malignancy. Lancet 1:111-115, 1983.

Additional References

Cooper, B.T., Holmes, G.K., Ferguson, R., and Cooke, W.T. Celiac disease and malignancy. Medicine (Baltimore) 59:249-261, 1980.

_____, Holmes, G.K., and Cooke, W.T. Lymphoma risk in celiac disease of later life. Digestion 23:89-92, 1982.

Filippa, D.A., Lieberman, P.H., Weingrad, D.N., DeCosse, J.J., and Bretsky, S.S. Primary lymphomas of the gastrointestinal tract. Am. J. Surg. Pathol. 7:363-372, 1983.

Freeman, H.J., Weinstein, W.M., Shnitka, T.K., Piercey, J.R., and Wensel, R.H. Primary abdominal lymphoma. Presenting manifestation of celiac sprue or complicating dermatitis herpetiformis. Am. J. Med. 63:585-594, 1977.

Holmes, G.K., Stokes, P.L., Sorahan, T.M., et al. Coeliac disease, gluten-free diet, and malignancy. Gut 17:612-619, 1976.

Morson, B.C., Dawson, I.M.P., and Spriggs, A.I. Gastrointestinal Pathology, pp. 344-358. 2nd ed. Oxford: Blackwell Scientific Publications, 1979.

Otto, H.F., Bettmann, I., Weltzien, J.V., and Gebbers, J.O. Primary intestinal lymphomas. Virchows Arch. [Pathol. Anat.] 391:9-31, 1981.

ALPHA-CHAIN DISEASE OR IMMUNOPROLIFERATIVE SMALL INTESTINAL DISEASE

Definition. This term refers to various benign and malignant conditions of the small intestine, usually seen in low socioeconomic groups, presumably because of attendant poor hygiene, poor nutrition, and high rates of intestinal infection.

Clinical Features. Patients with this disease are usually 10 to 30 years of age and present with weight loss, diarrhea, and abdominal pain. They have a history of poor hygiene, with high rates of parasitic infection and infantile enteritis. α-Heavy-chain is usually present in the serum in small quantities. The respiratory tract may be the principal site of disease in rare cases (Seligmann et al.).

Pathologic and Immunologic Features. A massive reactive plasma cell infiltrate of the lamina propria extends into the submucosa of the small intestine (Lewin et al.). Other patients may show florid follicular hyperplasia (Asselah et al.; Nassar et al.). Immunoblasts and atypical plasma cells increase over time, infiltrating the muscularis. Plasma cells contain α-heavy chain with no light chain, whereas immunoblasts contain small quantities of cytoplasmic IgA.

Differential Diagnosis. *Immunoblastic lymphoma, B cell type.* The borderline between reactive states and neoplasia, clinically and pathologically, is poorly defined in this disease. Neoplasia is indicated by an increasing density of the infiltrate, its penetration through the muscularis, the presence of dysplastic plasma cells, and aggregates of immunoblasts. Monotypism is difficult to assess because plasma cells may contain only the α–chain with no light chain, and immunoblasts often show scant amounts of cytoplasmic IgA.

References

Asselah, F., Slavin, G., Sowter, G., and Asselah, H. Immunoproliferative small intestinal disease in Algerians. I. Light microscopic and immunochemical studies. Cancer 52:227-237, 1983.

Lewin, K.J., Kahn, L.B., and Novis, B.H. Primary intestinal lymphoma of "Western" and "Mediterranean" type, alpha chain disease and massive plasma cell infiltration. Cancer 38:2511-2528, 1976.

Nassar, V., Salem, P.A., Shahid, M.J., et al. "Mediterranean abdominal lymphoma" or immunoproliferative small intestinal disease. Part II: Pathological aspects. Cancer 41:1340-1354, 1978.

Seligmann, M., Mihaesco, E., Preud'homme, J.L., Danon, F., and Brouet, J.C. Heavy chain diseases: current findings and concepts. Immunol. Rev. 48:145-167, 1979.

Additional References

Galian, A., Lecestre, M.J., Scotto, J., et al. Pathological study of alpha-chain disease, with special emphasis on evolution. Cancer 39:2081-2101, 1977.

Isaacson, P. Middle East lymphoma and alpha-chain disease. Am. J. Surg. Pathol. 3:431-441, 1979.

Khojasteh, A., Haghshenass, M., and Haghighi, P. Current concepts: immunoproliferative small intestinal disease. A "third-world lesion". N. Engl. J. Med. 308:1401-1405, 1983.

Rambaud, J.C., Galian, A., Danon, F.G., et al. Alpha-chain disease without qualitative serum IgA abnormality. Report of two cases, including a "nonsecretory" form. Cancer 51:686-693, 1983.

Salem, P.A., Nassar, V.H., Shahid, M.J., et al. "Mediterranean abdominal lymphoma" or immunoproliferative small intestinal disease. Part I: Clinical aspects. Cancer 40:2941-2947, 1977.

X-LINKED LYMPHOPROLIFERATIVE SYNDROME (DUNCAN'S SYNDROME)

Definition. The diagnosis of X-linked lymphoproliferative syndrome may be made if two or more maternally related males develop lymphoproliferative disorders (fatal mononucleosis/lymphoma) or failure of the marrow or immune systems. This syndrome has been reported in over

100 individuals in 25 kindreds. The precise immune defect has not been clearly established, but these patients may have unregulated killer and natural killer activity against Epstein-Barr virus-infected or uninfected cells (Sullivan et al.).

Clinical Features. Males usually develop clinical manifestations between the ages of 5 months and 23 years that consist of death from infectious mononucleosis, aplastic anemia, hypogammaglobulinemia, or malignant lymphoma (Barr et al.; Purtilo; Purtilo et al.; Rosen). Lymphadenopathy and hepatosplenomegaly are often massive in patients dying with infectious mononucleosis. Malignant lymphomas are seen in extranodal sites including the liver.

Pathologic and Immunologic Features. Node and spleen sections show florid immunoblastic proliferation separating and replacing lymphoid follicles with marked plasmacytosis. The portal areas of the liver are infiltrated by lymphocytes, plasma cells, and macrophages. Bone marrow is minimally involved early, although small granulomas may be present. Plasmacytoid cells are often present in the peripheral blood. T cells are usually decreased in nodes, and B cells are initially polytypic.

Differential Diagnosis. The X-linked lymphoproliferative syndrome is a relatively rare and subtle immunodeficiency easily recognized by the increased susceptibility to infectious mononucleosis. However, patients may also show increased susceptibility to bacterial, parasitic, and other viral infections. There is no specific way to diagnose the X-linked lymphoproliferative syndrome (except through the family history) until the susceptibility to infectious mononucleosis becomes apparent.

Malignant lymphoma, follicular center cell, small noncleaved cell type or immunoblastic lymphoma, B cell type. The proliferative reactions in patients with X-linked lymphoproliferative syndrome may be florid, extensive, and associated with considerable architectural distortion. Immunoblasts and plasma cells may be present in sufficiently large numbers to suggest neoplasia. The diagnosis of malignant lymphoma may be made with confidence by demonstrating monomorphic aggregates or actual tumorous masses.

References

Barr, R.S., DeLor, C.J., Clausen, K.P., et al. Fatal infectious mononucleosis in a family. N. Engl. J. Med. 290:363-367, 1974.

Purtilo, D.T. X-linked lymphoproliferative syndrome. An immunodeficiency disorder with acquired agammaglobulinemia, fatal infectious mononucleosis, or malignant lymphoma. Arch. Pathol. Lab. Med. 105:119 121, 1981.

_____, Yang, J.P., Allegra, S., et al. Hematopathology and pathogenesis of the X-linked recessive lymphoproliferative syndrome. Am. J. Med. 62:225-233, 1977.

Rosen, F.S. Lymphoma, immunodeficiency and the Epstein-Barr virus. (Editorial). N. Engl. J. Med. 297:1120-1121, 1977.

Sullivan, J.L., Byron, K.S., Brewster, F.E., Baker, S.M., and Ochs, H.D. X-linked lymphoproliferative syndrome. Natural history of the immunodeficiency. J. Clin. Invest. 71:1765-1778, 1983.

Additional References

Harada, S., Sakamoto, K., Seeley, J.K., et al. Immune deficiency in the X-linked lymphoproliferative syndrome. I. Epstein-Barr virus-specific defects. J. Immunol. 129:2532-2535, 1982.

Purtilo, D.T. Epstein-Barr virus-induced oncogenesis in immune-deficient individuals. Lancet 1:300-303, 1980.

_____. Immunopathology of infectious mononucleosis and other complications of Epstein-Barr virus infections. Pathol. Annu. 15(part 1):253-299, 1980.

_____. Immune deficiency predisposing to Epstein-Barr virus-induced lymphoproliferative diseases: the X-linked lymphoproliferative syndrome as a model. Adv. Cancer Res. 34:279-312, 1981.

Purtilo, D.T., DeFlorio, D., Jr., Hutt, L.M., et al. Variable phenotypic expression of an X-linked recessive lymphoproliferative syndrome. N. Engl. J. Med. 297:1077-1080, 1977.

_____ , Szymanski, I., Bhawan, J., et al. Epstein-Barr virus infections in the X-linked recessive lymphoproliferative syndrome. Lancet 1:798-801, 1978.

_____ , Paquin, L., DeFlorio, D., Virzi, F., and Sakhuja, R. Immunodiagnosis and immunopathogenesis of the X-linked recessive lymphoproliferative syndrome. Semin. Hematol. 16:309-343, 1979.

_____ , Sakamoto, K., Barnabei, V., et al. Epstein-Barr virus-induced diseases in boys with the X-linked lymphoproliferative syndrome (XLP): update on studies of the registry. Am. J. Med. 73:49-56, 1982.

TRANSPLANT PATIENTS ON IMMUNOSUPPRESSION WITH LYMPHOPROLIFERATIVE DISORDERS

Definition. Whole-organ transplant recipients have a higher risk (approximately 40 times higher) of developing a lymphoproliferative disorder that may occur in the transplanted organ (particularly the heart) or in native organs. Patients with multiple allotransplants are at an increased risk for this lymphoproliferative syndrome.

Clinical Features. After renal transplants, some patients develop infectious mononucleosis-like syndrome with pharyngitis, fever, and adenopathy. Lymphoproliferations in these patients are polymorphous and are potentially reversible. Approximately 5 years after transplantation, other patients may develop localized extranodal lymphomas, usually in the brain, liver, gastrointestinal tract, lung, soft tissue, or oropharynx. Epstein-Barr virus infections are implicated by serology and the presence of genomic DNA in lymphoproliferative lesions.

Pathologic and Immunologic Features. Polymorphic proliferations consist of extensive infiltrates of small and transformed lymphocytes, plasma cells, and occasional large multilobated and giant cells (Frizzera et al.). Extensive necrosis may be present. The polymorphic processes by flow, FSIP, and PIP show polyclonal processes. The presence of malignant lymphoma is indicated by masses of transformed lymphocytes or immunoblasts, some of which are plasmacytic. Typing of malignant lymphomas usually shows a monoclonal B process, but it may be null, polyclonal, and rarely T (Lippman et al.; Weintraub and Warnke). Gene rearrangement studies, even in polymorphous processes, indicate monoclonal B cell proliferations in some cases. One case in the mediastinum has marked as an immature cortical thymocyte. Various karyotypic abnormalities, including hyperdiploidy and translocations, have been described.

Differential Diagnosis. Biopsies of lymphocytic lesions in these cases are difficult to evaluate, and useful guidelines are not yet available. Lymphoproliferative processes developing shortly after a transplant are not likely to be neoplastic, although they may be associated with distressing symptoms and outcome. Such lesions are usually polymorphous and polytypic. Lymphoproliferative processes developing long after transplant may be easier to recognize as malignant lymphomas because they are often mass lesions, monomorphic in appearance, and clearly clonal. However, lesions of this type may regress after reduction of immunosuppression.

References

Frizzera, G., Hanto, D.W., Gajll-Peczalska, K.J., et al. Polymorphic diffuse B-cell hyperplasias and lymphomas in renal transplant recipients. Cancer Res. 41(11 part 1):4262-4279, 1981.

Lippman, S.M., Grogan, T.M., Carry, P., Ogden, D.A., and Miller, T.P. Post-transplantation T cell lymphoblastic lymphoma. Am. J.. Med. 82:814-816, 1987.

Weintraub, J. and Warnke, R.A. Lymphoma in cardiac allotransplant recipients. Transplantation 33:347-351, 1982.

Additional References

Cleary, M.L., Warnke, R., and Sklar, J. Monoclonality of lymphoproliferative lesions in cardiac-transplant recipients. Clonal analysis based on immunoglobulin-gene rearrangements. N. Engl. J. Med. 310:477-482, 1984.

Hanto, D.W., Gajl-Peczalska, K.J., Frizzera G., et al. Epstein-Barr virus (EBV) induced polyclonal and monoclonal B-cell lymphoproliferative diseases occurring after renal transplantation. Ann. Surg. 198:356-369, 1983.

_____ , Frizzera, G., Gajl-Peczalska, K.J., and Simmons, R.L. Epstein-Barr virus, immunodeficiency, and B cell lymphoproliferation. Transplantation 39:461-472, 1985.

Matas, A.J., Hertel, B.F., Rosai, J., Simmons, R.L., Najarian, J.S. Post transplant malignant lymphoma. Am. J. Med. 61:716-720, 1976.

LYMPHOMATOID PAPULOSIS

Definition. This lymphoproliferative disorder apparently affects only the skin. It has been traditionally considered a benign disease biologically because it may have a protracted clinical course with self-healing (Macaulay). The nature of lymphomatoid papulosis is in question because of the "malignant" histopathologic appearance and its apparent evolution to overt lymphoma in some cases.

Clinical Features. The age of onset ranges from 7 to 68 years, with an average age of 41 years. Females have an increased incidence. Patients have crops of papules and small nodules that ulcerate and then often spontaneously resolve with hyperpigmented or hypopigmented atrophic scars. Trunk and limbs are usually affected. The lesions last 3 to 8 weeks, with recurrences for many years. Ten percent of the patients develop malignant lymphoma (Weinman and Ackerman).

Pathologic and Immunologic Features. Infiltrates are usually dense, superficial and deep, wedge-shaped, and obscure the dermal-epidermal junction. Epidermal necrosis and ulceration are usually present. The epidermis near ulcers may be hyperplastic. Vasculitis has been described in approximately 10 percent of the cases. Predominant cells are large and hyperchromatic and have lobulated nuclei and scant cytoplasm (plate LXI). A small cell variant and cells with amphophilic cytoplasm and irregular nuclei containing prominent nucleoli have also been described. Reactive components consist of a mixed infiltrate with neutrophils, eosinophils, and histiocytes, whereas small lymphocytes may be interspersed among large cells. By frozen section immunoperoxidase, large cells mark as T cells, usually T helper cells, and are CD30 (Ki-1), CD2, and CD4 positive (Kadin et al.). On paraffin immunoperoxidase, CD30 (Ber H2) reactivity is noted (plate LXI-C), and CD15 (Leu-M1) positivity has been demonstrated in some cases.

Differential Diagnosis. The diagnosis of lymphomatoid papulosis may be suggested by the clinical story of recurrent crops of papular lesions that may self-heal. The histopathologic changes are often interpreted as neoplastic due to the density of large cells, their atypia, and numerous mitoses. The findings of epithelial hyperplasia or ulceration and a mixed inflammatory infiltrate are unusual in overtly lymphomatous processes involving the skin. Immunophenotypic analysis will be particularly helpful in diagnosis.

Leukemic infiltrates are usually homogeneous in appearance and rarely produce

A. This gross photograph shows a typical crop of lesions on the trunk of a patient with lymphomatoid papulosis. Some of the lesions are regressing, whereas others have recently formed.

B. In this illustration, there is marked epithelial proliferation associated with an extensive infiltrate of large cells in the upper dermis and extending into the subcutaneous tissue. X10.

C. With the CD30 antibody, numerous large positive cells were identified. This lesion subsequently regressed, and there have been no recurrences within a short period of follow-up. X40.

D. With α_1-antichymotrypsin, many cells deep in the dermis show distinct cytoplasmic positivity. Very few large cells of the type marking with CD30 are present. The large number of reacting histiocytes accounts for the presumably mistaken designation of "relapsing histiocytosis" for some cases of this type.

E. At high magnification, the predominant cell is large and has abundant cytoplasm. Some multinucleated cells are present. PAS. X600.

PLATE LXI

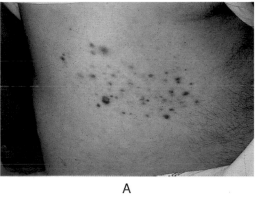

A

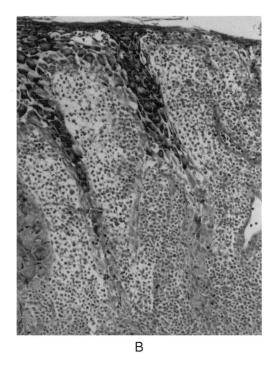

B

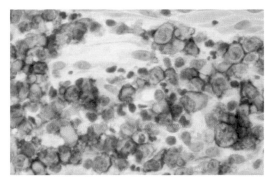

C

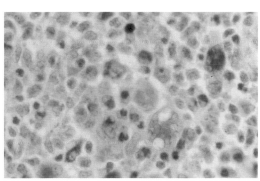

D

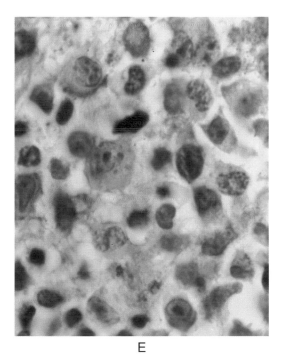

E

significant epithelial changes. Inflammatory dermatoses, and even drug reactions, usually contain few large cells.

References

Kadin, M.E., Nasu, K., Sako, D., Said, J., and Vonderheid, E. Lymphomatoid papulosis. Am. J. Surg. Pathol. 119:315-325, 1985.

Macaulay, W.L. Lymphomatoid papulosis. A continuing self-healing eruption clinically benign—histologically malignant. Arch. Dermatol. 97:23-30, 1968.

Weinman, V.F. and Ackerman, A.B. Lymphomatoid papulosis. Am. J. Dermatol. 3:129-163, 1981.

Additional References

Kadin, M.E., Vonderheid, E.C., Sako, D., Clayton, L.K., and Olbricht, S. Clonal composition of T cells in lymphomatoid papulosis. Am. J. Pathol. 126:13-17, 1987.

Sanchez, N.P., Pittelkow, M.R., Muller, S.A., Banks, P.M., and Winkelmann, R.K. The clinicopathologic spectrum of lymphomatoid papulosis: study of 31 cases. J. Am. Acad. Dermatol. 8:81-94, 1983.

Weiss, L.M., Wood, G.S., Trela, M., Warnke, R.A., and Sklar, J. Clonal T-cell populations in lymphomatoid papulosis. N. Engl. J. Med. 315:475-479, 1986.

Willemze, R., Meyer, C.J., van Vloten, W.A., and Scheffer, E. The clinical and histological spectrum of lymphomatoid papulosis. Br. J. Dermatol. 107:131-144, 1982.

LEUKEMOID REACTIONS

Definition. Leukemoid reactions refer to changes in the peripheral blood that resemble leukemia; neutrophilia is most common, but eosinophilia, basophilia, and monocytosis also occur.

Clinical Features. Patients with leukemoid reactions are usually adults with neoplasms or infections, particularly tuberculosis. Patients with leukemoid reactions are almost always symptomatic from underlying diseases, and the process may resolve with appropriate successful treatment.

Pathologic and Immunologic Features. In neutrophilic leukemoid reactions, mature granulocytes predominate in the peripheral blood; immature forms are rare,

and there is minimal eosinophilia and basophilia. Mature monocytes may be increased. Leukocyte alkaline phosphatase score is higher than normal. Marrow sections show moderate hypercellularity and obvious differentiation to mature forms. Marrows are rarely completely cellular, and the Philadelphia chromosome is absent.

Differential Diagnosis. Chronic myeloid leukemia may be ruled out by the rarity of immature forms in the peripheral blood, as well as minimal eosinophilia and basophilia. Normal or high leukocyte alkaline phosphatase score and the absence of the Philadelphia chromosome are confirmatory.

Chronic myelomonocytic leukemia usually has a marrow and peripheral monocytosis (often dramatically demonstrated by α-naphthyl acetate esterase positivity) and minimal basophilia and eosinophilia. Clinical findings in leukemoid reaction are also often more dramatic.

MYELODYSPLASTIC SYNDROMES

Patients with myelodysplasia usually have hypercellular marrows but peripheral cytopenias associated with characteristic morphologic abnormalities. These are clonal disorders, probably at the multi- or pluripotential stem cell level, as proven by karyotypic abnormalities and G6PD isotype. The clone retains a capacity to differentiate, but there is varied lineage penetrance with abnormalities in one or all cell lines. Clonal instability is manifest by culmination in acute leukemia in a significant percentage of patients.

Definition. The most widely used classification is that of the French-American-British group (Bennett; Bennett et al.), which has the following diagnostic categories: (1) refractory anemia; (2) refractory anemia with increased sideroblasts; (3) refractory anemia with excess blasts; and (4) refractory anemia with excess blasts in transformation. Chronic myelomonocytic leukemia is also included in the French-American-British classification of myelodysplastic syndrome, but chronic myelomonocytic leukemia is considered separately here because it seems to meet the criteria of a neoplasm. Tables 59 and 60 present the diagnostic criteria for these different types of myelodysplasia.

Clinical Features. Patients are usually elderly, and the diseases are very rare in individuals under the age of 60 years. Disease in the elderly is particularly likely to occur without a prior history of chemotherapy or radiotherapy, whereas the converse is true in those under 60 years. The incidence in people over 60 may be 1 per 1000 per year. This disease is found predominantly in males, although this preponderance may be obscured in the very elderly due to excess mortality of the male population. Patients often present with incidentally discovered cytopenias, marrow failure, or infections. The overall median survival is 27 months, although this is a prognostically diverse group. Progression to acute leukemia occurs in less than half of all patients. The natural history of these cases is fairly diverse (Hamblin and Oscier). Some patients show a gradual increase in marrow blasts with increasing pancytopenia, and their illness may terminate in either marrow failure or leukemia. Others show an abrupt transformation to acute leukemia, with this transformation occurring at any time and usually with a change in karyotypic abnormalities. Other patients, particularly those with a refractory anemia or refractory anemia with ringed sideroblasts, may follow a stable course for years.

Pathologic Features. Characteristic morphologic abnormalities may be noted in both peripheral blood and bone marrow (Tables 59, 60). Biopsies and marrow film should be evaluated to detect the morphologic abnormalities that may affect all hematopoietic lineages. The marrow biopsy is useful in evaluating the distorted marrow topography that may appear as a reversal of the usual location of myelopoiesis and erythropoiesis, with myelopoiesis being abnormally and centrally located in myelodysplastic syndromes (Tricot et al., 1984a,b). Marrow biopsies may also show stromal abnormalities such as areas of edema, ectatic sinuses, perivascular fibrosis, and increased reticulin. Diagnoses are most apparent when there is a trilineage myelodysplasia accompanied by hypercellular bone marrow but with peripheral cytopenia. However, single or bilineage myelodysplasia also occurs, and some patients have hypocellular bone marrows.

Karyotypic Features. Chromosomal abnormalities are detected in 40 to approximately 80 percent of patients with myelodysplastic syndromes, and survival may be partially predicted by chromosomal analysis (Yunis et al.). The most common chromosomal abnormalities are 5Q–, 20Q–, trisomy 8, monosomy 5, monosomy 7, and loss of the Y chromosome. The chromosomal abnormalities regularly seen in the acute myeloid leukemias are not seen in myelodysplastic syndrome, and the Philadelphia chromosome is very rare. Patients with refractory macrocytic anemia and morphologic abnormalities of megakaryocytes (small mononuclear forms) often have an interstitial deletion of the long arm of chromosome 5 (Niemer and Golde).

Other Studies. Bone marrow culture studies show that there are at least two

Table 59

FRENCH-AMERICAN-BRITISH CLASSIFICATION OF MYELODYSPLASTIC SYNDROMES*

Type	Peripheral Blood	Bone Marrow
Refractory anemia	< 1 percent blasts	< 5 percent blasts; dyspoiesis in one or all lineages; ringed sideroblasts are not to exceed 15 percent
Refractory anemia with ringed sideroblasts	< 1 percent blasts	As refractory anemia, with >15 percent of ringed sideroblasts
Refractory anemia with excess of blasts	< 5 percent blasts	As refractory anemia, with 5 to 20 percent blasts
Refractory anemia with excess blasts in transformation	< 5 percent blasts; blasts may contain Auer rods	As refractory anemia, with 20 to 30 percent blasts or 5 to 20 percent blasts with Auer rods

* Modified from Hamblin and Oscier

patterns of myeloid colony growth that may have prognostic significance (List et al.). These have been designated as leukemic and nonleukemic. The nonleukemic pattern is marked by persistent colony formation accompanied by small clusters with modest maturation impairment, whereas the leukemic growth shows absent or reduced colony growth. In patients studied serially, evolution from a nonleukemic to leukemic pattern has been demonstrated with disease progression.

Differential Diagnosis. The French-American-British criteria are based in part on numerical guidelines; few pathologists or hematologists are entirely comfortable with strict adherence to numeric criteria for purposes of making diagnoses in practice. The evaluation of chromosomal abnormalities may be the single most important prognostic factor in these patients and perhaps with time may become very specific

as a diagnostic criterion as well. Dysmyelopoiesis is not limited to the myelodysplastic syndromes because morphologically and clinically similar features may be seen in megaloblastic anemia, regenerating bone marrows after chemotherapy, and in the marrow after toxic injury such as alcohol.

References

Bennett, J.M. Classification of the myelodysplastic syndromes. Clin. Haematol. 15:909-923, 1986.

_____ , Catovsky, D., Daniel, M.T., et al. Proposals for the classification of the myelodysplastic syndromes. Br. J. Haematol. 51:189-199, 1982.

Hamblin, T.J. and Oscier, D.G. The myelodysplastic syndrome—a practical guide. Hematol. Oncol. 5:19-34, 1987.

List, A.F., Garewal, H.S., and Sandberg, A.A. The myelodysplastic syndromes: biology and implications for management. J. Clin. Oncol. 8:1424-1441, 1990.

Nimer, S.D. and Golde, D.W. The 5q– abnormality. Blood 70:1705-1712, 1987.

Table 60

MORPHOLOGIC ABNORMALITIES IN PERIPHERAL BLOOD AND BONE MARROW IN MYELODYSPLASTIC SYNDROMES*

Lineage	Peripheral Blood	Bone Marrow
Erythroid	Oval macrocytes; dimorphic picture; normoblasts; reticulocytopenia; polychromasia, punctate basophilia	Multinuclear erythroids or nuclear buds; Howell-Jolly bodies; megaloblasts; ringed sideroblasts; PAS+ normoblasts
Megakaryocytic	Giant platelets; agranular platelets	Variation in size, particularly with dwarf forms; single oval nuclei or multiple small nuclei
Leukocytic	Variation in granularity and lobation	Hypogranularity and increased blasts

* Modified from Hamblin and Oscier

Tricot, G., De Wolf-Peeters, C., Hendrickx, B., and Verwilghen, R.L. Bone marrow histology in myelodysplastic syndromes. I. Histological findings in myelodysplastic syndromes and comparison with bone marrow smears. Br. J. Haematol. 57:423-430, 1984a.

_____ , De Wolf-Peeters, C., Vlietinck, R., and Verwilghen, R.L.. Bone marrow histology in myelodysplastic syndromes. II. Prognostic value of abnormal localization of immature precursors in MDS. Br. J. Haematol. 58:217-225, 1984b.

Yunis, J.J., Rydell, R.E., Oken, M.M., et al. Refined chromosome analysis as an independent prognostic indicator in de novo myelodysplastic syndromes. Blood 67:1721-1730, 1986.

MYELOPROLIFERATIVE SYNDROMES

The term myeloproliferative disorder proposed by Damashek in 1951 brings together in a single broad group a variety of interrelated myeloid disorders with manifestations of ineffective or failing hematopoiesis. Morphologically, they exhibit features of combined dysplastic proliferation of all myeloid series, such as erythroid, granulocytic, and megakaryocytic, usually with a dominance of one series (plates LXII, LXIII). Commonly, there is a change in the dominant component during the evolution of the disease process. In addition, this combined proliferation is joined by the mesenchymal components in the marrow stroma, known as myelofibrosis, and bone, known as myelosclerosis.

Definition. The various terms used relate to the dominating marrow/soft tissue component and its peripheral blood expression. Myeloid metaplasia refers to the abnormal myeloid proliferations in extramedullary sites such as the liver, spleen, and bone marrow.

Agnogenic myeloid metaplasia is used for the syndrome of abnormal extramedullary proliferations in patients with large spleens and myelofibrosis (Ward and Block); the latter is a distinctive fibrillary

PLATE LXII

A. MYELOFIBROSIS, MARROW BIOPSY
(Plate LXII-A and B are from the same patient)

This low magnification photomicrograph shows marked replacement of the marrow space by hypocellular connective tissue, irregular thickening of the bony trabeculae, and absence of most of the hematopoietic elements. X8.

B. MYELOFIBROSIS, MARROW BIOPSY

A higher magnification illustration shows very few hematopoietic elements, with the exception of megakaryocytes. There is moderate connective tissue deposition. X80.

C. PANMYELOSIS, MARROW BIOPSY
(Plate LXII-C and D are from the same patient)

This photograph shows the cellular phase of agnogenic myeloid metaplasia. The marrow is moderately cellular, with a suggestion of increased connective tissue. X8.

D. PANMYELOSIS, MARROW BIOPSY

On higher magnification, a few foci of the marrow show connective tissue deposition, loss of hematopoietic tissue, and scattered megakaryocytes similar to those in plate LXII-B. X80.

E. PANMYELOSIS IN POLYCYTHEMIA RUBRA VERA, MARROW PARTICLE
(Plate LXII-E and F are from the same patient)

The marrow in this disorder is typically greater than 80 percent cellular and shows trilineage hyperplasia. X20.

F. PANMYELOSIS IN POLYCYTHEMIA RUBRA VERA, MARROW PARTICLE

A high magnification examination shows trilineage hyperplasia, numerous dysplastic hypersegmented megakaryocytes, and a rare mononuclear megakaryocyte. The erythroid hypercellularity and the megakaryocytic abnormalities are helpful in the recognition of polycythemia vera. X80.

G. PANMYELOSIS, IDIOPATHIC THROMBOCYTHEMIA, MARROW PARTICLE

The marrow in this disorder may closely resemble that of polycythemia vera. Megakaryocytes are usually clumped and moderately increased in number, whereas erythroid elements are not prominent. X30.

PLATE LXII

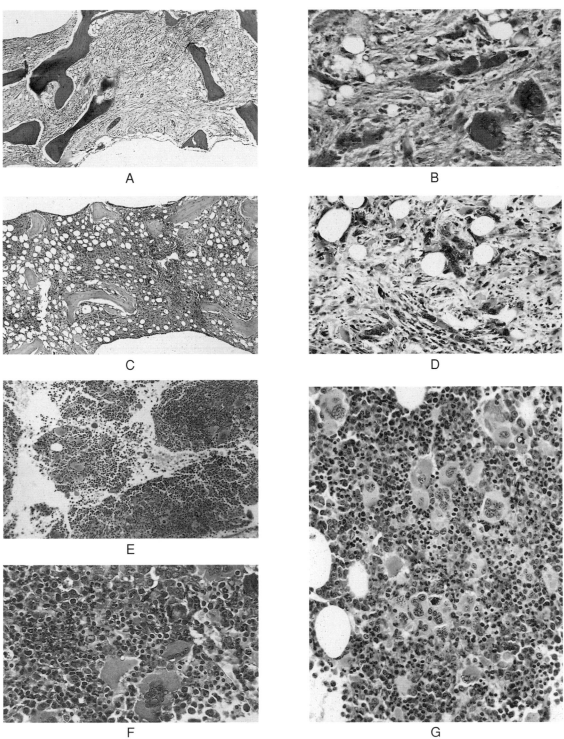

A

B

C

D

E

F

G

PLATE LXIII

A. MEGAKARYOCYTIC MYELOSIS, LYMPH NODE
(Plate LXIII-A–C are from the same patient)

A patient with marked leukocytosis has distorted lymph node architecture. Abnormal megakaryocytes are distributed throughout this node, principally in sinuses. X40.

B. MEGAKARYOCYTIC MYELOSIS, LYMPH NODE

At a higher magnification, the abnormal megakaryocytes are dramatically evident in the lymph node sinuses. X100.

C. MEGAKARYOCYTIC MYELOSIS, LYMPH NODE

The bizarre nuclear lobation features of the abnormal dysplastic megakaryocytes are demonstrated in this illustration. X400

D. MEGAKARYOCYTIC MYELOSIS WITH MYELOFIBROSIS, AUTOPSY BONE MARROW

Numerous dysplastic megakaryocytes are scattered through a hypocellular, somewhat fibrotic marrow. The bony trabeculae are unaltered. X50.

PLATE LXIII

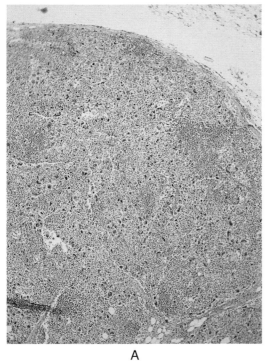

A

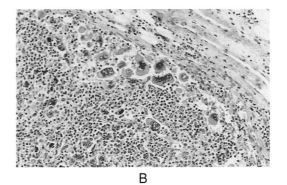

B

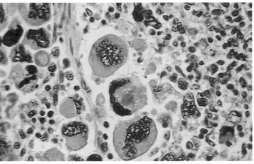

C

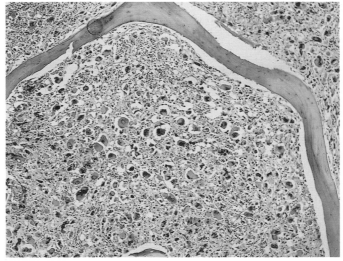

D

connective tissue replacement of the marrow in which dysplastic megakaryocytes occur in interlocking clusters. The term panmyelosis is used when all dysplastic myeloid series are found, whereas megakaryocytic myelosis is used when the megakaryocytic series is dominant. Polycythemia vera is considered a panmyelosis with absolute erythrocytosis. Essential thrombocythemia is a panmyelosis with marked megakaryocytic hyperplasia and thrombocytosis. Leukoerythroblastic anemia refers to the peripheral blood manifestations in which abnormal forms of each series are found in the peripheral blood in association with anemia.

Various terms have been used for the hyperleukocytosis associated with myeloproliferative disorders, including chronic myelogenous leukemia of the aged or Philadelphia chromosome negative leukemia. The marrow typically exhibits combined proliferations, often with myelofibrosis, dysplastic megakaryocytes, and even megakaryocytic myelosis in extramedullary sites.

Clinical Features. In agnogenic myeloid metaplasia, middle-aged and elderly patients slowly develop anemia and splenomegaly. The median survival rate is 4 to 5 years, and patients may develop acute leukemia (Pitcock et al.).

Polycythemia vera is a chronic disease with pruritus and hemorrhagic and thrombotic tendencies and is seen in middle-aged and elderly patients. The median survival is greater than 11 years, and patients may develop myelofibrosis or acute leukemia. In essential thrombocythemia, adults usually present with recurrent hemorrhages or thromboembolic phenomena. Platelet counts are routinely greater than $1 \times 10^6/\mu L$.

Pathologic and Immunologic Features. Agnogenic myeloid metaplasia has characteristic marrow changes consisting of trilineage hyperplasia with numerous megakaryocytes, progressing to hypocellularity, marrow fibrosis, and osteosclerosis (plate LXII-A–D). The peripheral blood shows leukoerythroblastic anemia with teardrop erythrocytes. Extramedullary hematopoiesis may be seen in the spleen, liver, lymph nodes, or soft tissue sites such as the retroperitoneum or mediastinum. Marrow changes in polycythemia vera are moderate to marked hypercellularity with trilineage hyperplasia (plate LXII-E,F). Myelofibrosis may develop. This is a clonal proliferation and there may be chromosomal abnormalities. In essential thrombocythemia, there is moderate hypercellularity with trilineage hyperplasia. Megakaryocytes are increased above 10 to 12 per high power field and are found in clusters (plate LXII-G). Megakaryocytes may be mononuclear or have unusually dense nuclear chromatin. Clumping of megakaryocytes is usually seen. Megakaryocytes may be particularly bizarre in some cases of panmyelosis, and the Philadelphia chromosome is not present (plate LXIII).

Differential Diagnosis. Leukemia may develop in any of the myeloproliferative disorders and is heralded by rising blast percentages in the peripheral blood or aggregates of blasts in the marrow. The development of acute leukemia in polycythemia vera may be treatment related. Chronic myeloid leukemia may closely resemble all of the myeloproliferative disorders and may be diagnosed by the demonstration of the Philadelphia chromosome.

References

Damashek, W. Some speculations on the myeloproliferative syndromes. Blood 6:372-375, 1951

Pitcock, J.A., Reinhard, E.H., Justus, B.W., and Mendelsohn, R.S. A clinical and pathological study of seventy cases of myelofibrosis. Ann. Intern. Med. 57:73, 1962.

Ward, H. and Block, M. The natural history of agnogenic myeloid metaplasia (AMM) and a critical evaluation of its relationship with the myeloproliferative syndrome. Medicine (Baltimore) 50:357-420, 1971.

Additional References

Ellis, J.T., Silver, R.T., Coleman, M., and Geller, S.A. The bone marrow in polycythemia vera. Semin. Hematol. 12:433-434, 1975.

Gunz, F.W. Hemorrhagic thrombocythemia: a critical review. Blood 15:706-723, 1960.

Kurnick, J.E., Ward, H.P., and Block, M.H. Bone marrow sections in the differential diagnosis of polycythemia. Arch. Pathol. 94:489-499, 1972.

Silverstein, M.N. Primary or hemorrhagic thrombocythemia. Arch. Intern. Med. 122:18-22, 1968.

_____. The evolution into and the treatment of late stage polycythemia vera. Semin. Hematol. 13:79-84, 1976.

_____ and Linman, J.W. Causes of death in agnogenic myeloid metaplasia. Mayo Clin. Proc. 44:36-39, 1969.

PROLIFERATIONS OF MONONUCLEAR PHAGOCYTES

The classification of these uncommon diseases is difficult. Functional subpopulations of histiocytes are imprecisely identified, specific criteria for mononuclear phagocyte identification have not been observed, and cases of fatal disseminated disease have often been accepted as malignant regardless of morphology.

Histiocytic infiltration and proliferation vary widely in degree, are ubiquitous in distribution, produce numerous disease states, and are described under a variety of terms. Most of these proliferations are obviously limited in malignant potential (plate LXV-C–E), or the malignant component is probably not histiocytic (i.e., malignant fibrous histiocytoma). One of the most dramatic processes simulating malignant lymphoma is sinus histiocytosis with massive adenopathy.

SINUS HISTIOCYTOSIS WITH MASSIVE ADENOPATHY

Definition. This is a reactive adenopathy, possibly infectious, associated with striking and characteristic architectural changes in nodes and soft tissue.

Clinical Features. Black children are usually affected and have bilateral, painless, massive cervical adenopathy; fever; leukocytosis; anemia; and polyclonal hypergammaglobulinemia. Occasionally, subcutaneous, central nervous system, kidney, or orbital lesions are noted. Deaths are rare, but no cases with transformation to malignant lymphoma or malignant histiocytosis have been reported.

Pathologic and Immunologic Features. Residual follicular centers are sparse or absent, whereas sinuses are packed with histiocytes with intervening islands of lymphoid tissue (plate LXIV-A) (Lampert and Lennert; Rosai and Dorfman). Capsular fibrosis may be a prominent feature. Plasmacytosis is seen in medullary areas and may be marked. Histiocytes show minimal to moderate nuclear atypia, but emperopolesis is prominent in typical cases, with lymphocytes and red cells in the histiocytes (plate LXIV-B,C). Otherwise typical cases may show minimal emperopolesis (plate LXV-A,B). Plasma cells are polytypic in this condition.

Differential Diagnosis. Malignant histiocytosis might be suspected if small biopsies were obtained from atypical sites (e.g., abdomen). Furthermore, histiocytic nuclei may show atypia. The extreme rarity of malignant histiocytosis and the occasional extranodal involvement of sinus histiocytosis warrant a conservative approach in these unusual circumstances (plate LXIV-D).

PLATE LXIV

A. SINUS HISTIOCYTOSIS WITH MASSIVE LYMPHADENOPATHY, LYMPH NODE
(Plate LXIV-A–C are from the same patient)
This patient was a 16 year old male with a 6 month history of a progressively enlarging nontender submandibular mass. There were no other symptoms. The patient had been treated with an antituberculous agent because of a positive tuberculin skin test. His complete blood count and protein electrophoresis were normal. Two lymph nodes were removed, each measuring 4.0x3.0x2.5 cm. In this photomicrograph, the lymph node architecture is markedly distorted by a dramatic population of large pale-staining cytoplasmic cells that expand the sinuses and compress the small amount of residual lymphoid tissue. X40. (Courtesy of Dr. R.F. Dorfman, Palo Alto, CA.)

B. SINUS HISTIOCYTOSIS, WITH MASSIVE LYMPHADENOPATHY, LYMPH NODE
This large dilated sinus contains numerous histiocytes with intact lymphocytes packed in their cytoplasm. X100. (Courtesy of Dr. R.F. Dorfman, Palo Alto, CA.)

C. SINUS HISTIOCYTOSIS, WITH MASSIVE LYMPHADENOPATHY, LYMPH NODE
The cytoplasm of most histiocytes is pale and markedly vacuolated. The frequency of histiocytes containing lymphocytes varies from area to area; here, they are less frequent. The histiocytes with cytoplasmic lymphocytes have acidophilic cytoplasm. X400. (Courtesy of Dr. R.F. Dorfman, Palo Alto, CA.)

D. HISTIOCYTOSIS, EYE
This 50 year old black male from Nigeria presented with multiple cutaneous and subcutaneous nodules and a mass in the left orbit. There was no palpable lymphadenopathy, and the patient was otherwise asymptomatic. It was necessary to remove the eye. The skin nodule was also biopsied. A section reveals the massiveness of the orbital lesion and extension to the cornea. At this magnification, the numerous pale-staining foci resemble the sinus histiocyte aggregates in the other case shown on this plate. X3. (Courtesy of Dr. R.F. Dorfman, Palo Alto, CA.)

PLATE LXIV

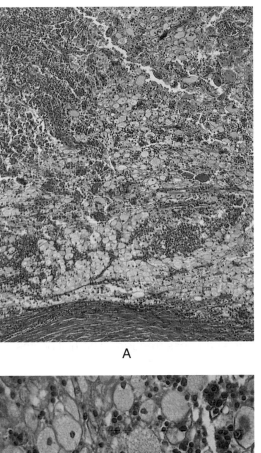

A

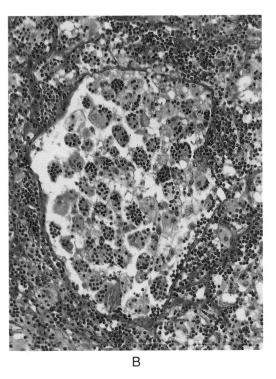

B

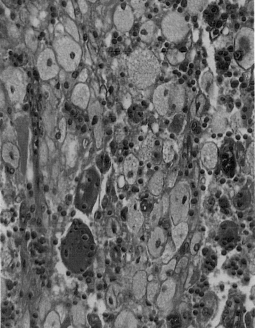

C

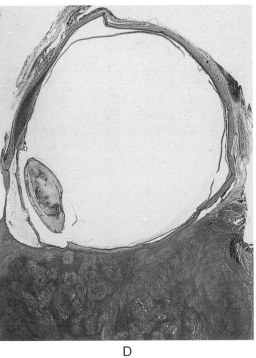

D

PLATE LXV

A. SINUS HISTIOCYTOSIS WITHOUT LYMPHOCYTE EMPEROPOLESIS, LYMPH NODE
(Plate LXV-A and B are from the same patient)

In this illustration, widely dilated sinuses packed with pale cytoplasmic cells distort the architecture and compress the remaining lymphoid tissue into narrow zones. H&E. X35.

B. SINUS HISTIOCYTOSIS WITHOUT LYMPHOCYTE EMPEROPOLESIS, LYMPH NODE

The cells filling these sinuses have a pale finely vacuolated cytoplasm, well-demarcated cellular borders, and round to oval small nuclei. The medullary tissue is packed with normal-appearing plasma cells. H&E. X400.

C. HISTIOCYTOSIS, SKIN (HISTIOCYTOMA)
(Plate LXV-C–E are from the same patient)

An 18 year old asymptomatic male discovered a scalp nodule that was 1.7 cm in diameter. No bone lesions were discovered. Acid phosphatase and nonspecific esterase (α-naphthyl butyrate) were both strongly positive (not shown). An infiltrate composed predominantly of large cytoplasmic histiocytes extends throughout the dermis and up to the epidermis. H&E. X100.

D. HISTIOCYTOSIS, SKIN (HISTIOCYTOMA)

The cytoplasm is more amphophilic in the periphery of the mononuclear and giant cells in this Giemsa stain. Giemsa. X400.

E. HISTIOCYTOSIS, SKIN (HISTIOCYTOMA)

In this illustration, the cytoplasm is lightly pyroninophilic in the mononuclear forms and heavily pyroninophilic in the giant cells, reflecting the variable RNA content of the cytoplasm. The nucleoli are clearly demonstrated in this MGP stain. The peripheral intensity of staining in both Giemsa and MGP stains differs from the staining of immunoblasts. MGP. X400.

PLATE LXV

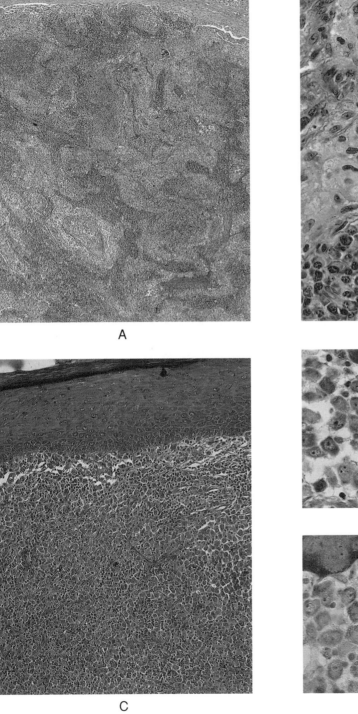

A

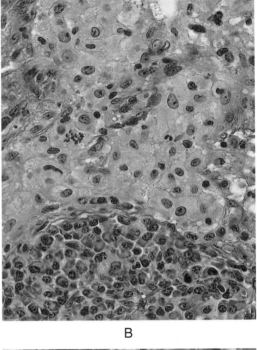

B

C

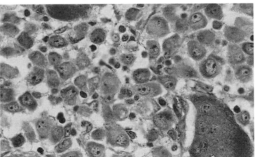

D

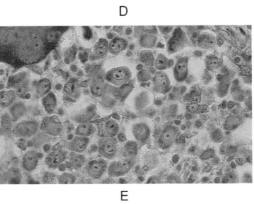

E

Marked proliferation of sinus macrophages may occur as an isolated phenomenon, apparently without clinical significance (fig. 133).

References

Lampert, F. and Lennert, K. Sinus histiocytosis with massive lymphadenopathy. Cancer 37:783-789, 1976.

Rosai, J. and Dorfman, R.F. Sinus histiocytosis with massive lymphadenopathy: a pseudolymphomatous benign disorder. Cancer 30:1174-1188, 1972.

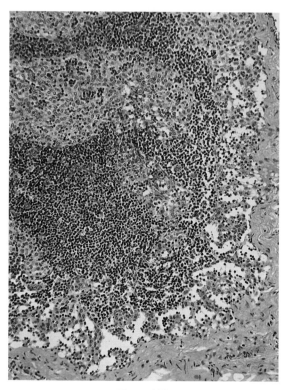

Figure 133
SINUS HISTIOCYTOSIS, LYMPH NODE
In this figure, a subcapsular sinus is slightly distended, and there is normal adjacent nodal tissue. The sieve-like arrangement of sinus macrophages is apparent. In the deeper portions of the node, the sinuses were packed by sinus lining cells. H&E. X80.

HISTIOCYTOSIS X, FOCAL AND DISSEMINATED

Diseases characterized by a proliferation of benign-appearing histiocytes containing Langerhans granules have usually been divided into three entities: eosinophilic granuloma, Hand-Schuller-Christian syndrome, and Letterer-Siwe disease. The nature of the proliferative process (i.e., neoplasm versus immunologic reaction) is unknown, and there is disagreement as to whether these entities represent a spectrum of one disease or distinct disorders. Farber and, later, Lichenstein (1953, 1964) proposed the former, whereas Daneshbod and Kissane (1976, 1978) and Lieberman and colleagues believed that at least two separate and distinct processes are involved, with Hand-Schuller-Christian syndrome being a type of polyostotic eosinophilic granuloma and Letterer-Siwe disease in a class by itself.

Most histiocytoses of cells with Langerhans granules fall into one of the above categories, but the classification remains incomplete. Some cases of fatal disseminated disease do not fit the clinical definition of Letterer-Siwe disease; for example, the patients are not infants with a skin rash and hepatosplenomegaly. Whether these patients have a form of "polyostotic eosinophilic granuloma" with visceral involvement or a modified type of Letterer-Siwe disease remains unclear and demonstrates the blurred clinical and pathologic features of these disorders.

Definition. Histiocytosis X is a proliferation of benign-appearing histiocytes containing Langerhans granules. There are several clinical expressions. Eosinophilic granuloma may be monostotic or polyostotic or present in the skin, lymph nodes, or lungs; Letterer-Siwe disease has skin rash and hepatosplenomegaly as its major manifestations.

Clinical Features. Eosinophilic granuloma (localized or widespread) is most common in the first decade. Involved sites are the skull, ribs, femur, skin, nodes, and, less frequently, lung. This disease has a good prognosis, and some lesions regress spontaneously. The triad of bony lesions, exophthalmos, and diabetes insipidus is called Hand-Schuller-Christian syndrome. Letterer-Siwe disease occurs in infants less than 3 years of age and causes hepatosplenomegaly and a generalized skin rash with accentuation in axillary and inguinal areas (plate LXVI-C).

Pathologic and Immunologic Features. Eosinophilic granuloma is charac-terized by masses of Langerhans histiocytes and eosinophils in varying numbers, usually in sinuses (plate LXVI-A,B). Giant cells and areas of necrosis may produce a granulomatous appearance. In Letterer-Siwe disease, the infiltrate of bland histiocytes is more monomorphous, and there are few eosinophils. In all cases, histiocyte nuclei have characteristic longitudinal grooving on touch imprints (plate LXVI-D,E; fig. 134) or tissue sections, with fine chromatin patterns. Electron microscopy shows Langerhans granules (fig. 135).

Differential Diagnosis. Eosinophilic granuloma involving the nodes may be confused with Hodgkin's disease because of the architectural distortion and granulomatous features with giant cells and eosinophils.

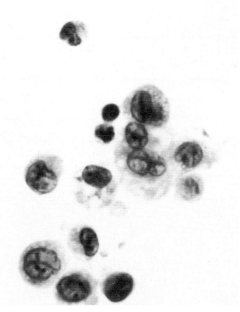

Figure 134
HISTIOCYTOSIS X, IMPRINT OF LYMPH NODE
The nuclear grooves are seen clearly in this touch imprint. H&E. X500.

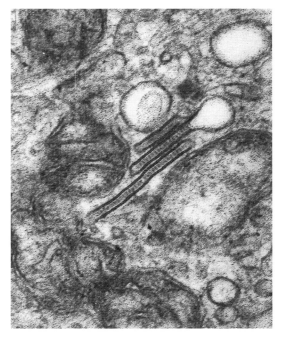

Figure 135
HISTIOCYTOSIS, EOSINOPHILIC GRANULOMA
At high magnification, a Langerhans granule is shown to be a rod- or flask-shaped structure with a central zipper-like component. X102,900.

PLATE LXVI

A. HISTIOCYTOSIS X, EOSINOPHILIC GRANULOMA, LYMPH NODE
(Plate LXVI-A and B are from the same patient)

This illustration shows partial architectural distortion due to infiltration of sinuses by histiocytes and eosinophils. Areas of necrosis are present. X27.

B. HISTIOCYTOSIS X, EOSINOPHILIC GRANULOMA, LYMPH NODE

At higher magnification, a sinus contains numerous histiocytes and eosinophils. Giant cells may be present in eosinophilic granuloma but are not shown in this illustration. X140.

C. HISTIOCYTOSIS X, LETTERER-SIWE DISEASE

This photograph shows emaciation, abdominal distension (due to hepatosplenomegaly), and hemorrhagic skin rash seen in some fatal cases of this disease.

D. HISTIOCYTOSIS X, LETTERER-SIWE DISEASE, LYMPH NODE
(Plate LXVI-D and E are from the same patient)

In this illustration, the lymph node architecture is replaced by a widely distributed histiocytic proliferation; the capsule is markedly thickened by the same process. X30.

E. HISTIOCYTOSIS X, LETTERER-SIWE DISEASE

At a higher magnification, the histiocytes have a variable amount of pale-staining acidophilic cytoplasm with ill-defined cellular borders. The nuclei are round to oval and often folded with a central linear groove, imparting a monocytoid appearance to the cell. X315.

PLATE LXVI

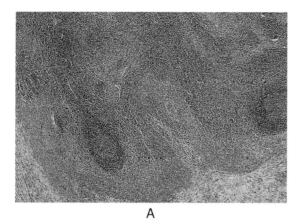

A

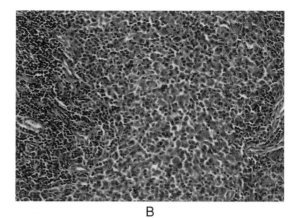

B

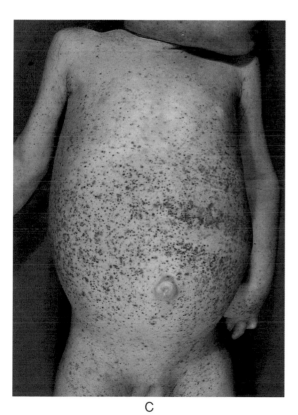

C

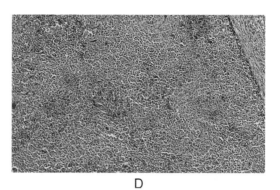

D

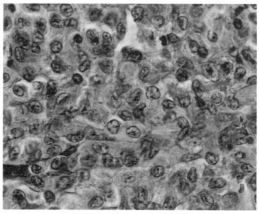

E

References

Daneshbod, K. and Kissane, J.M. Histiocytosis. The prognosis of polyostotic eosinophilic granuloma. Am. J. Clin. Pathol. 65:601-611, 1976.

_____ and Kissane, J.M. Idiopathic differentiated histiocytosis. Am. J. Clin. Pathol. 70:381-389, 1978.

Farber, S. The nature of "solitary or eosinophilic granuloma" of bone. Am. J. Pathol. 17:625-629, 1941.

Lichtenstein, L. Histiocytosis-X. Integration of eosinophilic granuloma of bone, "Letterer-Siwe disease" and "Schuller-Christian disease" as related manifestations of a single nosologic entity. Arch. Pathol. 56:84-102, 1953.

_____ . Histiocytosis X (eosinophilic granuloma of bone, Letterer-Siwe disease, and Schüller-Christian disease). J. Bone Joint Surg. 46A:76-90, 1964.

Lieberman, P.H., Jones, C.R., Haghbin, M., and Murphy, M.L. Further thoughts on the eosinophilic granuloma problem. Gann Monogr. Cancer Res. 15:305-315, 1973.

Additional References

Motoi, M., Helbron, D., Kaiserling, E., and Lennert, K. Eosinophilic granuloma of lymph nodes—a variant of histiocytosis X. Histopathology 4:585-606, 1980.

Newton, W.A. and Hamoudi, A.B. Histiocytosis: a histologic classification with clinical correlation. Perspect. Pediatr. Pathol. 1:251-283, 1973.

Vogel, J.M. and Vogel, P. Idiopathic histiocytosis. Semin. Hematol. 9:349-369, 1972.

VIRUS-ASSOCIATED HEMOPHAGOCYTIC SYNDROME

Definition. Virus-associated hemophagocytic syndrome is an immune deficiency associated with a serious and often fatal response to viral infections and is accompanied by prominent histiocytic proliferation and erythrophagocytosis (McKenna et al.; Risdall et al.). Familial hemophagocytic reticulosis may be an inherited immunodeficiency causing a predisposition to the hemophagocytic syndrome.

Clinical Features. Virus-associated hemophagocytic syndrome may affect children or adults. Most patients are on immunosuppressive therapy. Occasional previously healthy patients have developed symptoms after Epstein-Barr virus infections (Wilson et al.). The disease has a relatively abrupt onset with fever, severe constitutional symptoms, hepatosplenomegaly, diffuse pulmonary infiltrates, and skin rash. Leukopenia, thrombocytopenia, and disseminated intravascular coagulation are common. The mortality rate is estimated to be 30 to 40 percent.

Pathologic and Immunologic Features. Cellularity in the marrow may vary, partly due to the underlying diseases and their treatment. Histiocytes and macrophages are moderately increased but do not produce mass lesions and are uniformly bland in appearance (fig. 136). Phagocytosis of red cells, platelets, or

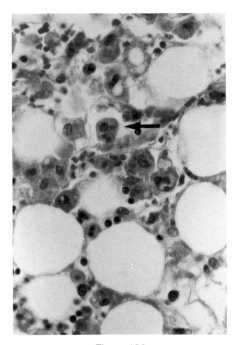

Figure 136
VIRUS-ASSOCIATED HEMOPHAGO-
CYTIC SYNDROME, MARROW
The histiocytes in this figure are bland in appearance. There is also slight erythrophagocytosis (arrow). PAS. X195.

nucleated cells may be demonstrated. Nodes show prominent sinus histiocytes with phagocytosis. There may be focal necrosis in the liver.

Differential Diagnosis. Mistaken diagnoses of malignant histiocytoses have been made because this disease process is serious or life threatening and because sections show histiocytic proliferation with erythrophagocytosis.

References

McKenna, R.W., Risdall, R.J., and Brunning, R.D. Virus-associated hemophagocytic syndrome. Hum. Pathol. 12:395-398, 1981.

Risdall, R.J., McKenna, R.W., Nesbit, M.E., et al. Virus-associated hemophagocytic syndrome. A benign histiocytic proliferation distinct from malignant histiocytosis. Cancer 44:993-1002, 1979.

Wilson, E.R., Malluh, A., Stagno, S., and Crist, W.M. Fatal Epstein-Barr virus-associated hemophagocytic syndrome. J. Pediatr. 98:260-262, 1981.

INDEX